# Lecture Notes in Computer Science     8159

Commenced Publication in 1973
Founding and Former Series Editors:
Gerhard Goos, Juris Hartmanis, and Jan van Leeuwen

## Editorial Board

T0183115

Li Shen   Tianming Liu   Pew-Thian Yap
Heng Huang   Dinggang Shen
Carl-Fredrik Westin (Eds.)

# Multimodal Brain Image Analysis

Third International Workshop, MBIA 2013
Held in Conjunction with MICCAI 2013
Nagoya, Japan, September 22, 2013
Proceedings

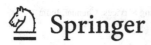

Springer

Volume Editors

Li Shen
Indiana University School of Medicine, Indianapolis, IN, USA
E-mail: shenli@iu.edu

Tianming Liu
University of Georgia, Athens, GA, USA
E-mail: tliu@cs.uga.edu

Pew-Thian Yap
The University of North Carolina at Chapel Hill, NC, USA
E-mail: ptyap@med.unc.edu

Heng Huang
The University of Texas at Arlington, TX, USA
E-mail: heng@uta.edu

Dinggang Shen
The University of North Carolina at Chapel Hill, NC, USA
E-mail: dgshen@med.unc.edu

Carl-Fredrik Westin
Harvard Medical School, Boston, MA, USA
E-mail: westin@bwh.harvard.edu

ISSN 0302-9743                              e-ISSN 1611-3349
ISBN 978-3-319-02125-6                      e-ISBN 978-3-319-02126-3
DOI 10.1007/978-3-319-02126-3
Springer Cham Heidelberg New York Dordrecht London

Library of Congress Control Number: 2013946482

CR Subject Classification (1998): I.4, I.5, H.3, I.3.5-8, I.2.10, J.3  LNCS Sublibrary:

SL 6 – Image Processing, Computer Vision, Pattern Recognition, and Graphics

*Typesetting:* Camera-ready by author, data conversion by Scientific Publishing Services, Chennai, India
Printed on acid-free paper
Springer is part of Springer Science+Business Media (www.springer.com)

# Preface

The 3$^{rd}$ international workshop on Multimodal Brain Image Analysis (MBIA) was held on September 22, 2013 in conjunction with the 16$^{th}$ international conference on Medical Image Computing and Computer Assisted Intervention (MICCAI) at the Toyoda Auditorium Complex, Higashiyama Campus, Nagoya University, Nagoya, Japan. The objective of MBIA 2013 was to move forward the state of the art in analysis methodologies, algorithms, software systems, validation approaches, benchmark datasets, neuroscience, and clinical applications.

Brain imaging techniques, such as structural MRI, functional MRI, diffusion MRI, perfusion MRI, EEG, MEG, PET, SPECT, and CT, are playing increasingly important roles in elucidating structural, functional and molecular properties in normal and diseased brains. It is widely believed that these different imaging modalities provide distinctive yet complementary information that is critical to the understanding of the working dynamics of the brain. These multimodal image data, when coupled with genetic, cognitive and other biomarker data, provide exciting opportunities to enhance our mechanistic understanding of brain function and behavior. However, effective processing, fusion, analysis, and visualization of images from multiple sources are still facing major computational challenges owing to the variation in imaging resolutions, spatial-temporal dynamics, and the fundamental biophysical mechanisms that determine the characteristics of the images. The MBIA workshop is a forum dedicated to the exchange of ideas, data, and software among researchers, with the goal of fostering the development of innovative technologies that will propel hypothesis testing and data-driven discovery in brain science.

This year the workshop received 35 submissions (including 4 invited papers). Based on the scores and recommendations provided by the Program Committee (PC), which consisted of 27 notable experts in the field, 24 papers were selected for poster presentations. Out of these 15 were selected for podium presentations.

We are enormously grateful to the authors for the high-quality submissions, the PC for evaluating the papers and providing valuable suggestions for improving the papers, the keynote speaker Dr. Polina Golland for her outstanding lecture on "Joint modeling of anatomical and functional connectivity for population studies", all the presenters for their excellent presentations, and the MICCAI organizers and MBIA 2013 attendees for their support.

July 2013

Li Shen
Tianming Liu
Pew-Thian Yap
Heng Huang
Dinggang Shen
Carl-Fredrik Westin

# Organization

## Program Committee

| | |
|---|---|
| John Ashburner | University College London, UK |
| Vince Calhoun | University of New Mexico, USA |
| Gary Christensen | University of Iowa, USA |
| Moo K. Chung | University of Wisconsin-Madison, USA |
| Rachid Deriche | INRIA, France |
| James Gee | University of Pennsylvania, USA |
| Xiaoping Hu | Emory University, USA |
| Xintao Hu | Northwestern Polytechnical University, China |
| Tianzi Jiang | Chinese Academy of Science, China |
| David N. Kennedy | University of Massachusetts Medical School, USA |
| Sungeun Kim | Indiana University School of Medicine, USA |
| Xiaofeng Liu | GE Global Research, USA |
| Kwangsik Nho | Indiana University School of Medicine, USA |
| Daniel Rueckert | Imperial College London, UK |
| Feng Shi | UNC Chapel Hill, USA |
| Paul M. Thompson | UCLA, USA |
| Qian Wang | UNC Chapel Hill, USA |
| Yongmei Wang | University of Illinois at Urbana-Champaign, USA |
| Yalin Wang | Arizona State University, USA |
| Yang Wang | Indiana University School of Medicine, USA |
| Simon K. Warfield | Harvard Medical School and Boston Children's Hospital, USA |
| Chong-Yaw Wee | UNC Chapel Hill, USA |
| Guorong Wu | UNC Chapel Hill, USA |
| Thomas Yeo | Duke-NUS Graduate Medical School, Singapore |
| Daoqiang Zhang | Nanjing University of Aeronautics and Astronautics, China |
| Gary Zhang | University College London, UK |
| Dajiang Zhu | University of Georgia, USA |

# Table of Contents

# Locally Weighted Multi-atlas Construction

Junning Li, Yonggang Shi, Ivo D. Dinov, and Arthur W. Toga*

Laboratory of Neuro Imaging, Department of Neurology
University of California, Los Angeles, CA, USA
{junningl,yonggang.shi}@gmail.com, dinov@ucla.edu, toga@usc.edu

**Abstract.** In image-based medical research, atlases are widely used in many tasks, for example, spatial normalization and segmentation. If atlases are regarded as representative patterns for a population of images, then multiple atlases are required for a heterogeneous population. In conventional atlas construction methods, the "unit" of representative patterns is images. Every input image is associated with its most similar atlas. As the number of subjects increases, the heterogeneity increases accordingly, and a big number of atlases may be needed. In this paper, we explore using region-wise, instead of image-wise, patterns to represent a population. Different parts of an input image is fuzzily associated with different atlases according to voxel-level association weights. In this way, regional structure patterns from different atlases can be combined together. Based on this model, we design a variational framework for multi-atlas construction. In the application to two T1-weighted MRI data sets, the method shows promising performance, in comparison with a conventional unbiased atlas construction method.

## 1 Introduction

In image-based medical researches, atlases are widely used to represent a population of images. They provide common spaces for spatial normalization, references for alignment, and propagation sources for segmentation.

One of the most widely used methods is registering input images to a pre-selected reference image, and then taking the average of the warped images as the atlas. Because all the images are transformed to be as similar as possible to the reference, the choice of the reference has significant impacts on the result. To avoid the bias introduced by arbitrary choice, the average image or the geometric mean of the input images can be used as the initial reference, as proposed by Joshi et al. (2004) [1] and Park et al. (2005) [2]. Instead of transforming input images toward a reference image, Seghers et al. (2004) [3] transformed them with the morphological mean of their transformations to all the other images. This method requires registration between all input image pairs.

In recent years, manifold-guided group registration methods are developed. Relationship between the input images is modeled with a manifold, and the input images are transformed gradually along the manifold to a center, instead of

---

* This work is supported by grants K01EB013633, R01MH094343, and P41EB015922 from NIH.

L. Shen et al. (Eds.): MBIA 2013, LNCS 8159, pp. 1–8, 2013.

directly "jump" to a reference image. This avoids inaccurate direct registration between dissimilar images. The manifold is usually represented by a $k$-nearest-neighbor graph whose vertices represent images and whose edges are weighted with the transformational metric between two images. Hamm et al. (2010) [4] employed the minimum spanning tree of the graph to guide the registration. Jia et al. (2010) [5] and Wang et al. (2010) [6] embedded a clustering procedure to merge images as intermediate centers when they become similar enough. Such a method not only reduces computation load but also builds a hierarchical structure for the inputs. Wu et al. (2011) [7] used directed graphs instead of undirected ones to optimize the registration procedure.

For a heterogeneous population, multiple atlases are required to represent it, as discussed in [8] by Blezek and Miller. Multi-atlases are usually constructed by partitioning the input images into sub-groups and then constructing an atlas for each of them. Aljabar et al. (2009) showed that the way of partitioning considerably impacts the result. Therefore, data-driven approaches should be employed. Sabuncu et al. (2009) [9] used Gaussian mixture models to cluster input images. Xie et al. (2013) [10] clustered input images according the manifold formed by them.

If atlases are regarded as representative patterns for a population of images, the "unit" of patterns used in the aforementioned methods is images. Every input image is associated with its most similar atlas. As the number of subjects increases, the heterogeneity among subjects increases accordingly. To represent a large population, we may need a big number of atlases. Let us assume the following not rigorously correct yet illustrating situation. Suppose the brain has $m$ anatomic structures, and each structure has $n$ possible patterns among a population. To represent all the possible combinations, we may need $m \times n$ atlases, if the pattern unit is images.

In this paper, we explore using region-wise, instead of image-wise, patterns to represent a population of images. We allow different parts of an input image to fuzzily associate with different atlases according to voxel-level association weights. In this way, structure patterns from different atlases can be combined together. In Section 2, we present a variational framework for constructing such a locally weighted multi-atlas. In Section 3, we demonstrate its application to two T1-weighted MRI data sets, where the proposed method show promising performance, in comparison with the group-mean method [1]. In Section 4, we briefly discuss possible future work.

## 2   Locally Weighted Multi-atlas

### 2.1   Generative Model

We assume that the input images are generated with voxel-level random sampling from a small number of template images and then they are randomly warped. Such a generative model is illustrated in Fig. 1 and the notations used in it is listed in Table 1. In the template space, the intensity value at point $x$ of a latent image $\bar{I}_s$ is randomly sampled from template images $\{T_k, k = 1, \ldots, K\}$, at the same point

**Table 1.** Notations

| | | | |
|---|---|---|---|
| $I_s$ | Image of subject $s$ | $T_k$ | The $k$th atlas image |
| $\varphi_s$ | Transformation for image $I_s$ | $x$ | Point in space |
| $\hat{I}_s = I_s \circ \varphi_s$ | Warped image of subject $s$ | $W_{sk}(x)$ | Weight of $\bar{I}_s(x)$'s association with $T_k$ |
| $\bar{I}_s$ | Latent image of $\hat{I}_s$ | $\Omega$ | Spatial domain |

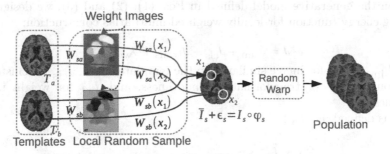

**Fig. 1.** Generative Model

location, where $K$ is the number of atlases. After noise $\varepsilon_s$ is added to it, $\bar{I}_s$ is randomly warped to be an input image $I_s$. The voxel-level probability distribution that intensity values of $\bar{I}_s$ are sampled from $T_k$s is configured with weight images $\{W_{sk}, k = 1, \ldots, K|s\}$. Such a generative process can be written as

$$\kappa_s(x) \sim \text{Multinomial}\{W_{sk}(x), k = 1, \ldots, K|s\} \tag{1}$$

$$\bar{I}_s(x) = T_{\kappa_s(x)}(x) \tag{2}$$

$$I_s = (\bar{I}_s + \varepsilon_s) \circ \varphi_s^{-1} \tag{3}$$

where $\text{Multinomial}\{W_{sk}(x), k = 1, \ldots, K|s\}$ denotes a multinomial distribution such that $P(\kappa = k) = W_{sk}(x)$ and $\{W_{sk}, k = 1, \ldots, K|s\}$ satisfies $\sum_k W_{sk}(x) = 1$ for any $s$ and $x$.

The intensity values of $\bar{I}_s$ at different points can be sampled from different template images. In this way, $\bar{I}_s$ is able to combine different patterns from different templates. To avoid abrupt transition between structure patterns, adjacent points should intend to be sampled from the same template image, and the weight images $W_{sk}$ should be spatially smooth.

Fig. 2 shows an example of such a generative process. Each of the images is composed of two parts, one from the images of either letter "A" or letter "B", the other from the images of either letter "C" or letter "D". In total, there are four image-level patterns: "AB", "AD", "CB" and "CD", as shown in the middle row of figure. Then the four patterns are randomly warped to be input images, as

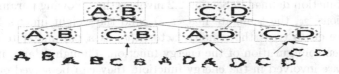

**Fig. 2.** Example of Image Generation Process

shown in the bottom row of the figure. If we represent the images with regional patterns, we just need two atlases: "AB" and "CD" (as shown in the top row of the figure), or "AD" and "CB", instead four atlases.

## 2.2 Atlas Construction Model

Based on the generative model defined in Eqs. (1), (2) and (3), we design the following energy function for locally weighted multi-atlas construction:

$$J = J_{\text{sim}} + J_{\text{cls}} + J_{\text{trans}} + J_{\text{wt}} \tag{4}$$

where $J_{\text{sim}}$ counts for image similarity in the template space, $J_{\text{cls}}$ for clustering dispersion, $J_{\text{trans}}$ for transformation smoothness, and $J_{\text{wt}}$ for weight image smoothness.

$J_{\text{sim}}$ is defined as

$$J_{\text{sim}} = \sum_s \int_{x \in \Omega} \sum_k W_{sk}(x) \left\| I_s \circ \varphi_s(x) - T_k(x) \right\|^2 dx \tag{5}$$

where the weight images satisfy $W_{sk}(x) \geqslant 0$ and $\sum_k W_{sk}(x) = 1$ for any $s$ and $x$.

$J_{\text{cls}}$ is defined as

$$J_{\text{cls}} = \sum_s \int_{x \in \Omega} h(x) \sum_k W_{sk}(x) \ln \frac{W_{sk}(x)}{Q_k(x)} dx \tag{6}$$

where $\{Q_k, k = 1, \ldots, K\}$ are prior weight images and $h(x)$ is a penalty factor. Being the integration of the Kullback–Leibler divergence between $\{W_{sk}\}$ and $\{Q_k\}$, $J_{\text{cls}}$ imposes similarity between $\{W_{sk}\}$ and $\{Q_k\}$. For simplicity, we used $Q_k(x) = 1/K$.

$J_{\text{wt}}$ is defined as

$$J_{\text{wt}} = \sum_s \int_{x \in \Omega} \sum_k \langle \nabla W_{sk}, \nabla W_{sk} \rangle \, dx \tag{7}$$

to model the smoothness of the weight images.

$J_{\text{trans}}$ is defined as

$$J_{\text{trans}} = \sum_s \int_{x \in \Omega} \langle D\varphi_s, D\varphi_s \rangle \, dx \tag{8}$$

where $D$ is a spatial difference operator. For diffusion regularization, $D$ is the gradient operator; for curvature regularization, $D$ is the Laplace operator.

## 2.3 Alternating Optimization

The energy function defined in Section 2.2 involves the following parameters: the transformations $\varphi_s$, the template images $T_k$, and the weight images $W_{sk}$ . For simplicity, we do to treat the penalty factor $h(x)$ as a parameter to optimize, but as a given configuration of the energy function. Though a large number of parameters are involved in the energy function, they can be solved one by one with alternating optimization.

**2.3.1  Optimizing $T_k$ Given $\varphi_s$ and $W_{sk}$:** $T_k$ is involved only in $J_{\text{sim}}$, as the center of weighted variances, as shown in Eq. (5). Given $\varphi_s$ and $W_{sk}$, the optimal value of $T_k$ is the locally weighed average of $I_s \circ \varphi_s$, as defined in the following equation:

$$T_k(x) = \frac{\sum_s W_{sk}(x) \times I_s \circ \varphi_{sk}(x)}{\sum_s W_{sk}(x)}$$

**2.3.2  Optimizing $W_{sk}$ Given $T_k$ and $\varphi_s$:** $W_{sk}$ is involved in $J_{\text{sim}}$, $J_{\text{cls}}$ and $J_{\text{wt}}$. Because $J_{\text{wt}}$ imposes smoothness on $W_{sk}$ and its Green's function is a Gaussian kernel, for simplicity, we first solve $W_{sk}$ with $J_{\text{sim}}$ and $J_{\text{cls}}$, and then smooth it with a Gaussian kernel. The method of Lagrange multipliers implies that to minimize $J_{\text{sim}}$ and $J_{\text{cls}}$ under the constraint $\sum_k W_{sk}(x) = 1$, $W_{sk}$ must satisfy

$$W_{sk}(x) \propto U_{sk}(x) := Q_k(x) e^{-\frac{\|I_s \circ \varphi_s(x) - T_k(x)\|^2}{h(x)}}$$

Therefore, the solution of $W_{sk}(x)$ without smoothing is $\frac{U_{sk}(x)}{\sum U_{sk}(x)}$.

**2.3.3  Optimizing $\varphi_s$ Given $T_k$ and $W_{sk}$:** $\varphi_s$ is involved in $J_{\text{sim}}$, and $J_{\text{trans}}$. The contribution of a particular $\varphi_s$ to the total energy function $J$ is

$$
\begin{aligned}
J_{\varphi_s} &= \int_{x \in \Omega} \sum_k W_{sk}(x) \|I_s \circ \varphi_s(x) - T_k(x)\|^2 \, dx + \int_{x \in \Omega} \langle D\varphi_s, D\varphi_s \rangle \, dx \\
&= \int_{x \in \Omega} \left\| I_s \circ \varphi_s(x) - \sum_k W_{sk}(x) T_k(x) \right\|^2 dx + C + \int_{x \in \Omega} \langle D\varphi_s, D\varphi_s \rangle \, dx
\end{aligned}
$$

where $C$ is a constant fully determined by $T_k$ and $W_{sk}$. As the equation implies, $\varphi_s$ can be optimized by registering $I_s$ to $\sum_k W_{sk} T_k$.

## 3  Experiments

The proposed method is applied to one synthetic data set (100 images) and two real MRI data sets (each of 40 images) for atlas construction, and compared with the conventional unbiased group-mean method [1]. The group-mean method registers input images to the average of their warped images, and iteratively repeats this procedure. Before atlas construction, we linearly align all the input images. For multi-atlas construction, we set the number of atlases $K$ to two.

The Dice label overlap index is used to measure the performance of the methods. The template label images $L_k$s are derived from the warped input label images, with weighted majority vote according to weights $\{W_{sk}, s = 1, \ldots, S|k\}$. The predicted label image for a warped image $\hat{I}_s$ in the template space, is derived from the template label images by fusing them together with weighted majority vote according to weights $\{W_{sk}(x), k = 1, \ldots, K|s\}$.

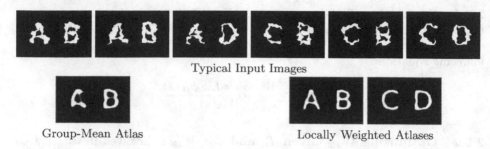

Typical Input Images

Group-Mean Atlas                    Locally Weighted Atlases

**Fig. 3.** ABCD100

## 3.1    Synthetic Data

We generate 100 images according the model illustrated in Figs. 1 and 2. For the description of the generative procedure, please refer to Section 2.1. We expect the proposed method to recover the underlying region-level patterns "A", "B", "C", "D" as two atlas images, for example "AB" and "CD", or "AD" and "CB", instead using four atlases. As shown in Fig. 3, the proposed method satisfactorily recovers the underlying regional patterns as two images "AB" and "CD".

## 3.2    OASIS Data Set

The OASIS data set contains T1-weighted MR brain images of 416 subjects at ages ranging from 18 to 96. The images are at the resolution of $1 \times 1 \times 1$ mm$^3$ and of voxel size $176 \times 208 \times 176$. For each subject, a label image indicating the segmentation of white matter (WM), gray matter (GM) and cerebrospinal fluid (CSF) is also provided. We randomly sampled 40 images from the data set, one half with ages ranging from 20 to 30, and the other half ranging from 70 to 80.

As shown in Fig. 4, the proposed method constructs one atlas with a large ventricle and the other with a smaller one. The proposed method achieves better tissue overlap than the group-mean method (86.9% vs. 81.4%), as shown in the table in Fig. 4.

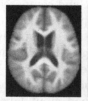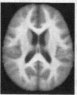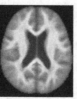

|            | Overall | CSF  | GM   | WM   |
|------------|---------|------|------|------|
| Group-Mean | 81.4    | 64.9 | 84.3 | 84.5 |
| LWM        | 86.9    | 74.4 | 88.1 | 91.2 |

Group-Mean    Locally Weighted Atlases

Dice Indices of Tissue Overlap

**Fig. 4.** OASIS40. "LWM" means locally weighted multi-atlas.

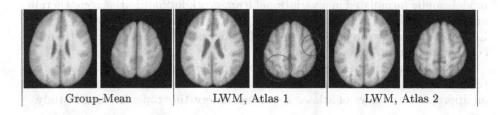

| Group-Mean | LWM, Atlas 1 | LWM, Atlas 2 |

**Fig. 5.** LPBA40: Constructed Atlases. "LWM" means locally weighted multi-atlas.

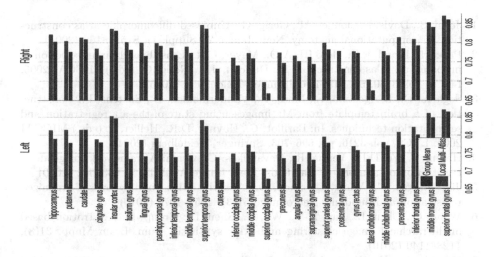

**Fig. 6.** LPBA40: Dice Overlap Indices of 54 ROIs

## 3.3   LPBA40 Data Set

The LPBA40 data set [11] has T1 images of 40 subjects and 54 regions are
manually segmented for each of them. The proposed method is applied to it,
with the number of atlases $K$ set to two. As shown in Fig. 5, the two atlases
produced by the proposed method show different patterns in the upper part of
the brain, and are visually sharper than that by the group-mean method. The
overall Dice overlap indices of the proposed method and the group-mean method
are 80.4% and 78.5% respectively. Overlap indices of the 54 regions are shown
in Fig. 6.

## 4   Conclusion and Discussion

In this paper, we exploring using region-wise, instead of image-wise, patterns to
represent a population of images. Different parts of an input image are fuzzily
associated with different atlases according to voxel-level association weights. In
this way, structure patterns in different atlases can be combined together. Such a

model can be formulated in a variational framework for multi-atlas construction, and solved with alternating optimization. In the applications to the OASIS and LPBA40 data sets, the proposed method achieves better label overlap than the conventional group-mean method [1].

It worths further investigation to use morphological difference, instead of intensity difference, for determining the voxel-level association weights. Choosing an appropriate number of atlases is another interesting topic for future study.

# References

1. Joshi, S., Davis, B., Jomier, M., Gerig, G.: Unbiased diffeomorphic atlas construction for computational anatomy. NeuroImage 23(Suppl. 1), S151–S160 (2004)
2. Park, H., Bland, P.H., Hero III, A.O., Meyer, C.R.: Least biased target selection in probabilistic atlas construction. In: Duncan, J.S., Gerig, G. (eds.) MICCAI 2005. LNCS, vol. 3750, pp. 419–426. Springer, Heidelberg (2005)
3. Seghers, D., D'Agostino, E., Maes, F., Vandermeulen, D., Suetens, P.: Construction of a brain template from Mr images using state-of-the-art registration and segmentation techniques. In: Barillot, C., Haynor, D.R., Hellier, P. (eds.) MICCAI 2004. LNCS, vol. 3216, pp. 696–703. Springer, Heidelberg (2004)
4. Hamm, J., Ye, D.H., Verma, R., Davatzikos, C.: Gram: A framework for geodesic registration on anatomical manifolds. Med. Image Anal. 14(5), 633–642 (2010)
5. Jia, H., Wu, G., Wang, Q., Shen, D.: Absorb: Atlas building by self-organized registration and bundling. Neuroimage 51(3), 1057–1070 (2010)
6. Wang, Q., Chen, L., Yap, P.-T., Wu, G., Shen, D.: Groupwise registration based on hierarchical image clustering and atlas synthesis. Hum. Brain Mapp. 31(8), 1128–1140 (2010)
7. Wu, G., Jia, H., Wang, Q., Shen, D.: Sharpmean: groupwise registration guided by sharp mean image and tree-based registration. Neuroimage 56(4), 1968–1981 (2011)
8. Blezek, D.J., Miller, J.V.: Atlas stratification. Med. Image Anal. 11(5), 443–457 (2007)
9. Sabuncu, M.R., Balci, S.K., Shenton, M.E., Golland, P.: Image-driven population analysis through mixture modeling. IEEE Transactions on Medical Imaging 28(9), 1473–1487 (2009)
10. Xie, Y., Ho, J., Vemuri, B.: Multiple atlas construction from a heterogeneous brain MR image collection. IEEE Transactions on Medical Imaging PP(99), 1 (2013)
11. Shattuck, D.W., Mirza, M., Adisetiyo, V., Hojatkashani, C., Salamon, G., Narr, K.L., Poldrack, R.A., Bilder, R.M., Toga, A.W.: Construction of a 3D probabilistic atlas of human cortical structures. Neuroimage 39(3), 1064–1080 (2008)

# Assessing Structural Organization and Functional Interaction in Gyral, Sulcal and Cortical Networks

Xiaojin Li[1], Xintao Hu[1], Xi Jiang[2], Lei Guo[1], Junwei Han[1], and Tianming Liu[2]

[1] School of Automation, Northwestern Polytechnical University, Xi'an, China
{lxj9173,xintao.hu,guolei.npu,junweihan2010}@gmail.com
[2] Cortical Architecture Imaging and Discovery Lab, Department of Computer Science and Bioimaging Research Center, The University of Georgia, Athens, GA
{superjx2318,tianming.liu}@gmail.com

**Abstract.** Literature studies showed that the fibers connected to gyri are significantly denser than those connected to sulci. Therefore, we hypothesize that gyral, sulcal and cortical brain networks might exhibit different graph properties and functional interactions that reflect the organizational principles of cortical architecture. In this way, we evaluated the graphical properties of the structural brain networks and the functional connectivities among brain networks which are composed of gyral regions of interest (ROI) (G-networks), sulcal ROIs (S-networks) and mixed gyral and sulcal ROIs (C-networks). The results demonstrated that G-networks have the highest global and local economical properties and the strongest small-worldness. In contrast, S-networks have the lowest global and local economical properties and the weakest small-worldness. Meanwhile, the overall functional connectivity strength among G-networks is stronger than those in S-networks, and those in C-networks are in between. The results indicate that gyri may play a hub role in human brains.

**Keywords:** gyri, sulci, wiring cost, efficiency, small-worldness, fMRI.

## 1 Introduction

It has been of great interest in the neuroimaging field to study properties of structural connectivity patterns and brain networks recently. Prior literature studies [1-3] showed that the white matter fibers connected to gyri are significantly denser than those connected to sulci. This finding has been replicated in a range of primate brains including human, chimpanzee, and macaque monkey via diffusion tensor imaging (DTI) and high-angular resolution diffusion imaging (HARDI) [1, 2], and might suggest the different roles of gyri and sulci in structural and functional brain networks.

Inspired by the above finding, we hypothesize in this paper that structural and functional brain networks constructed from gyral, sulcal and cortical regions might exhibit different graph properties and functional interaction patterns that reflect the fundamental organization of the cortical architecture. To test this hypothesis, based on multimodal DTI and resting-state functional magnetic resonance imaging (R-fMRI) data, we evaluated the graph-theoretical properties related to wiring cost

L. Shen et al. (Eds.): MBIA 2013, LNCS 8159, pp. 9–17, 2013.

[4], efficiency [4] and small-worldness [5] of the structural brain networks, which are composed of gyral regions of interest (ROI) (G-networks), sulcal ROIs (S-networks) and mixed cortical gyral and sulcal ROIs (C-networks), and further examined whether there exist significantly different graph properties and functional interaction among these three groups of structural brain networks. The underlying rationale of this study is two-fold: 1) The possible measured significant differences of those graph properties which depict the global organization of the structural brain networks and functional brain networks could reveal the different roles that gyri and sulci may play, thus providing novel insight into the structural and functional principles of the brain architecture and potentially offering meaningful guidance for neuroimage analysis methodologies; 2) The multimodal assessments of structural properties and functional interaction patterns of different brain networks could potentially elucidate the close relationship between brain structure and function, which has been a major research topic in neuroimaging.

## 2    Materials and Methods

### 2.1    Data Acquisition and Pre-processing

DTI and R-fMRI datasets of 10 healthy young adult subjects were acquired on a 3T GE MRI scanner under IRB approvals. Acquisition parameters for the scans were as follows. DTI: 256×256 matrix, 2 mm slice thickness, 240 mm FOV, 50 slices, 15 DWI volumes, b-value 1000; R-fMRI: 64×64 matrix, 4 mm slice thickness, 220 mm FOV, 30 slices, TR = 2s, total scan length = 400s. The preprocessing steps of DTI data included brain skull removal, motion correction, and eddy current correction. After preprocessing, streamline fiber tracks were reconstructed via MEDINRIA [6]. Brain tissue segmentation was performed based on DTI data [7]. Based on the white matter tissue map, the gray matter (GM)/white matter (WM) cortical surface was reconstructed using the marching cubes algorithm [8]. Cortical folding patterns were analyzed using a method based on surface profiling similar to [9], in which the cortical surface was divided into sulcal and gyral regions. More details are referred to [9]. The preprocessing of the R-fMRI data included brain skull removal, motional correction, spatial smoothing, slice time correction, global drift removal and band pass filtering (0.01~0.1Hz).

### 2.2    Brain Network Construction

The structural brain network is represented as a weighted undirected graph $\mathbf{G}=(\mathbf{V},\mathbf{E})$ in which $\mathbf{V}=\{v_i, i=1, 2, ..., N\}$ is the set of nodes and $\mathbf{E}=\{e_{ij}, i, j=1, 2, ..., N\}$ is the set of edges. In this paper, in order to achieve the desired spatial resolution and functional specificity, we identify each graph node as an ROI on the reconstructed cortical surface, and use the number of DTI-derived fiber connections between a pair of nodes as their edge, which has been a common and widely-used method to measure the connectivity of structural brain networks in the literature [10].

Since the focus of this study is on the global graph property difference of structural brain networks and global interaction difference of functional networks that are constructed with ROIs in different cortical regions, we do not necessarily need the correspondences of network nodes across individuals. In addition, given the current algorithms and methods for brain image registration, it is difficult to seek accurate correspondences among brain ROIs across individual brains due to the tremendous cortical anatomy variability. Thus, the G-networks and S-networks are composed of a group of ROIs randomly selected from gyral or sulcal regions in the whole brain, respectively. C-networks are composed of a combination of balanced G-network nodes and S-network nodes. Here, the edge between an ROI-pair is defined as the number of fibers connecting the ROI-pair [11]. Thus, a structural connectivity matrix $A_{N \times N}$ is obtained for a brain network with $N$ nodes. Notably, the self-loops are currently ignored in this work. In this paper, the traditional thresholding process was not necessary because the weighted adjacency matrix of structural network is intrinsically sparse, in that many node pairs are not interconnected [10]. Fig. 1 shows exemplar brain networks of three different types such as G-network, C-network and S-network. It is noteworthy that our reconstruction method ensured that most of the surface voxels are in the GM, and the ROIs have the same size.

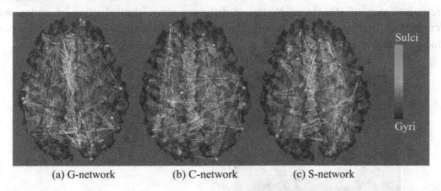

(a) G-network          (b) C-network          (c) S-network

**Fig. 1.** Examples of brain networks of three different types. (a)-(c): (a) G-network; (b) C-network; (c) S-network. The nodes are represented by yellow spheres and the edges are represented by the white lines. The constructed structural brain networks are overlaid on the corresponding cortical surfaces (divided into gyri and sulci) reconstructed from DTI data.

Next, the functional interaction between a pair of nodes ROIs is measured by the method based on cross wavelet transform (XWT) [12, 13], which is a powerful tool in assessing the multi-scale time-frequency interactions between R-fMRI time series. By combining the wavelet transforms of two time series, the XWT uncovers the regions in the time-frequency domain where both time series share high co-power, which is considered and defined as functional interaction strength of ROIs in this work. We used the Morlet kernel [13] and statistical significance test of 95% significance level [12, 13] to derive the functional interaction strength. With this configuration, we obtained a weighted matrix $Sig$ that represents significance level of XWT for each pair of R-fMRI time series, denoted as a significance map. The matrix representation enables us to focus on regions in the time-frequency domain where the co-power of the time series are significant [14]. The higher values in the significance map are of special interest since it contains stronger functional interactions at various scales. Fig. 2 shows an exemplar significance map. The red regions in significance map are of special interest since it contains stronger interactions. In this case, we derive a matrix $IM_{N \times N}$ to represent the interaction matrix between all the network node ROI pairs. $IM$ is calculated as:

$$IM(R_i, R_j) = \sum_{Sig_{R_iR_j} \geq 0.95} Sig_{R_iR_j} \tag{1}$$

where $R_i$ and $R_j$ are two ROIs. We also consider the average of $IM$ as the overall functional interaction strength among the network that is given by:

$$Q = \frac{2}{N(N-1)} \sum_{1 \leq i < j \leq N} IM(R_i, R_j) \tag{2}$$

where $N$ is the number of all nodes ROIs.

For statistical analysis of brain networks with different sizes, the number of the nodes in the constructed structural brain networks varied from 100 to 800 with the incremental step of 100. In each step of different sizes, the selection of nodes was independently repeated for 10 times. The network construction procedure was performed for each subject separately.

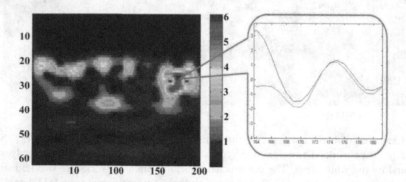

**Fig. 2.** An exemplar significance map. The $x$-axis is time, and the $y$-axis is period. The unit of $x$- and $y$-axes is second. The red regions indicate stronger interaction domains between the two ROIs and the R-fMRI signals in the example red area are shown in the zoomed window on the right.

## 2.3   Graph Properties

In this work, we employed and designed several graph theoretic properties related to wiring cost [4], network efficiency [4] and small-worldness [5] as the metrics to assess the organization of structural brain networks.

In graph theory, the shortest path length plays an important role in charactering the internal structure of a graph. The shortest path length between a pair of nodes is defined as the path between the two nodes that the number of its constituent edges is minimized. The characteristic path length is the average of the shortest paths over all possible pairs of nodes [4]. The global efficiency is to consider the harmonic mean of the shortest lengths. The average inverse shortest path length is a related measure that is known as global efficiency, i.e. $E_{glob}$ [4]:

$$E_{glob} = \frac{1}{N}E_i = \frac{1}{N}\sum_{i \in G} \frac{\sum_{j \in G, j \neq i} d_{ij}^{-1}}{(N-1)}$$ (3)

where $N$ is the number of the graph nodes, and the $d_{ij}$ is the shortest path length between node $i$ and $j$. It has been shown in the literature that this definition may make $E_{glob}$ a superior measure of functional integration [15]. Unlike characteristic path length, $E_{glob}$ can be meaningfully measured for disconnected networks, as paths between disconnected nodes are defined to have infinite length, and correspondingly zero efficiency. The local efficiency was defined as the average efficiency of the local sub- graphs [4]:

$$E_{loc} = \frac{1}{N}\sum_{i \in G} E_{loc,i} = \frac{1}{N}\sum_{i \in G} \frac{\sum_{j,h \in G, j \neq i} a_{ij}a_{jh}[d_{jh}(G_i)]^{-1}}{k_i(k_i - 1)}$$ (4)

where $E_{loc,i}$ is the local efficiency of node $i$, and $d_{jh}$ is the length of the shortest path between $j$ and $h$. Here, $k_i$ is the degree of node $i$. $a_{ij}$ is the connection status between $i$ and $j$: $a_{ij}=1$ when $e_{ij}$ exists, $a_{ij}=0$ otherwise.

The simplest measure of the wiring cost of a network is defined as follows, and $L$ is the number of the edges in the network [4]:

$$cost = \frac{L}{N \times (N-1)/2}$$ (5)

For the purpose of more compact measurement of economical property of a network, we defined two parameters in order to integrate wiring cost and network efficiency, namely, *Ratio* and *Diff* for the global and local properties. Higher *Ratio* or *Diff* indicates that a network is more economical. They are calculated as follows:

$$Ratio_{glob} = E_{glob} / cost, \quad Diff_{glob} = E_{glob} - cost$$ (6)

$$Ratio_{loc} = E_{loc} / cost, \quad Diff_{loc} = E_{loc} - cost$$ (7)

Also, the small-worldness has been widely reported and used as one of the most important properties of both functional and structural human brain networks [9]. Small-world networks are formally defined as networks that are significantly more clustered than random networks, yet have approximately the same characteristic path length as random networks. More generally, small-world networks should be simultaneously highly segregated and integrated. Small-worldness is often analyzed by considering the fraction of nodes in the network that have a particular number of connections going into them [16]. It is calculated as [4]:

$$\gamma = C_p / C_{rand} > 1, \quad \lambda = L_p / L_{rand} \approx 1, \quad small\text{-}worldness: \sigma = \gamma / \lambda > 1$$ (8)

where $C_p$ and $C_{rand}$ are the average clustering coefficient [4], and $L_p$ and $L_{rand}$ are the characteristic path lengths of brain network and random network, respectively.

## 3    Results

The result figures of 5 randomly selected subjects are shown in Figs. 3(a)-3(e). Specifically, Fig. 3(a) shows $Ratio_{glob}$ for G-, S- and C-networks of various sizes; $Diff_{glob}$ is shown in Fig. 3(b); $Ratio_{loc}$ is shown in Fig. 3(c); $Diff_{loc}$ is shown in Fig. 3(d), and small-worldness is shown in Fig. 3(e). In general, it is clearly seen that G-network has the highest value of each property and S-network has the lowest ones, while those of C-network are in-between. This observation is reproduced and confirmed with the increase of the numbers of nodes. When the number of nodes is over 500, G-network holds overwhelming superiority. The group averaged $Ratio_{glob}$, $Ratio_{loc}$, $Diff_{glob}$, $Diff_{loc}$ and small-worldness for G-, C- and S-networks of all the 10 subjects when the number of nodes varies from 100 to 800 are shown in Figs. 4(a)-4(e), respectively. The trends are very similar to those in a single subject. These results demonstrate that G-network is the most economical compared with C- and S-networks. These results are also reproducible in other independent groups of subjects.

The functional interaction strengths of G-, C- and S-networks with 100-400 nodes has no significant difference. However, there are substantial differences when the brain networks contain more than 500 nodes. Figs. 5(a)-5(e) show the average functional interaction strengths of 5 subjects with nodes varying from 500 to 800. Although a few cases do not exhibit obvious difference on specific numbers of nodes among G-, C- and S-networks, most of the subjects' results indicate that the G-networks have stronger functional interaction strengths than others, especially higher than S-networks. Quantitative group-averaged functional interaction strengths for G-, C- and S-networks when the number of ROIs varies from 500 to 800 are shown in Table 1. It shows the trend that the functional interaction in G-network is stronger than that in S-network, and the functional interaction in C-network is in-between.

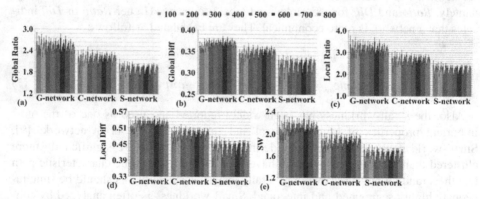

**Fig. 3.** The structural graph properties of 5 randomly selected subjects' G-, C- and S-networks when the number of nodes varies from 100 to 800. In each sub-group, color bar clusters in different colors correspond to different network sizes, and each 5-bar cluster in the same color represents 5 subjects. The error bars are derived from the 10-times repeats of random nodes selection. (a) $Ratio_{glob}$; (b) $Diff_{glob}$; (c) $Ratio_{loc}$; (e) $Diff_{loc}$; (f) Small-worldness.

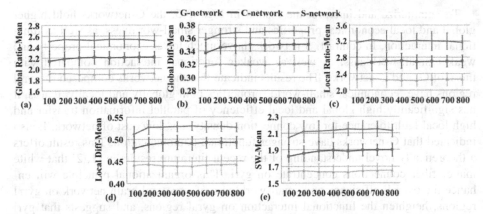

**Fig. 4.** Group-averaged $Ratio_{glob}$, $Ratio_{loc}$, $Diff_{glob}$, $Diff_{loc}$ and small-worldness for G-, C- and S-networks when the number of nodes varies from 100 to 800 are shown in (a)-(e), respectively. The horizontal-axis is the number of nodes. The vertical axis represents the graph property metrics.

**Table 1.** The group-average functional interaction strengths of G-, C- and S-networks when the number of nodes varies from 500 to 800

| Nodes | G-network | C-network | S-network |
|-------|-----------|-----------|-----------|
| 500 | 6698 ± 5.4% | 6655 ± 5.6% | 6603 ± 5.9% |
| 600 | 6702 ± 5.4% | 6652 ± 5.6% | 6613 ± 6.0% |
| 700 | 6695 ± 5.4% | 6648 ± 5.5% | 6611 ± 5.9% |
| 800 | 6707 ± 5.4% | 6652 ± 5.7% | 6609 ± 6.0% |

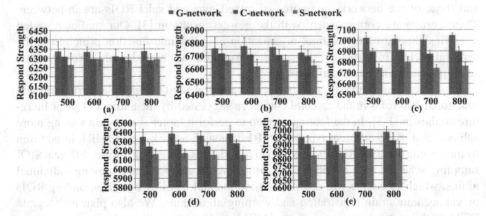

**Fig. 5.** The functional interaction responds strength of G-, C- and S-networks for each subject (5 selected randomly), when the number of nodes varies from 500 to 800, is shown in (a)-(e), respectively. The x-axis is the number of nodes.

To summarize and interpret the results in Figs. 3-5, the G-networks hold higher global and local economical properties and stronger small-worldness, as well as functional interaction. In contrast, S-networks have much lower economical property and weaker small-worldness, as well as weaker functional interaction compared with those of G- and C-networks. The results indicate that the networks composed of gyral regions have 'economical small-world' properties both globally and locally, that is, it has significantly high global and local efficiency of parallel information transfer and high local fault tolerance for low connection density, i.e., low cost of network. It also indicated that G-networks have stronger functional communication. This result offers a theoretically novel understanding of the recent literature results in [1, 2] that white matter fiber connections concentrate on gyri. This organizational principle will enhance the overall efficiency and small-worldness of structural brain network on gyral regions, heighten the functional interaction on gyral regions, and suggests that gyri might be the structural and functional hubs of the cerebral cortex. The results in Figs. 3-5 also suggest the close relationship between brain network structure and function. That is, G-networks of higher structural connection strength exhibit higher functional interaction strength, and structural connection hubs tend to be functional integration centers too.

## 4    Discussion and Conclusion

Inspired by the recent literature findings that there exist significant different white matter fiber connection patterns between sulci and gyri [1, 2], in this paper, we examined the organization of the structural and functional brain networks that are composed of gyri, sulci and mixed cortical ROIs. Our experimental results demonstrated that brain networks composed of gyri ROIs have the highest global and local economical properties and the strongest small-worldness, and also have the strongest functional interaction. Those of the networks composed of sulci ROIs are on the opposite, and those of the networks composed of mixed gyri and sulci ROIs are in-between. These results are correspondent with the newest results in [3]. Our studies revealed novel insights into the structural organization and dynamic function principle of the cerebral cortex. In particular, the revealed principles are reproducible across random sampling cases and among different subjects.

Altogether, our analysis results suggest that gyral regions may play structural and functional hub roles in the cerebral cortex, as suggested by the authors of prior literature studies in [1-3]. In the future, we plan to perform larger scale studies using more subjects and using different types of fMRI data such as task-based fMRI, in addition to the resting state fMRI data used in this work. Also, we plan to use different ROI sampling schemes such as those ROIs with rough correspondences among individual brains, which of course will entail extensive manual labeling of corresponding ROIs or via accurate brain registration and warping algorithms. We also plan to integrate DTI based structural connectivity into fMRI based connectivity analysis.

# References

[1] Nie, J., Guo, L., Li, K., Wang, Y., et al.: Axonal Fiber Terminations Concentrate on Gyri. Cerebral Cortex 22(12), 2831–2839 (2011)

[2] Chen, H., Zhang, T., Guo, L., Liu, T., et al.: Coevolution of Gyral Folding and Structural Connection Patterns in Primate Brains. Cerebral Cortex 23(5), 1208–1217 (2013)

[3] Deng, F., Jiang, X., Zhu, D., Zhang, T., Li, K., Guo, L., Liu, T.: A Functional Model of Cortical Gyri and Sulci. Brain Structure and Function (in press, 2013)

[4] Rubinov, M., Sporns, O.: Complex network measures of brain connectivity: Uses and interpretations. NeuroImage 52(3), 1059–1069 (2010)

[5] Humphries, M.D., Gurney, K.: Network 'small-world-ness': a quantitative method for determining canonical network equivalence. PLoS ONE 3(4), e0002051(2008)

[6] http://www-sop.inria.fr/asclepios/software/MedINRIA/

[7] Liu, T., Li, H., Wong, K., Tarokh, A., Guo, L., Wong, S.T.C.: Brain Tissue Segmentation Based on DTI Data. NeuroImage 38(1), 114–123 (2007)

[8] Liu, T., Nie, J., Tarokh, A., Guo, L., Wong, S.: Reconstruction of Central Cortical Surface from MRI Brain Images: Method and Application. NeuroImage 40(3), 991–1002 (2008)

[9] Li, K., Guo, L., Li, G., Nie, J., Faraco, C., Zhao, Q., Miller, L.S., Liu, T.: Gyral folding pattern analysis via surface profiling. NeuroImage 52(4), 1202–1214 (2010)

[10] Zalesky, A., Fornito, A., Harding, I.H., Cocchi, L., Yücel, M.: Whole-brain anatomical networks: Does the choice of nodes matter? NeuroImage 50, 970–983 (2010)

[11] Hagmann, P., Kurant, M., Gigandet, X., Thiran, P., et al.: Mapping human whole-brain structural networks with diffusion MRI. PLoS ONE 2(7), e597 (2007)

[12] Torrence, C., Compo, G.P.: A practical guide to wavelet analysis. Bull. Amer. Meteor. Soc. 79(1), 61–78 (1998)

[13] Chang, C., Glover, G.H.: Time-frequency dynamics of resting-state brain connectivity measured with fMRI. NeuroImage 50(1), 81–98 (2010)

[14] Deng, F., Zhu, D., Liu, T.: Optimization of fMRI-derived ROIs based on coherent Functional Interaction Patterns. In: Ayache, N., Delingette, H., Golland, P., Mori, K. (eds.) MICCAI 2012, Part III. LNCS, vol. 7512, pp. 214–222. Springer, Heidelberg (2012)

[15] Achard, S., Bullmore, E.: Efficiency and cost of economical brain functional networks. PLoS Comput. Biol. 3(2), e17 (2007)

[16] Bullmore, E., Sporns, O.: Complex brain networks: graph theoretical analysis of structural and functional systems. Nat. Rev. Neurosci. 10(3), 186–198 (2009)

# Quantification and Analysis of Large Multimodal Clinical Image Studies: Application to Stroke

Ramesh Sridharan[1,*], Adrian V. Dalca[1,*], Kaitlin M. Fitzpatrick[2],
Lisa Cloonan[2], Allison Kanakis[2], Ona Wu[2], Karen L. Furie[3],
Jonathan Rosand[2], Natalia S. Rost[2], and Polina Golland[1]

[1] Computer Science and Artificial Intelligence Lab, MIT
[2] Department of Neurology, Massachusetts General Hospital, Harvard Medical School
[3] Department of Neurology, Rhode Island Hospital,
Alpert Medical School of Brown University

**Abstract.** We present an analysis framework for large studies of multimodal clinical quality brain image collections. Processing and analysis of such datasets is challenging due to low resolution, poor contrast, misaligned images, and restricted field of view. We adapt existing registration and segmentation methods and build a computational pipeline for spatial normalization and feature extraction. The resulting aligned dataset enables clinically meaningful analysis of spatial distributions of relevant anatomical features and of their evolution with age and disease progression. We demonstrate the approach on a neuroimaging study of stroke with more than 800 patients. We show that by combining data from several modalities, we can automatically segment important biomarkers such as white matter hyperintensity and characterize pathology evolution in this heterogeneous cohort. Specifically, we examine two sub-populations with different dynamics of white matter hyperintensity changes as a function of patients' age. Pipeline and analysis code is available at http://groups.csail.mit.edu/vision/medical-vision/stroke/.

## 1 Introduction

We present a framework to summarize and quantify large multimodal collections of clinical images in population studies of neurological disease. We use registration and segmentation algorithms to build robust computational pipelines that handle variable image quality and large image set sizes. Large population studies with clinical quality multimodal images present many challenges, including poor resolution, varying slice acquisition directions and orientations across modalities, poor contrast, limited field of view, and misalignment of scans of different modalities. In this work, we develop insights for adapting existing algorithms to clinical images, and use these insights to build a robust and scalable framework. We demonstrate the application of the methods on a preliminary study of over 800 patients with the goal of expanding the study by an order of magnitude in the near future by including images from multiple sites.

---

* Ramesh Sridharan and Adrian V. Dalca contributed equally to this work.

L. Shen et al. (Eds.): MBIA 2013, LNCS 8159, pp. 18–30, 2013.
© Springer International Publishing Switzerland 2013

Our work is motivated by a large scale imaging study of stroke. The brain scans are acquired within a few hours of stroke onset, which limits scanning time and requires fast imaging protocols. Due to the acquisition constraints, scans of different modalities are not only low resolution (with greater than 5mm slice thickness), but are also anisotropic in different directions as illustrated in Figure 1. Distinguishing between white and gray matter is challenging in the resulting T1 images, even for an expert, due to poor tissue contrast. To assess susceptibility to cerebral ischemia (insufficient blood flow to the brain) and predict stroke severity, image features such as white matter hyperintensity (WMH) [17] and stroke lesions were labeled manually in T2-FLAIR and DWI scans respectively. WMH burden is found to be higher in patients who develop a cerebral infarct compared to those with less damaging transient ischemic attacks, and is also associated with small vessel stroke subtypes [18]. The segmentation and analysis of WMH is therefore important for understanding mechanisms underlying stroke. Manual segmentation by an expert takes 10 to 30 minutes per patient. Segmentation of 1089 patients in the study took over three years. With the project poised to receive thousands more scans from other participating sites in the near future, the need for automatic segmentation and analysis tools is clear.

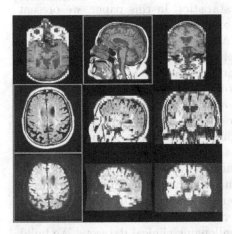

**Fig. 1.** T1 (top), T2-FLAIR (middle), and DWI (bottom) images from a patient in the stroke study. Three orthogonal slices are shown for each modality; in plane slices are highlighted in blue. Note the cropped field of view and large slice thickness.

Enabled by increasingly more affordable imaging technology and collaborative acquisition efforts [7,16], the trend of large scale multimodal multi-site clinical studies with lower quality images is bound to continue. Population genetics studies that typically require large patient cohorts are starting to include imaging data, creating large scale imaging datasets. In contrast to high quality research scans in studies that commonly motivate method development, such as ADNI [29] and Predict-HD [14], we focus on lower quality clinical images. As our results demonstrate, existing algorithms can be adapted to handle clinical quality scans by carefully investigating the properties of the input images and using the insights to optimize the application of the methods.

Our framework consists of three main components: registration, segmentation, and analysis. Our ultimate goal is in-depth analysis of disease progression in large clinical datasets, which will deliver insights into the structural and functional changes associated with a disorder from noisy, low quality images. Accurate registration is a critical prerequisite for such analysis, as it brings all imaging modalities into a common coordinate frame and enables data fusion across subjects and modalities [19]. Quantifying regions

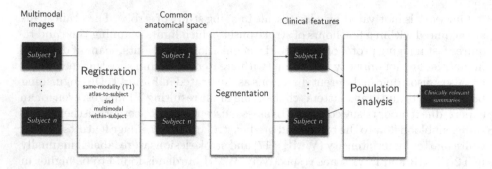

**Fig. 2.** A flowchart of our computational pipeline. Registration of all modalities for all patients into a common space and segmentation of clinical features enable large scale population analysis.

of interest requires accurate segmentation. Manual segmentation is infeasible for larger datasets with thousands of images, motivating the development of automatic methods. Population analysis of heterogeneous data requires improved models to capture trends, variability, and statistics. In this paper, we present steps and insights toward the goal of large scale analysis for clinical studies.

Prior work in registration, segmentation, and population analysis has often focused on high quality images. Registration of clinical images is often constrained to rigid or affine alignment to atlas reference frames such as Talairach coordinates [23]. However, accurate alignment of relevant brain structures requires nonlinear deformations [2,26]. For example, atrophy of the cortex and growth of the ventricles are of interest in many neuroimaging studies. In stroke imaging, white matter hyperintensity is typically found close to the ventricles. Therefore, an accurate deformable registration of the white matter near the ventricles is important for spatial analysis of white matter hyperintensity distribution in the population. Although recent registration algorithms have enjoyed success in many medical imaging applications, a better understanding of the interactions between the algorithms and relevant properties of images is essential for such algorithms to function properly on large, challenging clinical datasets. We build on the work of Klein *et al.* [12], which evaluates a variety of different registration algorithms on high resolution scans of slice thicknesses below 1.5mm with no visible pathologies. Methods for segmentation and analysis of medical images have been researched in depth [1,20], but their utility for large scale clinical studies of pathology is yet to be fully characterized. Previous work in population analysis has often focused on higher quality datasets [6,20], while analysis of larger datasets has been naïve [21]. In this paper, we address the key challenges of building a robust computational pipeline for registration and segmentation in a common reference frame, enabling analysis and summary of a pilot study of over 800 patients. We employ regression mixture modeling [8,15] and kernel regression for imaging [4,13,28] to identify and characterize different modes of white matter hyperintensity evolution as a function of age. Fig. 2 presents a flowchart of the proposed computational framework.

The remainder of this paper is organized as follows. In Section 2, we introduce our approach to registration of images within each patient in a study and to spatial alignment of all patients into a common coordinate frame. In Section 3, we discuss the challenges of automatic segmentation and outline our solutions. In Section 4, we describe the population analysis methods in further detail. Section 5 illustrates our approach on a cohort of stroke patients. We conclude with a discussion of directions for future research suggested by our experience and results.

## 2    Registration

Given a multimodal set of scans for a patient, we aim to align all patient images into the common anatomical space of an atlas. In this section, we briefly review image registration, and motivate the necessity of proper initialization, brain masking, and intensity correction for successful registration of clinical images. We perform spatial normalization into the atlas space using T1 images, followed by alignment of all other modalities (T2-FLAIR, DWI, etc.) via intra-patient multimodal registration. However, the methods we describe can be used with any atlas modality that enables accurate anatomical alignment.

Image registration techniques have been widely studied, and generally include a distance or similarity metric, a transformation model, and an optimization procedure [5,19,27]. Three of the most popular metrics used in registration are sum of squared differences (SSD), cross correlation (CC), and mutual information (MI). SSD and CC are used when the intensity distributions are directly comparable between the two images. MI is typically used for multimodal registration when the intensity profiles differ between scans (e.g., when registering a T1-weighted image to a T2-weighted image) [27]. Optimizing over nonrigid transformations is usually only effective after an accurate initialization based on simpler rigid or affine alignment. Registration between clinical images of patients and an atlas image is difficult in large, potentially multi-site studies for two main reasons. First, the patient images contain many irrelevant structures: our goal is brain analysis, but the images include the skull and large portions of the neck, and may even crop structures of interest, as illustrated in Fig. 1. The optimization procedure treats all regions uniformly, and aligning these bright, highly variable structures may drive the registration and result in an inaccurate transformation of the brain. Second, since images in large clinical studies are often acquired at multiple sites with different scanners and different acquisition parameters, the range of values and the intensity distributions across tissue classes varies greatly across images of the same modality. We address these challenges by proposing general strategies for each registration step. Algorithm 1 summarizes the steps of our registration pipeline. All registration steps are performed using the ANTS [2] software package.

*Intra-modal initialization with MI.* When registering images of the same modality, the standard practice of first computing an initial rigid registration (i.e., rotation and translation only) is relatively insensitive to the problem of

---

**Algorithm 1.** Registration pipeline of Section 2

---

1: INITIAL RIGID REGISTRATION: Rigidly register the atlas T1 image to the patient
    T1 image, using MI as a metric to handle intensity profile differences.
2: APPROXIMATE BRAIN MASK PROPAGATION: Use the estimated rigid transformation
    from Step 1 to transfer the brain mask from the atlas space to the patient T1 space
    to use for intensity correction and to guide nonrigid registration.
3: PATIENT T1 INTENSITY CORRECTION: Use the approximate brain mask from Step 2
    to estimate the white matter intensity mode in the patient T1 image. Scale patient
    T1 intensities so that the mode of white matter intensity matches that of the atlas,
    enabling the use of intensity-based metrics in registration.
4: NONRIGID T1 REGISTRATION: Nonrigidly register the atlas T1 image to the
    intensity-corrected patient T1 image from Step 3 using CC as a metric, with
    the transformation from Step 1 for initialization and the approximate brain mask
    from Step 2 to restrict the region where the metric is computed.
5: BRAIN MASK PROPAGATION: Use the estimated nonrigid transformation from Step 4
    to obtain a more accurate brain mask in the patient T1 space.
6: MULTIMODAL REGISTRATION: Rigidly register the patient T2-FLAIR/DWI images
    to the T1 image of the same patient using MI as a metric, with the final brain
    mask from Step 5 to restrict the region where the metric is computed.

---

extraneous structures. Inconsistent intensity distributions in images of the same
modality in clinical datasets render the usual intra-modality metrics such as
CC and SSD ineffective for alignment since the assumption of direct intensity
matching for the same tissue type across different images is violated. Standard
methods for matching intensity profiles, such as histogram equalization, cannot
be used either, since they would be dominated by non-brain regions such as the
neck. We employ MI in performing this rigid registration since the difference
of tissue intensities between these images is more similar to the difference of
tissue intensities between images of different modalities. We build on this initial
registration to solve the problems of inconsistent field of view and intensity
profiles described above.

*Skull stripping and brain masking.* Since we are typically only interested
in the brain in neuroimaging studies, we seek an accurate transformation in
the brain, and restrict the region where the registration metric is evaluated accordingly. In research-quality images, skull stripping or brain mask extraction is
achieved via watershed methods that assume that the brain consists of a single
connected component separated from the skull and dura by CSF [22]. Unfortunately, such techniques are highly dependent on image quality, and require
high resolution and reliable contrast. As a result, they often fail when applied
to clinical images. Instead, we propagate a brain mask from the atlas via the
estimated rigid transformation. While not a perfect brain mask, it enables intensity correction and constrains the final nonrigid registration to a region that
reasonably approximates the brain.

*Intensity correction.* In our experiments with clinical images of stroke patients, MI failed when used in nonrigid registration, resulting in inconsistent deformations that did not match the images. Differences in intensity profiles of patient images prevent us from using intensity-based measures such as CC and SSD directly. Using the approximate brain mask, we adjust the intensity separately for each image to solve this problem. Histogram equalization still cannot be used due to the approximate nature of the brain mask and variable intensity profiles (see Fig. 3). We choose to restrict our intensity correction to global scaling. Specifically, we match the intensity of the white matter while not altering the shape of the intensity profiles. As one of the largest structures in the brain, the white matter is important to match well between the two images in registration. We estimate the mode of white matter intensity for each patient as the mode of the component with higher intensity in a two-component mixture model for intensity values within the brain mask.

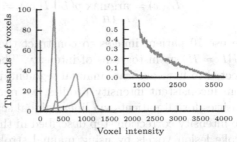

*Final non-rigid registration.* Once the image intensity distribution of the patient image has been matched to that of the atlas image, non-rigid registration can then be performed with CC as a metric. In order to prevent non-brain structures from dominating the optimization, we continue to use the approximate brain mask in computing this registration. Once the registration is concluded, we propagate a more accurate mask of the brain to be used for multimodal registration within each patient.

**Fig. 3.** Voxel intensity histograms from three different patients (shown in three different colors), illustrating typical differences in intensity distributions within the approximate brain mask obtained via rigid registration from the atlas. The inset highlights the difference at the high end of intensity values.

*Intra-patient multimodal registration.* In order to align other modalities (such as T2-FLAIR and DWI in the stroke study) into the atlas coordinate system, we first estimate the rigid transformation to the atlas-modality image (in our case, this is T1) using MI, and compose it with the final nonrigid transformation between the patient and the atlas.

*Evaluating registration quality.* Since visual inspection is not feasible for thousands of patients, we employ automatically computed measures of registration quality to detect when registration failed. We construct a (voxelwise) median image of registered patients for each modality in the atlas space, compute SSD of each intensity-corrected patient image from this median image within the brain mask, and isolate patients whose measures are substantially higher than the rest using the Tukey fence (more than 1.5 times the interquartile range above the third quartile) [24].

# 3   White Matter Hyperintensity (WMH) Segmentation

WMH is characterized by high intensity in T2-FLAIR MRI, but so are other brain structures such as the ventricle lining (ependyma) and the skull. Stroke lesions, both acute and chronic, can sometimes appear bright in T2-FLAIR as well. As a result, manual segmentation of WMH is typically performed via thresholding followed by expert editing to restrict the segmentation to the relevant regions of white matter and exclude areas with stroke lesions.

We create an expert-defined region of interest for WMH in the atlas space and take advantage of the registration pipeline to propagate this region to the patient's T2-FLAIR image. We employ MAP classification to label WMH voxels within the region of interest. Given intensity $I(x)$ at voxel $x$, we choose label $L(x) \in \{H, \bar{H}\}$ (where $H$ represents WMH and $\bar{H}$ represents healthy tissue) to maximize the posterior probability of the label $p(L(x)|I(x))$:

$$L^*(x) = \underset{L \in \{H, \bar{H}\}}{\mathrm{argmax}}\, p(L \mid I(x)) = \underset{L \in \{H, \bar{H}\}}{\mathrm{argmax}}\, p(I(x) \mid L)\, p(L). \tag{1}$$

We use 10 patient images to construct the likelihood models $p(I|L = H)$ and $p(I|L = \bar{H})$ as histograms of intensity. These training images were visually inspected to have accurate manual segmentations. As T2-FLAIR scans also suffer from inconsistent intensity profiles, we match the T2-FLAIR white matter intensities for all patients via linear global scaling before segmentation, similar to the intensity correction step described in the previous section. We exclude acute stroke lesion voxels by using manual stroke segmentations derived from DWI scans, which are aligned to T2-FLAIR scans as part of the registration pipeline. To estimate the prior $p(L)$, we use the proportion of voxels in the 10 training images with the corresponding label within the region of interest specified in the atlas space.

As with training data, we use DWI stroke lesion segmentations to exclude acute stroke voxels when performing WMH labeling in new patients. Future directions of research include developing automatic methods for stroke lesion segmentation.

# 4   Progression of WMH Spatial Distribution

WMH burden and its evolution with respect to clinical variables, such as age, is important for understanding cerebrovascular mechanisms related to stroke [17,18]. While the overall WMH *volume* of each patient can be compared and analyzed from just the manual segmentations for each patient, we use the registration framework to evaluate and visually inspect the *spatial distribution* of WMH and to understand its evolution across the brain as a function of age. Since WMH volume varies dramatically across different patients, we choose to first cluster the patients into more homogeneous sub-populations and then investigate the change of WMH distribution with age separately in each sub-population.

We use a two-component regression mixture model to capture variability in WMH volume growth [8,15]. Each component is characterized by a different

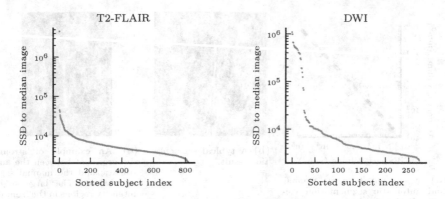

**Fig. 4.** Distances from patient images to median image for T2-FLAIR and DWI modalities, ranked in descending order. Outliers are shown in red, and are removed from subsequent analysis.

dependency of WMH burden on age. To determine the assignment of patients to sub-populations associated with components, we alternate between assigning the cluster membership of each patient and estimating the regression coefficients for WMH volume as a function of age in each cluster, until convergence.

Formally, let $v_i$ and $z_i$ be the scalar total WMH volume and cluster assignment of patient $i$ ($i \in \{1, \ldots, N\}$) respectively. We let $X_i$ be a $p$-dimensional feature vector associated with patient $i$. Specifically, we use age and a constant to account for the intercept (i.e., $p = 2$). Let $v$ be the vector of all volume values and $X$ be the $N \times p$ matrix of features. We assume i.i.d. multinomial priors for cluster membership. Given $p$-dimensional regression coefficient vectors $\beta_c$ for each cluster $c$ and fixed variance $\sigma^2$, we assume that WMH volume $v_i$ in patient $i$ is normally distributed with mean $X_i\beta_c$ and fixed variance $\sigma^2$:

$$v_i = X_i\beta_c + \epsilon_i, \quad \text{where } \epsilon_i \sim \mathcal{N}(0, \sigma^2).$$

In order to estimate the parameters $\beta$, we use a hard-assignment EM variant, alternating until convergence between the E-step that computes the cluster assignments:

$$z_i = \operatorname*{argmin}_c \|v_i - X_i\beta_c\|_2^2, \tag{2}$$

and the M-step that solves for each $\beta_c$ using standard least-squares linear regression:

$$\beta_c = (X^T Z_c X)^{-1} X^T Z_c v, \tag{3}$$

where $Z_c$ is a diagonal binary matrix; $Z_c(i,i) = 1$ if $z_i = c$. The resulting algorithm is similar to $k$-means clustering.

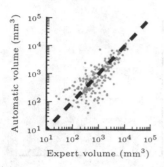

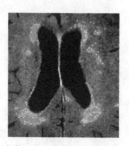

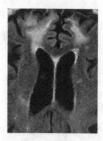

(a) Agreement between manual and automatic segmentation volumes. Each point represents one patient, and the dashed line ($y = x$) corresponds to perfect agreement.

(b) A typical segmentation result.

(c) An example of strong disagreement between the automatic and the manual segmentations. The large high intensity regions in the frontal lobe (translucent red) bilaterally represent chronic territorial infarcts that, although hyperintense, are excluded by the expert since they are not of interest in WMH volume calculations.

**Fig. 5.** Left: comparison of automatic and manual WMH segmentation volumes. Right: example segmentations. Manual segmentation (translucent red), automatic segmentation (yellow), and overlap (orange) are overlaid on axial slices.

Within each cluster, we use Nadaraya-Watson kernel regression [4,13,28] on the WMH label maps to visualize representative images $I_c(t)$ for each cluster $c$:

$$I_c(t) = \frac{\sum_{i=1}^{N} Z_c(i,i)K_h(t - t_i)I_i}{\sum_{i=1}^{N} Z_c(i,i)K_h(t - t_i)},\qquad(4)$$

where $t$ is the age of interest, $N$ is the number of patients, $I_i$ is the WMH label map of patient $i$ warped into atlas space, and $K_h(\cdot)$ is a Gaussian kernel function with standard deviation $h$ and mean 0. Intuitively, a representative WMH image is a weighted average of all WMH label maps, with patients close to age $t$ contributing more to the average. Visualizing representative images helps understand the progression of the disease with age.

## 5    Results

We illustrate our framework in the context of a stroke dataset which currently includes 1089 patients, with T1 ($1 \times 1$mm in-plane, slice thickness 5-7mm), T2-FLAIR ($1 \times 1$mm in-plane, slice thickness 5-7mm, PROPELLER sequence sometimes used if the patient moved), and DWI (at least 6 directions, b-value 1000 s/mm$^2$, 1mm $\times$ 1mm in-plane, slice thickness 5-7mm). Acquisition TR and TE varied depending on image protocol. T1 images were bias-field corrected [25] prior to analysis. In 819 patients, both T1 and manually segmented T2-FLAIR images were available. In 515 of these, DWI was also available, and in 276 of these, manual stroke lesion segmentations were available.

***Registration.*** For atlas-to-patient registration, we use the atlas constructed from 39 T1-weighted brain MRI scans and corresponding manual delineations that are part of the Freesurfer brain atlas [3,9,11]. The 39 subjects span a wide age range, reflect significant anatomical variation, and include some Alzheimer's patients.

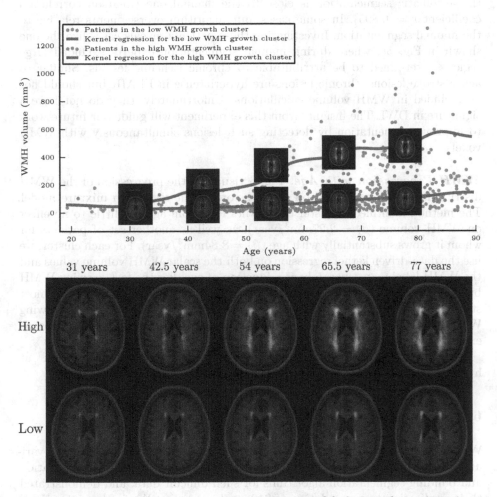

**Fig. 6.** Top: the two-component regression mixture model clusters the patients into those with high WMH growth as a function of age (red) and those with low WMH growth as a function of age (blue). The lines show a kernel regression of WMH volume as a function of age in each cluster. The representative images shown are obtained via kernel regression of the WMH label maps as a function of age. Bottom: the two sets of representative images in more detail.

After using our registration pipeline, the quality evaluation procedure identified 86 of 819 T2-FLAIR scans and 39 of 275 segmented DWI scans as outliers, leading us to exclude them from subsequent analysis (Fig. 4). Most outliers contain severe artifacts. We also verified that images that were close to the threshold but were included in the analysis were accurately registered by the method.

*WMH Segmentation.* Fig. 5 illustrates the volume agreement between the automatic and manual WMH segmentation. We observe that in most patients the automatic segmentation is close to the manual one (Pearson correlation coefficient $r = 0.895$). In some cases, our algorithm oversegments relative to the manual segmentation. Investigating these patients reveals cases like the one shown in Fig. 5c, where during manual segmentation experts excluded large regions determined to be attributable to chronic ischemic lesions. Similar to acute stroke lesions, chronic lesions are hyperintense in FLAIR but should not be included in WMH volume calculations. Unfortunately, they do not have a signature in DWI. The insights from this experiment will guide our future work to improve segmentation by detecting such lesions simultaneously with WMH voxels.

*WMH Progression with Age.* Fig. 6 visualizes the progression of the WMH distributions with age based on the two-component regression mixture model. The method identified a cluster of patients for whom age has little to no effect on WMH volume ($\beta_1 = 2.27\text{mm}^3/\text{year}$), as well as another set of patients for whom it grows substantially with age ($\beta_2 = 8.84\text{mm}^3/\text{year}$). For each cluster, we use the data-driven kernel regression on both the scalar WMH volume values and the WMH label map separately as a function of age. For the fast-growing WMH burden cluster, WMH tends to spread throughout the white matter, and most strongly in the posterior regions of the white matter. In the other, slow-growing WMH burden cluster, the white matter remains confined near the ventricles, as expected.

We provide code that implements all steps of our framework at http://groups.csail.mit.edu/vision/medical-vision/stroke/.

## 6    Conclusion

We presented a framework for analysis of large-scale studies with highly variable clinical images. We discussed necessary decisions in adapting registration and building segmentation algorithms for such difficult data, and demonstrated their application to a population of 819 stroke patients. We further introduced analysis to characterize WMH progression as a function of age, enabled by the multimodal registration and segmentation framework. In registration of clinical images, initialization, choice of cost function, automatic data-driven brain masking, intensity correction, and automatic evaluation are critical steps which we discussed in detail.

In the future, we will extend our segmentation methodology to include automatic segmentation of acute stroke lesions from DWI [10], and chronic stroke lesions from T2-FLAIR. This will enable completely automatic segmentation of white matter hyperintensity and provide more features for the clinical analysis. Additionally, richer analyses using more sophisticated models and additional clinical features such as stroke severity promise to lead to interesting clinical findings.

As large, multimodal, multicenter datasets of highly variable quality come online, fully automatic data-driven methods become a crucial part of the analysis. We have demonstrated a robust, scalable framework that enables such analysis for stroke studies.

**Acknowledgments.** We acknowledge the following funding sources: NSF GRFP, NSERC CGS-D, Barbara J. Weedon Fellowship, NIH NCRR NAC P41-RR13218 and NIH NIBIB NAC P41-EB-015902, NIH NIBIB NAMIC U54-EB005149, NIH-NINDS K23 NS064052, NINDS U01NS069208, and the American Stroke Association-Bugher Foundation Centers for Stroke Prevention Research.

# References

1. Admiraal-Behloul, F., et al.: Fully automatic segmentation of white matter hyperintensities in MR images of the elderly. Neuroimage 28(3), 607–617 (2005)
2. Avants, B.B., Tustison, N.J., Song, G., Cook, P.A., Klein, A., Gee, J.C.: A reproducible evaluation of ANTs similarity metric performance in brain image registration. Neuroimage 54(3), 2033–2044 (2011)
3. Daly, E., et al.: Predicting conversion to Alzheimer disease using standardized clinical information. Archives of Neurology 57(5), 675 (2000)
4. Davis, B.C., Fletcher, P.T., Bullitt, E., Joshi, S.: Population shape regression from random design data. In: IEEE International Conference on Computer Vision, pp. 1–7. IEEE (2007)
5. Hartkens, T., Rohr, K., Stiehl, H.S.: Evaluation of 3D operators for the detection of anatomical point landmarks in MR and CT images. Computer Vision and Image Understanding 86(2), 118–136 (2002)
6. Hinrichs, C., Singh, V., Xu, G., Johnson, S.C.: Predictive markers for AD in a multi-modality framework: an analysis of MCI progression in the ADNI population. Neuroimage 55(2), 574–589 (2011)
7. Hubert, H.B., Feinleib, M., McNamara, P.M., Castelli, W.P.: Obesity as an independent risk factor for cardiovascular disease: a 26-year follow-up of participants in the Framingham Heart Study. Circulation 67(5), 968–977 (1983)
8. Jacobs, R.A., Jordan, M.I., Nowlan, S.J., Hinton, G.E.: Adaptive mixtures of local experts. Neural Computation 3(1), 79–87 (1991)
9. Johnson, K.A., et al.: Preclinical prediction of Alzheimer's disease using SPECT. Neurology 50(6), 1563–1571 (1998)
10. Kabir, Y., Dojat, M., Scherrer, B., Garbay, C., Forbes, F.: Multimodal MRI segmentation of ischemic stroke lesions. In: International Conference of the IEEE Engineering in Medicine and Biology Society (EMBC), pp. 1595–1598. IEEE (2007)
11. Killiany, R.J., et al.: Use of structural magnetic resonance imaging to predict who will get Alzheimer's disease. Annals of Neurology 47(4), 430–439 (2000)
12. Klein, A., et al.: Evaluation of 14 nonlinear deformation algorithms applied to human brain MRI registration. Neuroimage 46(3), 786 (2009)

13. Nadaraya, E.A.: On estimating regression. Theory of Probability & Its Applications 9(1), 141–142 (1964)
14. Paulsen, J.S., et al.: Detection of Huntingtons disease decades before diagnosis: the Predict-HD study. Journal of Neurology, Neurosurgery & Psychiatry 79(8), 874–880 (2008)
15. Quandt, R.E., Ramsey, J.B.: Estimating mixtures of normal distributions and switching regressions. Journal of the American Statistical Association 73(364), 730–738 (1978)
16. Regan, E.A., et al.: Genetic epidemiology of COPD (COPDGene) study design. COPD: Journal of Chronic Obstructive Pulmonary Disease 7(1), 32–43 (2011)
17. Rost, N.S., et al.: White matter hyperintensity burden and susceptibility to cerebral ischemia. Stroke 41(12), 2807–2811 (2010)
18. Rost, N.S., et al.: White matter hyperintensity volume is increased in small vessel stroke subtypes. Neurology 75(19), 1670–1677 (2010)
19. Rueckert, D., Schnabel, J.A.: Medical image registration. Biomedical Image Processing, 131–154 (2011)
20. Sabuncu, M.R., Balci, S.K., Shenton, M.E., Golland, P.: Image-driven population analysis through mixture modeling. IEEE Transactions on Medical Imaging (TMI) 28(9), 1473–1487 (2009)
21. Salton, C.J., et al.: Gender differences and normal left ventricular anatomy in an adult population free of hypertension. A cardiovascular magnetic resonance study of the Framingham Heart Study Offspring cohort. Journal of the American College of Cardiology 39(6), 1055–1060 (2002)
22. Segonne, F., et al.: A hybrid approach to the skull stripping problem in MRI. Neuroimage 22(3), 1060–1075 (2004)
23. Talairach, J., Tournoux, P.: Co-planar stereotaxic atlas of the human brain. 3-Dimensional proportional system: an approach to cerebral imaging (1988)
24. Tukey, J.W.: Exploratory data analysis. Pearson (1977)
25. Tustison, N.J., Gee, J.C.: N4ITK: Nicks N3 ITK implementation for MRI bias field correction. Insight Journal (2009)
26. Vercauteren, T., Pennec, X., Perchant, A., Ayache, N., et al.: Diffeomorphic demons: Efficient non-parametric image registration. NeuroImage 45(1) (2008)
27. Viola, P., Wells III, W.M.: Alignment by maximization of mutual information. International Journal of Computer Vision 24(2), 137–154 (1997)
28. Watson, G.S.: Smooth regression analysis. Sankhyā: The Indian Journal of Statistics, Series A, 359–372 (1964)
29. Weiner, M.W., et al.: The Alzheimers Disease Neuroimaging Initiative: a review of papers published since its inception. Alzheimer's & Dementia 8(1), S1–S68 (2012)

# Modeling 4D Changes in Pathological Anatomy Using Domain Adaptation: Analysis of TBI Imaging Using a Tumor Database

Bo Wang[1,2,*], Marcel Prastawa[1,2], Avishek Saha[1,2], Suyash P. Awate[1,2],
Andrei Irimia[3], Micah C. Chambers[3], Paul M. Vespa[4], John D. Van Horn[3],
Valerio Pascucci[1,2], and Guido Gerig[1,2]

[1] Scientific Computing and Imaging Institute, University of Utah
[2] School of Computing, University of Utah
[3] Institute for Neuroimaging and Informatics, University of Southern California
[4] Brain Injury Research Center, University of California at Los Angeles
bowang@sci.utah.edu

**Abstract.** Analysis of 4D medical images presenting pathology (i.e., lesions) is significantly challenging due to the presence of complex changes over time. Image analysis methods for 4D images with lesions need to account for changes in brain structures due to deformation, as well as the formation and deletion of new structures (e.g., edema, bleeding) due to the physiological processes associated with damage, intervention, and recovery. We propose a novel framework that models 4D changes in pathological anatomy across time, and provides explicit mapping from a healthy template to subjects with pathology. Moreover, our framework uses transfer learning to leverage rich information from a known source domain, where we have a collection of completely segmented images, to yield effective appearance models for the input target domain. The automatic 4D segmentation method uses a novel domain adaptation technique for generative kernel density models to transfer information between different domains, resulting in a fully automatic method that requires no user interaction. We demonstrate the effectiveness of our novel approach with the analysis of 4D images of traumatic brain injury (TBI), using a synthetic tumor database as the source domain.

## 1 Introduction

Traumatic brain injury (TBI) is a critical problem in healthcare that impacts approximately 1.7 million people in the United States every year [3]. The varying cause and degree of injury (falls, car accidents, etc.) presents significant challenges in the interpretation of image data but also in quantitative assessment of brain pathology via image analysis. Determining effective therapy and intervention strategies requires the ability to track the image changes over time, which motivates the development of segmentation and registration methods for longitudinal 4D Magnetic Resonance (MR) images. Such methods need to account

---

* Corresponding author.

L. Shen et al. (Eds.): MBIA 2013, LNCS 8159, pp. 31–39, 2013.
© Springer International Publishing Switzerland 2013

for changes in brain structures due to deformation, as well as the formation and deletion of new structures (e.g., edema, bleeding) due to physiological processes associated with damage, therapeutical intervention, and recovery.

In 4D image analysis, researchers have proposed methods [9,2,5,6] to register images with lesions over time accounting for appearance of new structures. However, these methods have not been evaluated for mapping healthy subjects to a patient with lesions. Niethammer et al. proposed a registration method for TBI images using geometric metamorphosis that maps TBI over time using known, pre-segmented lesion boundaries defined manually [5]. Wang et al. [14] proposed a registration-segmentation method for 4D TBI images using personalized atlas construction that combines information from multiple time points, accounting for diffeomorphic changes (smooth deformation) and non-diffeomorphic changes (creation/deletion of lesions) over time. However, their method requires manual initialization in the form of user-defined spheres covering the lesions and only provides modeling of intra-patient changes without providing explicit mapping to normative healthy brain anatomy.

We propose a novel framework that models changes in 4D pathological anatomy across time and provides explicit mapping from a healthy template to TBI subject images. This aids analysis of TBI patients by enabling the mapping of parcellation labels describing anatomical regions of interest and quantitative comparison against a common reference space defined by the normative template. Moreover, our framework uses *transfer learning* [7] to leverage rich information from a "known source" domain, where we have a large collection of fully segmented images, to yield effective models for the "input target" domain (TBI images). This is essential as such a database does not exist for TBI imaging, and thus we explore and demonstrate the use of an existing database of multi-modal tumor imaging that serves as a well-studied source domain. The information in the learned tumor model are transferred to the domain of TBI images using *importance weighting based domain adaptation* [12], a well known transfer learning technique, resulting in a fully automatic method that does not require user input. In this paper, we propose importance weighting based domain adaptation for generative kernel density models, thus extending its applications beyond standard discriminative models available in machine learning literature [1].

## 2    Method

We propose a framework that constructs 4D models of pathological anatomy starting from a healthy template, to describe changes at different time points accounting for the complete 4D information. Our framework also leverages known domains, such as brain tumors, where we have a rich collection of information in the form of segmented tumor images with varying size, shape, deformations, and appearance. The database of tumor images is obtained by using the brain tumor simulator[1] developed by Prastawa et al.[11]. It is capable of generating synthetic

---

[1] http://www.nitrc.org/projects/tumorsim

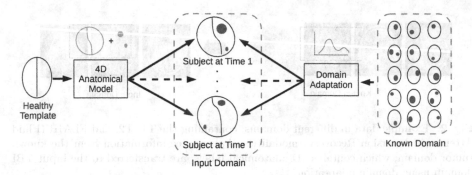

**Fig. 1.** Conceptual overview of the proposed framework. Our framework maps a healthy template to input TBI images at different time points using a 4D anatomical model which provides spatial context. The model leverages information from a different known domain, in this case tumor images that are fully segmented. Data from the known domain with lesions (indicated in red) at different locations with varying size, shape, and deformations are used to estimate an appearance model for the input TBI images.

images for a large variety of tumor cases with complete 3D segmentations. Fig. 1 shows a conceptual overview of our mathematical framework.

## 2.1  4D Modeling of Pathological Anatomy

We model the anatomical changes over time as a combination of diffeomorphic image deformation and non-diffeomorphic changes of probabilities for lesion categories, accounting for temporally smooth deformations and abrupt changes, e.g., due to lesions appearing and disappearing over time. Specifically, the spatial prior $P_t^c$ for each class $c$ at time point $t$ is modeled as

$$P_t^c = A^c \circ \phi_t + Q_t^c \qquad (1)$$

where $A$ is the tissue class probability that is initially associated with the healthy template, $\phi_t$ is the diffeomorphic deformation from time $t$ to the atlas, and $Q_t$ is the non-diffeomorphic probabilistic change for time $t$. This approach follows the metamorphosis framework of Trouvé and Younes [13]. Our method estimates a common subject-specific atlas $A$ for all time points.

Given the model and 4D multimodal images $I_t$ at timepoints $t$, we estimate model parameters that minimize the following functional:

$$\operatorname{argmin}_{A,\phi_t,Q_t,\theta_t} \mathcal{F}(A,\phi_t,Q_t,\theta_t) + \mathcal{R}_1(Q) + \mathcal{R}_2(A) + \mathcal{R}_3(\phi) \qquad (2)$$

s. t. $A^c \in [0,1], \quad \sum_c A^c = 1, \quad (A^c \circ \phi_t + Q_t^c) \in [0,1], \quad \sum_c (A^c \circ \phi_t + Q_t^c) = 1$

where $\mathcal{F}$ represents the data functional (the negative total log-likelihood)

$$\mathcal{F}(A,\phi_t,Q_t) = -\sum_{t=1}^{T} \sum_{x=1}^{N} \log \left( \sum_{c=1}^{C} P_t^c(x)\, p(I_t(x)|c,\theta_t^c) \right), \qquad (3)$$

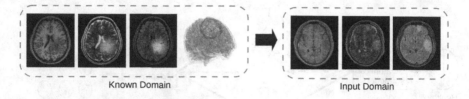

Known Domain                    Input Domain

**Fig. 2.** Example data in different domains, containing the T1, T2, and FLAIR (Fluid Attenuated Inversion Recovery) modalities. Appearance information from the known tumor domain, which contains 3D anatomical labels, are transferred to the input TBI domain using domain adaptation.

and $\mathcal{R}$ represents the regularity terms:

$$\mathcal{R}_1(Q) = \alpha \sum_t \| Q_t \|_{L_1}, \quad \mathcal{R}_2(A) = \beta \| A - A^{(0)} \|_{L_2}, \quad \mathcal{R}_3(\phi) = \gamma \sum_t d(id, \phi_t).$$
(4)

$T$ denotes the number of observed time points, $C$ denotes the number of tissue classes, $p(I_t | c, \theta_t^c)$ is the image likelihood function for class $c$ with parameter $\theta_t^c$, $A^{(0)}$ is the initial atlas $A$ obtained from the healthy template, and $d(id, \cdot)$ is the distance to the identity transform. $\mathcal{R}_1$ enforces the sparsity of $Q$, $\mathcal{R}_2$ prevents extreme deviations in $A$ from the initial model, and $\mathcal{R}_3$ enforces the smoothness of the deformations $\phi_t$. These regularization functionals are weighted by user-defined parameters $\alpha$, $\beta$, $\gamma$ respectively.

## 2.2   Image Appearance Model Using Domain Adaptation

We compute our image appearance model $p(I_t | c, \theta_t^c)$ using the well-known domain adaptation technique, where we adapt an appearance model from a known domain (tumor images) to the input domain (TBI images). We use a simulator [11] to generate a large collection of synthetic tumor images that resemble TBI images, and we use the rich information in this database to automatically compute the likelihood density model and then transfer this model to the TBI domain. Fig. 2 shows examples of fully segmented synthetic tumor images from the known domain and unsegmented TBI images in the input domain.

We select a tumor image from the database that has the smallest earth mover's distance [8] compared to the input TBI images. We then obtain training samples in the known or "source" domain as a subset of the completely segmented tumor data $\{\hat{I}(\hat{x}), \hat{\ell}(\hat{x}), \hat{P}_c(\hat{x})\}$, with $\hat{I}$ representing the tumor intensities, $\hat{\ell}$ representing the discrete segmentations, $\hat{P}_c$ representing the probabilistic segmentations, and $\hat{x}$ representing the coordinates in the tumor image domain. The transfer of learned appearance models is accomplished via domain adaptation that incorporates importance weighting. We weight intensity observations $I$ using the weights $w(I) = \frac{p(I)}{\hat{p}(I)}$ with $\hat{p}$ being the density in the source domain. In practice, $w$ is estimated using KLIEP (Kullback-Leibler Importance Estimation Procedure) [12]

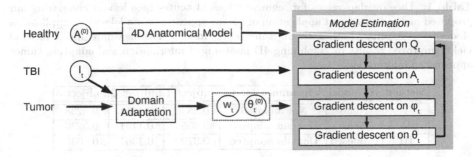

**Fig. 3.** Model parameter estimation process. The healthy template provides the initial personalized atlas $A$ in the 4D anatomical model. Input images together with the tumor database are used to generate densities represented by importance weights $w_t$ and kernel width parameter $\theta_t$. All parameters are updated using alternating gradient descent, where initially $Q_t$ is zero and $\phi_t$ is the identity transform.

which minimizes the Kullback-Leibler divergence between the density of the input domain and the weighted density of the source domain $KL(p(I) \parallel w(I)\,\hat{p}(I))$.

Using the estimated weights $w$, we compute the density parameter $\hat{\theta}$ that maximize the data likelihood in the tumor domain:

$$\underset{\hat{\theta}}{\operatorname{argmax}} \sum_{\hat{x}} w(\hat{I}(\hat{x})) \, \log \left( \sum_{c} \hat{P}_c(\hat{x})\,\hat{p}(\hat{I}(\hat{x})|c,\hat{\theta}_c) \right). \tag{5}$$

We use the kernel density model for the image appearance, parametrized by the kernel bandwidths for each class $\hat{\theta} = \{\hat{h}^{c=1}, \cdots, \hat{h}^{c=C}\}$. The image likelihood in the TBI domain is modeled in the same fashion, where we initialize TBI parameter $\theta$ using the "domain adapted" tumor parameter $\hat{\theta}$ from Eq. (5).

## 2.3   Model Parameter Estimation

We perform model parameter estimation by minimizing the overall objective function (Eq. 2) with respect to each parameter. Fig. 3 provides a conceptual view of the parameter estimation process, which incorporates gradient descent updates that are effectively image registration and segmentation operations. In particular, we use these gradient equations to optimize the data functional $\mathcal{F}$:

$$\nabla_{Q_t^c}\mathcal{F}(x) = -\frac{p(I_t(x)|c,\theta_t^c)}{\sum_{c'} P_t^{c'}(x)\,p(I_t(x)|c',\theta_t^{c'})}, \tag{6}$$

$$\nabla_{A^c}\mathcal{F}(x) = -\sum_{t} \frac{|D\,\phi_t(x)|\,p(I_t(\phi_t^{-1}(x))|c,\theta_t^c)}{\sum_{c'} [A^{c'}(x) + Q_t^{c'}(\phi_t^{-1}(x))]\,p(I_t(\phi_t^{-1}(x))|c',\theta_t^{c'})}, \tag{7}$$

$$\nabla_{\phi_t}\mathcal{F}(x) = -\sum_{c} \frac{p(I_t(x)|c,\theta_t^c)}{\sum_{c'} P_t^{c'}(x)\,p(I_t(x)|c',\theta_t^{c'})}\,\nabla(A^c \circ \phi_t(x)), \tag{8}$$

**Table 1.** Dice overlap values for segmentations of acute-stage lesions comparing our proposed method to a direct application of tumor appearance model and an application of domain adaption, both without using a 4D model. The new integrated method yields improved results by combining 4D anatomical information and adapting tumor appearance information.

| Method | 4D Model | Appearance Model | Subject 1 | Subject 2 | Subject 3 |
|--------|----------|------------------|-----------|-----------|-----------|
| I | None | Not adapted | 0.2536 | 0.1211 | 0.5238 |
| II | None | Domain adapted | 0.3053 | 0.1131 | 0.5238 |
| III | Proposed | Domain adapted | 0.3792 | 0.1367 | 0.6035 |

where $|D\phi|$ denotes the determinant of the Jacobian of $\phi$. The updates show that $Q_t$ moves to the data likelihood specific to time $t$, $A$ moves to the average data likelihood over time, and $\phi_t$ deforms $A$ to match the boundaries between data and atlas. Constraints are enforced using projected gradient descent [10]. The image likelihood model $p(I_t|c, \theta_t^c)$ obtained from domain adaptation is fitted to the input image data using gradient descent update $\nabla_{h_t^c} \mathcal{F}$, which finds the set of widths that best matches data to the current estimate of the atlas at timepoint $t$, $P_t^c = A^c \circ \phi_t + Q_t^c$.

## 3   Results

We evaluate the performance of our new approach on 4D TBI image data containing two time points: acute and chronic ($\approx$ 3 days and $\approx$ 6 months post-surgery). The performance of our proposed method is shown in Tab. 1, where

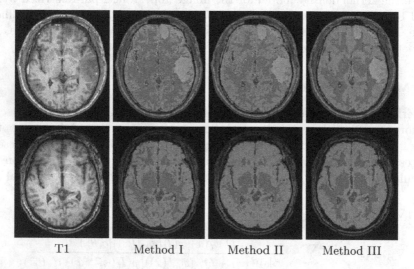

T1             Method I         Method II        Method III

**Fig. 4.** Segmentation results for subject 1 at acute (top) and chronic (bottom) stages using different methods. Our proposed method (III) has the best segmentation quality overall. Red: white matter, green: gray matter, blue: cerebrospinal fluid, and yellow: lesion.

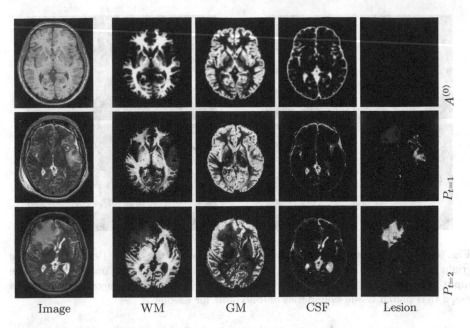

|  Image  |  WM  |  GM  |  CSF  |  Lesion  |
|---|---|---|---|---|

**Fig. 5.** Estimated 4D anatomical priors for TBI subject 3. First row shows the initial atlas $A^{(0)}$ in the template space, with the healthy T1 image as a reference. Second and third row show the personalized atlas $P_t = A \circ \phi_t + Q_t$ for acute and chronic stages, with input T2 images shown. Our method is able to account for changes in the left-frontal and mid-frontal regions across time.

we compare our method against those that do not use 4D modeling, with and without domain adaptation. Dice overlap values comparing automatic lesion segmentations against a human expert rater are relatively low, which is a well known fact when dealing with small objects with complex and fuzzily defined boundaries. However, our method not only provides improved lesion segmentation but also better overall segmentation, as shown qualitatively in Fig. 4.

The estimated 4D spatial priors for TBI subject 3 are illustrated in Fig. 5, incorporating template deformation to match image boundaries and non-diffeomorphic changes due to lesions. Subject 3 provides an interesting and revealing example of longitudinal pathology progression. The acute scan reveals gross pathology in the left frontal region, which results in considerable atrophy in this region at the chronic stage. However, the subject's chronic scan features an additional large lesion in the mid-frontal region due to the occurrence of a large abscess between acute and chronic scans. This is an excellent example of the dynamic and complex longitudinal changes that can occur in TBI patients.

The proposed method brings the advantage of providing a mapping from a normative template to a TBI subject. In Fig. 6, we show a parcellation label image, provided by the International Consortium for Brain Mapping (ICBM), that has been mapped to a TBI subject. The mapping of a normal anatomy to pathological anatomy will be potentially important to compare type, locality and

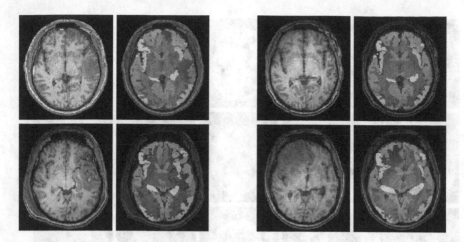

**Fig. 6.** Example brain parcellation labels mapped to the acute (left) and chronic (right) time points of subject 1 (top) and 3 (bottom). For each time point, we show the input T1 image and the overlaid parcellation labels. Our method generates parcellation maps that match tissue boundaries and account for lesions.

spatial extent of brain damages in the context of anatomically relevant regions with associated brain function information.

## 4    Conclusions

We demonstrate work in progress towards a framework that estimates 4D anatomical models from longitudinal TBI images. Our framework is fully automatic and leverages information from a different domain (brain tumor) to generate appearance models via domain adaptation. In addition to the new 4D anatomical modeling, we also presented a new domain adaptation method for generative kernel density models, integrated with our anatomical model in a single objective function (Eq. 2). Results on 3 TBI subjects show that our automatic method yields segmentations that match ground truth of manual segmentations. Furthermore, our method generates diffeomorphic deformation models as well as non-diffeomorphic probabilistic changes that have potential for analyzing and characterizing changes of normal appearing tissue and lesions. In the future, we will quantify temporal brain changes across a large set of TBI patients which were exposed to different treatment strategies. Our approach has potential to significantly improve regional and connectivity analysis of individuals relative to a population [4], by making use of the mapping of a normative template with associated parcellation labels to TBI subjects, without tedious manual input.

**Acknowledgments.** This work has been supported by National Alliance for Medical Image Computing (NA-MIC) U54 EB005149 (Guido Gerig) and the Utah Science Technology and Research (USTAR) initiative at the University of Utah.

# References

1. Beijbom, O.: Domain adaptations for computer vision applications. Tech. rep., University of California San Diego, arXiv:1211.4860 (April 2012)
2. Chitphakdithai, N., Duncan, J.S.: Non-rigid registration with missing correspondences in preoperative and postresection brain images. In: Jiang, T., Navab, N., Pluim, J.P.W., Viergever, M.A. (eds.) MICCAI 2010, Part I. LNCS, vol. 6361, pp. 367–374. Springer, Heidelberg (2010)
3. Faul, M., Xu, L., Wald, M., Coronado, V.: Traumatic brain injury in the United States: Emergency department visits, hospitalizations and deaths, 2002-2006. CDC, National Center for Injury Prevention and Control, Atlanta, GA (2010)
4. Irimia, A., Wang, B., Aylward, S., Prastawa, M., Pace, D., Gerig, G., Hovda, D., Kikinis, R., Vespa, P., Van Horn, J.: Neuroimaging of structural pathology and connectomics in traumatic brain injury: Toward personalized outcome prediction. NeuroImage: Clinical 1(1), 1–17 (2012)
5. Niethammer, M., Hart, G.L., Pace, D.F., Vespa, P.M., Irimia, A., Van Horn, J.D., Aylward, S.R.: Geometric metamorphosis. In: Fichtinger, G., Martel, A., Peters, T. (eds.) MICCAI 2011, Part II. LNCS, vol. 6892, pp. 639–646. Springer, Heidelberg (2011)
6. Ou, Y., Sotiras, A., Paragios, N., Davatzikos, C.: DRAMMS: Deformable registration via attribute matching and mutual-saliency weighting. Medical Image Analysis 15(4), 622–639 (2011)
7. Pan, S.J., Yang, Q.: A survey on transfer learning. IEEE Transactions on Knowledge and Data Engineering 22(10), 1345–1359 (2010)
8. Pele, O., Werman, M.: Fast and robust earth mover's distances. In: 2009 IEEE 12th International Conference on Computer Vision, pp. 460–467. IEEE (2009)
9. Periaswamy, S., Farid, H.: Medical image registration with partial data. Medical Image Analysis 10(3), 452–464 (2006)
10. Prastawa, M., Awate, S., Gerig, G.: Building spatiotemporal anatomical models using joint 4-D segmentation, registration, and subject-specific atlas estimation. In: 2012 IEEE Workshop on Mathematical Methods in Biomedical Image Analysis (MMBIA), pp. 49–56. IEEE (2012)
11. Prastawa, M., Bullitt, E., Gerig, G.: Simulation of brain tumors in MR images for evaluation of segmentation efficacy. Medical Image Analysis 13(2), 297–311 (2009)
12. Sugiyama, M., Nakajima, S., Kashima, H., Von Buenau, P., Kawanabe, M.: Direct importance estimation with model selection and its application to covariate shift adaptation. In: Advances in Neural Information Processing Systems, vol. 20, pp. 1433–1440 (2008)
13. Trouvé, A., Younes, L.: Metamorphoses through lie group action. Foundations of Computational Mathematics 5(2), 173–198 (2005)
14. Wang, B., Prastawa, M., Awate, S., Irimia, A., Chambers, M., Vespa, P., van Horn, J., Gerig, G.: Segmentation of serial MRI of TBI patients using personalized atlas construction and topological change estimation. In: 2012 9th IEEE International Symposium on Biomedical Imaging (ISBI), pp. 1152–1155 (2012)

# Bi-modal Non-rigid Registration of Brain MRI Data Based on Deconvolution of Joint Statistics

David Pilutti, Maddalena Strumia, and Stathis Hadjidemetriou

University Medical Center Freiburg, 79106 Freiburg, Germany
david.pilutti@uniklinik-freiburg.de

**Abstract.** Images of different contrasts in MRI can contain complementary information and can highlight different tissue types. Such datasets often need to be co-registered for any further processing. A novel and effective non-rigid registration method based on the restoration of the joint statistics of pairs of such images is proposed. The registration is performed with the deconvolution of the joint statistics and then with the enforcement of the deconvolved statistics back to the spatial domain to form a preliminary registration. The spatial transformation is also regularized with Gaussian spatial smoothing. The registration method has been compared to B-Splines and validated with a simulated Shepp-Logan phantom, with the BrainWeb phantom, and with real datasets. Improved results have been obtained for both accuracy as well as efficiency.

**Keywords:** Non-rigid registration, joint statistics restoration, brain registration, multi-contrast registration.

## 1 Introduction

In brain imaging different MRI contrasts can provide complementary information for tissue properties. The resulting images often need to be co-registered for any further analysis. The registration can be intra-subject or inter-subject and can also be achieved effectively with a non-rigid representation.

To address this problem B-Splines methods have been widely used [8]. They represent misregistration with splines centered on grid node pixels. To make this method robust even in the case of contrast change, it has been combined with a distance measure such as the mutual information [9]. An alternative and commonly used registration method has been the Demons method [11]. It is based on a variational formulation and assumes constancy in image contrast. The Demons method has been combined with the normalized mutual information and has been applied to the registration of multi-modal brain MRI [6].

Mutual information is an extensively used distance measure for multi-modal registration [7, 12]. However the mutual information is a scalar quantity that under-constrains the registration. This contributes to making the methods using it computationally intensive particularly for volumetric datasets. In practice such methods must be combined with considerable spatial subsampling and/or multiresolution [4–6, 8, 9].

L. Shen et al. (Eds.): MBIA 2013, LNCS 8159, pp. 40–50, 2013.

The approach presented in this work is shown to be able to register brain images of different as well as similar MRI contrasts. The spatial misregistration is represented in terms of its effect on the joint statistics. It is assumed that the misregistration smooths the joint statistics. We propose a novel systematic non-rigid registration method that is based on the restoration of the joint statistics. The problem is approached as a statistical restoration, where the effect of the misregistration is represented as a convolution of the statistics with a Gaussian filter. The statistics are restored with a Wiener filter [13] that is used adaptively. The deconvolved statistics are enforced to the registration between the images to obtain an initial spatial transformation. Then, the transformation is regularized for smoothness.

The implementation of the proposed method is iterative and interleaves between the two constraints. The method has been compared with the Slicer3D implementation of the B-Splines registration. They have been compared over a variable contrast extension of the 3D Shepp-Logan simulated phantom [10], a modified BrainWeb phantom [1], and on several real datasets. It has been performed in full image resolution with significantly reduced computational requirements. The proposed method improves performance in terms of spatial resolution, computational efficiency, as well as accuracy.

## 2  Method

The misregistration between images distorts their joint statistics. In this work the distortion is considered as Gaussian smoothing of the joint statistics, which is deconvolved with adaptive Wiener filtering. This assumes a smoothness of anatomy in space and a larger size for anatomic structures compared to that of the extent of the misregistration. Misregistration is also assumed to be spatially smooth. As a pre-processing step, the two images are normalized in terms of resolution if necessary as well as in terms of their dynamic range. The method then performs an additional pre-processing step concatenating a rigid and an affine registration. The result is then used to initialize the subsequent non-rigid registration.

The problem of the non-rigid registration of pairs of images is formulated with two priors. The first results from the deconvolution of the joint intensity statistics with the adaptive Wiener filter. The second results from the spatial regularization of the registration with a Gaussian filter. The method interleaves between the two priors iteratively, $k = 0, ..., K - 1$ for a total of $K$ iterations. An overview of the registration is given with the diagram shown in Fig. 1. A pairwise registration is between a reference image $I_{ref}$ and a moving image $I_{mov}$. A spatial transformation $\mathbf{T} = (u_x, u_y, u_z)$ from $I_{ref}$ to $I_{mov}$ is estimated to obtain the registered image $I_{reg} = I_{mov}(\mathbf{T}^{-1}(\mathbf{x}))$ where $\mathbf{x} = (x, y, z)$ are the spatial coordinates. The registration can accommodate a variable contrast. The method allows the registration over a limited Region Of Interest (ROI) over the image for which the contrast is intended for and is meaningful.

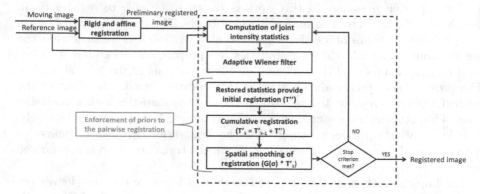

**Fig. 1.** Diagram describing the registration of two images with the proposed registration method. A preliminary rigid and affine registration is performed and the result is used to initialize the iterative non-rigid registration step until the stop criterion is met.

## 2.1   Computation of the Joint Intensity Statistics and Their Wiener Restoration

Two images $I_{ref}$ and $I_{mov}$ under assumed perfect alignment give rise to the joint histogram $H_{ideal}$. The joint statistics $H_0$ of the misregistered images are considered to result from the convolution of $H_{ideal}$ with a 2D Gaussian filter $G_{Hi,j}(\sigma_H)$:

$$H_0 = H_{ideal} * G_{Hi,j}(\sigma_H) + n_H, \tag{1}$$

where $\sigma_H$ is the standard deviation of the Gaussian convolution, $*$ is the convolution, $n_H$ is the noise and $i, j$ are the indices for the dynamic ranges of $I_{ref}$ and $I_{mov}$, respectively. The statistics $H_0$ are deconvolved with a 2D adaptive Wiener filter

$$f_{i,j} = \frac{G_{Hi,j}}{||G_{Hi,j}||_2^2 + \epsilon}, \tag{2}$$

where $\epsilon$ assumes a small value. The filter $f_{i,j}$ is convolved with $H_0$ to obtain an estimate of the restored deconvolved statistics with:

$$H_{rest} = f_{i,j} * H_0. \tag{3}$$

Fig. 2 shows two images and their joint statistics at different iterations before the Wiener deconvolution. The deconvolved statistics are used as a prior to constrain the estimation of the registration.

## 2.2   Adaptive Wiener Filter

The distortion in the joint statistics is assumed to be non-stationary throughout the dynamic ranges, depending on properties of different tissues. This has been modeled with an adaptive Wiener filter to preserve the distributions corresponding to different tissue types. The focus has been given to the estimation

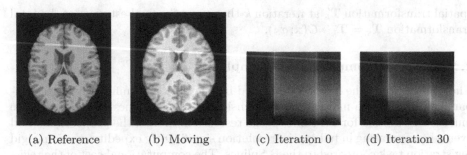

(a) Reference        (b) Moving        (c) Iteration 0        (d) Iteration 30

**Fig. 2.** Joint statistics for initial images (a) and (b) before Wiener deconvolution at the initial iteration (c) and after 30 iterations (d). The joint statistics in (d) become sharper.

of the local mean $\mu_{H_0}(i,j)$ and variance $\sigma^2_{H_0}(i,j)$ over a moving window of size $(2r+1) \times (2s+1)$. The local mean $\mu_{H_0}(i,j) = \langle H_0 \rangle_{r,s}$ and the local variance $\sigma_{H_0}{}^2(i,j) = \langle H_0^2 \rangle_{r,s} - \langle \mu_{H_0} \rangle^2_{r,s}$ are estimated over the observed joint statistics $H_0$ of the misregistered images. The standard deviation $\sigma_W(i,j) \propto \sqrt{\frac{1}{\sigma^2_{H_0}(i,j)}}$, where $\sigma_W$ is the standard deviation of the Wiener filter, used to represent the local variance of the Gaussian distortion and in turn to appropriately adjust the Wiener filter. Thus, the Wiener filter width becomes smaller as the distributions become steeper and is able to preserve their sharpness.

### 2.3  Enforcement of Priors to the Pairwise Registration

The two considered images $I_{ref}$ and $I_{mov}$ are used to construct a graph $R = (V, E)$. Each voxel of the image corresponds to a vertex in $V$. The edges in $E$ are connecting each node in $I_{ref}$ to nodes in a 6-connected spatial neighborhood $\mathcal{N}$ in $I_{mov}$, $\mathcal{N}(\mathbf{x}) = \mathbf{x} + \Delta\mathbf{x}$, where $\Delta\mathbf{x} = (\pm\Delta x, \pm\Delta y, \pm\Delta z)$ and $\Delta x, \Delta y, \Delta z$ are the sizes of a voxel along the axes. The voxel anisotropy is accounted for by using an edge weight $w_d = 1/(d+1)$ for a distance $d$.

The intensities of the edge between $I_{ref}(\mathbf{x})$ and $I_{mov}(\mathbf{x} + \Delta\mathbf{x})$ form an index for the restored joint histogram $H_{rest}$ to retrieve the second edge weight $w_H = H_{rest}(I_{ref}(\mathbf{x}), I_{mov}(\mathbf{x} + \Delta\mathbf{x}))$. The product $w_{tot}(\mathbf{x}, \Delta\mathbf{x})$, $w_{tot} = w_d \cdot w_H$ gives the total weight of an edge. The linear expectation of the direction of the edges connecting $\mathbf{x}$ over their weights gives an initial displacement $\mathbf{T}''(\mathbf{x})$ for voxel at $\mathbf{x}$. At iteration $k$ the displacements over the entire image give an initial transformation

$$\mathbf{T}''_k(\mathbf{x}) = \mathbf{x} + E_{w_{tot}}(\mathbf{x}, \Delta\mathbf{x}) = \mathbf{x} + \frac{\Sigma_{\mathcal{N}} w_{tot}(\mathbf{x}, \Delta\mathbf{x})(\Delta\mathbf{x})}{\Sigma_{\mathcal{N}} w_{tot}(\mathbf{x}, \Delta\mathbf{x})}. \tag{4}$$

This is accumulated to obtain $\mathbf{T}'_k = \mathbf{T}'_{k-1} + \mathbf{T}''_k$. The second prior is the spatial regularization. To regularize the estimation of the transformation $\mathbf{T}'_k$, the gradient magnitude $\|\nabla \mathbf{T}'_k\|_2$ over the image is penalized, that is equivalent to the application of a 3D Gaussian filter $G(\mathbf{x}; \sigma_S)$ with standard deviation $\sigma_S$ to the spatial transformation $\mathbf{T}'_k$ at iteration $k$ that gives the final estimate of the total transformation $\mathbf{T}_k = \mathbf{T}'_k * G(\mathbf{x}; \sigma_S)$.

## 2.4   Order of Computational Complexity

The complexity of the method developed in this work is significantly lower compared to that of the multicontrast extension of the B-Splines method with the mutual information for the same spatial resolution. In fact, the proposed method even when operating in full spatial resolution significantly expedites the non-rigid registration task compared to the B-Splines. The computational cost of the registration is expressed as a function of: $K$-number of iterations, $m$-effective size for each of the image dimensions, $n$-size of a neighborhood window $n = |\mathcal{N}|$ around a pixel, $p$-spatial subsampling factor between nodes, and $\sigma_S$ of the regularizer. In the proposed method the pairwise registration requires the computation and deconvolution of the joint statistics as well as the spatial smoothing only once per iteration. This is in contrast to the B-Splines method extended with the MI that requires the joint statistics estimation and the spatial smoothing $|\mathcal{N}|$ times for each of the $(m/p)^3$ nodes in every iteration to cover the entire image. The complexity of our method is $O([m^3n + m^3 3\sigma_S]K)$, while that of the B-Splines method with the MI is $O((m/p)^3 n[m^3n + m^3 3\sigma_S]K)$.

The cost of the Demons method extended with the MI can be even higher than that of the B-Splines depending on the levels $l$ of the multiresolution pyramids it is often combined with. Assuming that the image widths are halved at every level, the cost is $O\left(\left(\sum_{l'=0}^{l'=l-1}\left(\frac{m}{2^{l'}}\right)^3\right)n[m^3n + m^3 3\sigma_S]K\right)$.

## 3   Experiments and Results

### 3.1   Implementation of Method and End Condition of Iterations

The method has been implemented in $C++$. To improve performance the adaptive Wiener filter for the statistics has been implemented separably and is approximated as $f_{i,j} = \frac{G_{Hi}}{||G_{Hi}||_2^2 + \epsilon} * \frac{G_{Hj}}{||G_{Hj}||_2^2 + \epsilon}$ assuming that $G_{Hi,j} = G_{Hi} * G_{Hj}$, where $G_{Hi}$ and $G_{Hj}$ are 1D Gaussian filters. The value of the inverse signal to noise ratio $\epsilon$ for the adaptive Wiener filter has been set to 0.1. The spatial regularization $G(\mathbf{x}; \sigma_S)$ of the transformation has been performed using the ITK [2] implementation of the 3D recursive separable Gaussian filter along each of the components of the displacements $u_x, u_y$ and $u_z$ along the three axes. The pairwise non-rigid registration method developed is preceded by the rigid and affine registration methods provided by ITK [2]. The method processes 3D images.

The optimization iteratively alternates between the constraints arising from the statistical restoration and from the spatial regularization. The convergence of the registration is evaluated at every iteration. It uses the average $L_2$ norm of the spatial transformation $||T_k||$. The stop condition $s$ of the iterations is $s = \frac{||T_k||}{||T_0||} - 1 < -1\%$. A maximum number of $s_{max} = 50$ iterations is also enforced.

## 3.2  Validation Methodology

To evaluate the quality of the registration obtained from phantom datasets with the method presented, the voxelwise Sum of Absolute Differences $SAD = ||I_{true}(\mathbf{x}) - I_{reg}(\mathbf{x})||_2$, where $I_{true}$ is the true reference image in case of phantoms, has been calculated within a ROI between the true and the registered image. The percent improvement ($Imp$) of SAD is defined as $Imp_{SAD\%} = \frac{SAD_{bef} - SAD_{aft}}{SAD_{bef}} 100\%$, where $SAD_{bef}$ and $SAD_{aft}$ represent the SAD calculated before and after the registration, respectively. The registration of the bi-contrast real datasets has been evaluated by observation and by calculating the percent improvement in MI $Imp_{MI\%} = \frac{MI_{aft} - MI_{bef}}{MI_{aft}} 100\%$ before and after registration.

The method has been compared with the pairwise B-Splines based non-rigid registration method provided by Slicer3D [3]. The configuration of Slicer3D includes also a rigid and affine pre-registration steps as does the proposed method. MI has been used as a metric for all the registration steps. The tests were performed on a workstation with an Intel Core2 Duo 3.0 GHz CPU and 16GB of RAM. Our non-optimized implementation of the proposed method for a typical image can be further improved to achieve a high upper bound of speedup and had a 260% lower working memory requirement compared to the B-Splines method as shown in Table 1. It also operates in full image resolution as opposed to the B-Spline method that in practice requires subsampling. The B-Splines method tested operates in a grid of size $20 \times 20 \times 20$, which in the case of the BrainWeb phantom dataset gives a resolution of $9 \times 10.8 \times 9mm^3 = 875mm^3$ as subsampling. The presented method operates in full spatial resolution of $1 \times 1 \times 1mm^3 = 1mm^3$, which provides a resolution 875 times higher. The quantitative results and comparisons of the proposed method to those of the B-Splines method are shown in Table 1.

## 3.3  Shepp-Logan Phantom Data

A dataset for the validation of the proposed method has been a multicontrast simulation from the 3D Shepp-Logan phantom with a full resolution of $128 \times 128 \times 128$ pixels as displayed in Fig. 3 which shows an obvious improvement in alignment. The phantom has been modified to simulate the contrast change and a 3D sinusoidal function over the spatial image coordinates in all dimensions has been applied to simulate a non-rigid transformation. The value of $\sigma_S$ for the spatial smoothing has been set to 6 voxels. The registration has been performed within a manually specified ROI shown in Fig. 3d. After 8 iterations it can be seen in Fig. 3 that the phantom is properly registered. The registration between $I_{ref}$ and $I_{mov}$ gives an $Imp_{SAD\%}$ of about 68%. A performance comparison with the B-Splines method is shown in row 1 of Table 1, where it is shown that the proposed method improves the accuracy.

## 3.4  BrainWeb Phantom Data

Another validation phantom data has been obtained from the BrainWeb database as shown in Fig. 4. The phantom data consists of two images with a full resolution

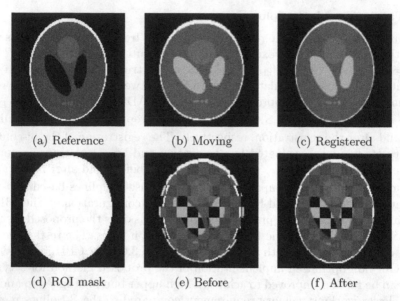

(a) Reference          (b) Moving          (c) Registered

(d) ROI mask          (e) Before          (f) After

**Fig. 3.** A 2D axial slice from the 3D Shepp-Logan phantom. (a) is the reference image, (b) is the misregistered image, (c) is the registered image obtained with the proposed method, and (d) is the ROI used. In (e) and (f) are the checkerboard compositions interleaving $I_{ref}$ and $I_{mov}$ before and after the registration.

of $180 \times 216 \times 180$ pixels taken using a $T_1$ and a $T_2$ sequences. The $T_1$ image has been used as reference. A non-linear misregistration has been simulated with a 3D sinusoid and has been applied to the $T_2$ image. The images were subsequently registered and the results are shown in the images in Fig. 4 and in row 2 of Table 1.

## 3.5   Real Brain Data

The real brain data in this study is composed of 5 young healthy volunteers. The study was approved by the local internal review board and the volunteers provided informed consent. The images were acquired with a 3T Siemens Trio MRI system equipped with head coils. The acquisition protocol consisted of a 3D $T_1$ and FLAIR sequences. The $T_1$ and FLAIR sequences give a matrix of size $512 \times 512 \times 160$ with a voxel of resolution $0.5 \times 0.5 \times 1mm^3$.

All real datasets were placed in the same anatomic space and the BrainWeb $T_1$ dataset has been chosen as the reference image. Fig. 5 shows an example of the registration between the $T_1$ BrainWeb phantom and a $T_1$ image from a volunteer. In Fig. 6 is an example of the registration between the $T_1$ BrainWeb phantom and a FLAIR image from a volunteer. The misregistered images shown in Fig. 5b and 6b are the results of the rigid and affine registration steps and are used as input for the non-rigid registration method proposed. The red arrows highlight the effect of the registration on significant brain structures.

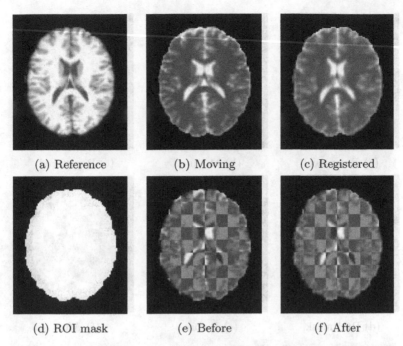

(a) Reference        (b) Moving        (c) Registered

(d) ROI mask        (e) Before        (f) After

**Fig. 4.** A 2D axial slice from the 3D BrainWeb phantom. (a) is the reference image, (b) is the misregistered image, and (c) is the registered image obtained with the proposed method. (d) is showing the ROI used, and (e) and (f) are the checkerboard compositions interleaving $I_{ref}$ and $I_{mov}$ before and after the registration.

**Table 1.** Performance and comparison of the proposed method with that of the Slicer3D optimized implementation of B-Splines

| Datasets | Method | Imp (SAD%) | Imp (MI%) | Resol. (voxels) | Exec. time | Memory Space |
|---|---|---|---|---|---|---|
| Shepp-Logan Phantom | B-Splines | 65.13% | | 1/262 | ~1min | 730MB |
| | Proposed | 68.54% | | 1 | ~18min | 450MB |
| BrainWeb Phantom | B-Splines | 47.39% | | 1/875 | ~2min | 4GB |
| | Proposed | 64.11% | | 1 | ~90min | 2GB |
| Volunteer 1 | B-Splines | | 52.06% | 1/875 | ~2min | 4GB |
| | Proposed | | 57.35% | 1 | ~90min | 2GB |
| Volunteer 2 | B-Splines | | 29.30% | 1/875 | ~2min | 4GB |
| | Proposed | | 32.31% | 1 | ~90min | 2GB |
| Volunteer 3 | B-Splines | | 44.65% | 1/875 | ~2min | 4GB |
| | Proposed | | 58.39% | 1 | ~90min | 2GB |
| Volunteer 4 | B-Splines | | 38.54% | 1/875 | ~2min | 4GB |
| | Proposed | | 56.13% | 1 | ~90min | 2GB |
| Volunteer 5 | B-Splines | | 19.28% | 1/875 | ~2min | 4GB |
| | Proposed | | 31.93% | 1 | ~90min | 2GB |

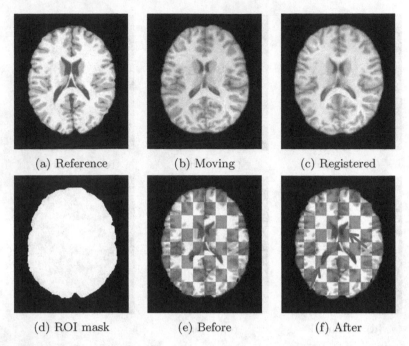

(a) Reference          (b) Moving          (c) Registered

(d) ROI mask          (e) Before          (f) After

**Fig. 5.** A 2D axial slice of a 3D real patient $T_1$ dataset registered to the $T_1$ BrainWeb phantom. (a) is the reference image, (b) is the misregistered image, (c) is the registered image obtained with the proposed method, and (d) is the ROI used. In (e) and (f) are the checkerboard compositions interleaving $I_{ref}$ and $I_{mov}$ before and after the registration. The red arrows highlight the effect of the registration on significant brain structures.

## 4  Summary and Discussion

Almost all the parameters of the method are held fixed for all the datasets. The only variable parameter is the $\sigma_S$ of the spatial regularizer, which should be at most equal to the spatial variation of the displacement field. The parameter $\sigma_W$ of the adaptive Wiener filter has been set with a proportionality constant so that its value is less than than of the width of the distributions of the tissues to preserve them. As shown analytically the order of computational complexity is lower than that of both the B-Splines and of the Demons method. The overall speedup is a power of the dimensionality of the considered datasets. The total time performance of the methods is shown in Table 1 and includes the common cost of the rigid and affine pre-processing steps. The relatively high time performance obtained by B-Splines in Slicer3D is due to the optimized software implementation and use of hardware such as multicore CPUs. However, it was not possible to test Slicer3D B-Splines with full resolution because of its excessive memory requirements.

The method developed significantly improves efficiency and accuracy of non-rigid registration of multi-modal brain datasets while operating at full spatial resolution. The method shows an improvement qualitatively in terms of visual comparison as well as quantitatively in terms of $Imp_{SAD\%}$, and $Imp_{MI\%}$. The method is based on a systematic model of the misregistration and its removal. It has accurately compensated the misregistration in phantoms as well as in several multi-modal real brain datasets. The non-rigid registration can accommodate both same as well as different image contrasts. It is iterative and results in an effective deconvolution of the joint statistics that only requires a single estimation of the joint statistics and the spatial smoothing per iteration that covers the entire image. The registration method proposed does not involve the MI distance measure. The MI allows more degrees of freedom than necessary and can lead to a significantly higher computational cost. The performance of this method as well as of all methods based on image statistics is improved if an ROI of meaningful contrast is considered.

An advantage of the method proposed is that it is robust to the anisotropic resolution present in the clinical imaging data of this study. The method developed in this work performs a dense spatial registration robust against contrast changes and anisotropy. The presented method can be extended to 4D data for an even higher expected comparative upper bound in speedup.

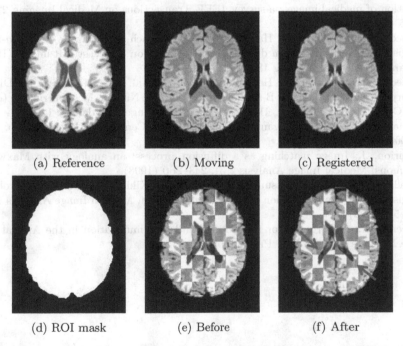

(a) Reference          (b) Moving          (c) Registered

(d) ROI mask          (e) Before          (f) After

**Fig. 6.** A 2D axial slice of a 3D real patient FLAIR dataset registered to the $T_1$ BrainWeb phantom. (a) is the reference image, (b) is the misregistered image, (c) is the registered image obtained with the proposed method, (d) is the ROI used. In (e) and (f) are the checkerboard compositions interleaving $I_{ref}$ and $I_{mov}$ before and after the registration. The red arrows highlight the effect of the registration on significant brain structures.

# References

1. Collins, D.L., Zijdenbos, A.P., Kollokian, V., Sled, J.G., Kabani, N.J., Holmes, C.J., Evans, A.C.: Design and construction of a realistic digital brain phantom. IEEE Trans. on Medical Imaging 17(3), 463–468 (1998)
2. Ibanez, L., Schroeder, W., Ng, L., Cates, J.: The ITK Software Guide, 2nd edn. Kitware, Inc. (2005) ISBN 1-930934-15-7
3. Johnson, H., Harris, G., Williams, K.: Brainsfit: Mutual information registrations of whole-brain 3D images, using the Insight Toolkit. Insight J. (2007), http://www.slicer.org
4. Lu, H., Reyes, M., Serifovic, A., Weber, S., Sakurai, Y., Yamagata, H., Cattin, P.: Multi-modal diffeomorphic Demons registration based on point-wise mutual information. In: Proc. of IEEE ISBI, pp. 372–375. IEEE (2010)
5. Martel, A., Froh, M., Brock, K., Plewes, D., Barber, D.: Evaluating an optical-flow-based registration algorithm for contrast-enhanced magnetic resonance imaging of the breast. Physics in Medicine and Biology 52, 3803 (2007)
6. Modat, M., Vercauteren, T., Ridgway, G., Hawkes, D., Fox, N., Ourselin, S.: Diffeomorphic Demons using normalised mutual information, evaluation on multi-modal brain MR images. SPIE-The International Society for Optical Engineering (2010)
7. Pluim, J.P.W., Maintz, J.B.A., Viergever, M.A.: Mutual-information-based registration of medical images: a survey. IEEE Transactions on Medical Imaging 22(8), 986–1004 (2003)
8. Rueckert, D., Sonoda, L., Hayes, C., Hill, D., Leach, M., Hawkes, D.: Non-rigid registration using free-form deformations: application to breast MR images. IEEE Trans. on Medical Imaging 18(8), 712–721 (1999)
9. Rueckert, D., Aljabar, P., Heckemann, R.A., Hajnal, J.V., Hammers, A.: Diffeomorphic registration using B-splines. In: Larsen, R., Nielsen, M., Sporring, J. (eds.) MICCAI 2006. LNCS, vol. 4191, pp. 702–709. Springer, Heidelberg (2006)
10. Schabel, M.: 3D Shepp-Logan phantom. MATLAB Central File Exchange, pp. 1–35 (2006)
11. Thirion, J.: Image matching as a diffusion process: an analogy with Maxwell's Demons. Medical Image Analysis 2(3), 243–260 (1998)
12. Wells III, W., Viola, P., Atsumi, H., Nakajima, S., Kikinis, R.: Multi-modal volume registration by maximization of mutual information. Medical Image Analysis 1(1), 35–51 (1996)
13. Wiener, N.: Cybernetics: or the Control and Communication in the Animal and the Machine, vol. 25. MIT Press (1965)

# Atlas Based Intensity Transformation of Brain MR Images

Snehashis Roy, Amod Jog, Aaron Carass, and Jerry L. Prince

Image Analysis and Communication Laboratory,
Department of Electrical and Computer Engineering,
The Johns Hopkins University

**Abstract.** Magnetic resonance imaging (MRI) is a noninvasive modality that has been widely used to image the structure of the human brain. Unlike reconstructed x-ray computed tomography images, MRI intensities do not possess a calibrated scale, and the images suffer from wide variability in intensity contrasts due to scanner calibration and pulse sequence variations. Most MR image processing tasks use intensities as the principal feature and therefore the results can vary widely according to the actual tissue intensity contrast. Since it is difficult to control the MR scanner acquisition protocols in multi-scanner cross-sectional studies, results achieved using image processing tools are often difficult to compare in such studies. Similar issues can happen in longitudinal studies, as scanners undergo upgrades or improvements in pulse sequences, leading to new imaging sequences. We propose a novel probabilistic model to transform image contrasts by matching patches of a subject image to a set of patches from a multi-contrast atlas. Although the transformed images are not for diagnostic purpose, the use of such contrast transforms is shown for two applications, (a) to improve segmentation consistency across scanners and pulse sequences, (b) to improve registration accuracy between multi-contrast image pairs by transforming the subject image to the contrast of the reference image and then registering the transformed subject image to the reference image. Contrary to previous intensity transformation methods, our technique does not need any information about landmarks, pulse sequence parameters or imaging equations. It is shown to provide more consistent segmentation across scanners compared to state-of-the-art methods.

**Keywords:** magnetic resonance imaging (MRI), intensity transformation, intensity normalization, histogram matching, brain.

## 1 Introduction

Magnetic resonance (MR) imaging is widely used to image the structure of human brains. MR image processing techniques, such as segmentation, have been used to understand normal aging [1]. Unfortunately, most image processing algorithms use image intensities as the primary feature, which is undesirable as MR image intensities are not calibrated to any specific underlying tissue properties.

L. Shen et al. (Eds.): MBIA 2013, LNCS 8159, pp. 51–62, 2013.
© Springer International Publishing Switzerland 2013

In addition to this, intensity contrast between brain tissues depends on non-biological factors—scanner calibration, the pulse sequence, and pulse-sequence specific imaging parameters.

One of the objectives of many brain segmentation algorithms is to segment a 3D structural MR image into three tissue classes, cerebro-spinal fluid (CSF), gray matter (GM), and white matter (WM). It has been shown that the variations in image intensities give rise to inconsistencies in the segmentation of the tissues [2]. This is of course exacerbated in large multi-site multi-scanner datasets, where either portions of the data are acquired with differing sequences (e.g., $T_1$-w SPGR, spoiled gradient recalled, and MPRAGE, magnetization prepared rapid gradient echo) or some contrasts are not available for a part of the data, preventing consistent longitudinal analysis.

Some previous approaches to MR intensity transformation have depended on the underlying tissue properties—proton density ($P_D$) and relaxation times ($T_1$, $T_2$, and $T_2^*$)—as it is possible to estimate these at every voxel and apply the imaging equation of the unobserved pulse sequence to obtain the desired tissue contrast [3]. However, these methods require multiple acquisitions as well as good knowledge of the imaging equations and other imaging parameters, which are often not known and difficult to estimate. Another solution is to match the histogram of the subject to the atlas with the desired tissue contrast by matching intensity landmarks [4] or minimizing some information theoretic criteria [5] between histograms. Individual histograms of segmented sub-cortical structures can also be matched to the corresponding histograms of an atlas of different contrast [6]; however this requires a detailed segmentation of the images which can itself be dependent on the contrast.

There has been recent work [7,8] on intensity transformation that requires neither estimation of any tissue parameters nor any atlas-to-subject registration. Using a co-registered pair of atlases with contrast $C_1$ and $C_2$, a patch from the subject $C_1$ image is matched to a sparse linear combination of atlas $C_1$ patches, and the corresponding atlas $C_2$ patches are linearly combined to estimate the subject $C_2$ patch [7]. However, no information from the atlas $C_2$ image is used in the matching process, unlike a joint dictionary learning approach to registration [9]. Fig. 1 shows the effect of not using atlas $C_2$ patches, where an MPRAGE contrast image is obtained from a $T_2$-w image with some obvious failures around the globus pallidus, our method by incorporating information from the C2 contrast does not suffer from this problem.

In this paper, we propose a probabilistic model for the image intensity transformation problem by taking into account information from both contrasts by incorporating the idea of coherent point drift [10]. The subject and the atlas images are decomposed into patches, and the subject patch collection is matched to the atlas patch collection using a number of Gaussian mixture models. Then the $C_2$ contrast of the $C_1$ subject patches is obtained as a maximum likelihood estimate from the model. We emphasize the point that the transformed images are not to be used by radiologists for any diagnostic purpose and are only used for image processing. The applications of such an intensity transformation method

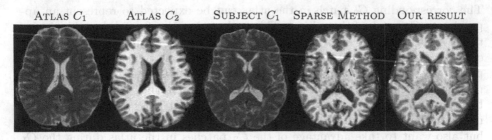

**Fig. 1.** While transforming $T_2$-w ($C_1$) to MPRAGE ($C_2$) contrast, if the information from $C_2$ image patches are not used, such as [7], it leads to artifacts in the transformed $C_2$ image (e.g., red arrow in the fourth column), which are not present in our result

are shown on two case-studies. (a) In large cross-sectional datasets [11,1], if the data is acquired with different scanners or pulse-sequences (e.g., SPGR and MPRAGE), the segmentation consistency between scans with variable intensity scale can be improved by intensity transformation to a common scale. (b) In diffusion-weighted imaging, $b_0$ images are required to be registered to the $T_1$-w structural MRI. The registration can be improved by a transformed $T_2$-w image as an intermediate step.

## 2 Method

### 2.1 Atlas and Patch Description

We define the atlas as a pair of co-registered images $\{a_1, a_2\}$ having the same pixel resolution and contrasts $C_1$ and $C_2$, respectively. The subject, also having the same pixel resolution, is denoted by $b_1$ and is of contrast $C_1$. Both $b_1$ and $a_1$ are scaled such that their WM peak intensities are at unity. WM peak intensity is found from the corresponding histogram. Both atlas and subject are assumed to be normal, i.e., they do not contain any pathologies such as tumor, white matter hyper-intensities, multiple sclerosis plaques, microbleeds etc. At each voxel of an image, 3D patches—size $p \times q \times r$—are stacked into 1D vectors of size $d \times 1$, with $d = pqr$. Atlas $C_1$ and $C_2$ patches are denoted by $\mathbf{y}_j$ and $\mathbf{v}_j$, respectively, where $j = 1, \ldots, M$. Subject $b_1$ yields $C_1$ contrast patches which are denoted by $\mathbf{x}_i, i = 1, \ldots, N$. The unobserved $C_2$ contrast subject patches of $b_1$ are denoted by $\mathbf{u}_i$. $N$ and $M$ are the number of non-zero voxels in the subject and the atlas, respectively. We combine the patch pairs as $2d \times 1$ vectors $\mathbf{p}_i = [\mathbf{x}_i^T \mathbf{u}_i^T]^T$ and $\mathbf{q}_j = [\mathbf{y}_j^T \mathbf{v}_j^T]^T$. The subject and atlas patch collections are defined as the collection of patches and patch-pairs $\mathbf{X} = \{\mathbf{x}_i\}$, $\mathbf{Y} = \{\mathbf{y}_i\}$, $\mathbf{P} = \{\mathbf{p}_i\}$, and $\mathbf{Q} = \{\mathbf{q}_j\}$.

### 2.2 Algorithm

If an atlas $C_1$ patch has a pattern of intensities that is similar to a given subject $C_1$ patch, it is likely that they arise from the same distribution of tissues.

The corresponding $C_2$ patch in the atlas can be expected to represent an approximate $C_2$ patch of the subject. This is the principle of patch-based intensity transformation. One could naively find a single patch within the atlas that is close (or closest) to the subject patch and then use the corresponding $C_2$ atlas patch directly. A slightly more complex way is to find a sparse collection of atlas patches that can better reconstruct the subject patch, then use the same combination of $C_2$ patches as the transformed $C_2$ subject patch [7]. In the present method, we want to retain the property of combining a small number of patches, but also want to take advantage of the $C_2$ patches in the atlas during the $C_1$ patch selection in an global optimization so as to minimize error propagation, that can arise in a directional (such as top-to-bottom left-to-right of the image) estimation process using partially estimated patches, e.g., in [8].

We propose a probabilistic model that relates subject patch collection to the atlas patch collection. Since atlas patches may not be plentiful enough to closely resemble all subject patches, we consider all convex combinations of $n$-tuples of atlas patches. We then postulate that a subject patch is a random vector whose probability density is Gaussian with mean given by an unknown convex combinations of $n$ nearby atlas patches and with unknown covariance matrix. This framework captures the notion that a small $n$ number of atlas patches could be used to describe a subject patch. In order to tie the $C_1$ and $C_2$ contrasts together, we further assume that the subject's unknown $C_2$ patch is a random vector whose mean lies in the (same) convex hull of the same $n$ atlas patches associated with the $C_1$ contrast, with a covariance matrix that can be different.

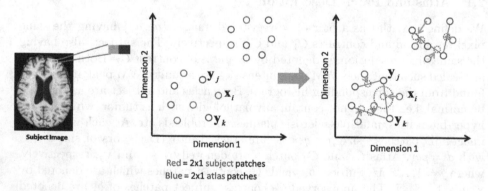

Red = 2x1 subject patches
Blue = 2x1 atlas patches

**Fig. 2.** Illustration of patch matching: a subject patch is modeled by a convex combination of two atlas patches

This can be summarized succinctly by considering a subject patch $\mathbf{p}_i$ and $n$ associated atlas patches $\mathbf{q}_{j_1}, \ldots, \mathbf{q}_{j_n}$. Then $\mathbf{p}_i$ is assumed to arise from the Gaussian distribution,

$$\mathbf{p}_i \sim \mathcal{N}(\alpha_{i,j_1}\mathbf{q}_{j_1} + \ldots + \alpha_{i,j_n}\mathbf{q}_{j_n}, \Sigma), \quad \sum_{\ell=1}^{n} \alpha_{i,j_\ell} = 1, \ \alpha_{i,j_\ell} \in (0,1). \quad (1)$$

where $\Sigma$ is a covariance matrix associated with the atlas patches. Fig. 2 illustrates this concept for patches of dimension $2 \times 1 \times 1$, i.e. two neighboring voxels in an image. The subject patches, shown in red, are to be matched to the atlas patches, in blue, where each $\mathbf{x}_i$ is modeled as a convex combination of $n = 2$ atlas patches $\mathbf{y}_j$ and $\mathbf{y}_k$. For computational and mathematical ease, we use $n = 2$ for the remainder of this paper. Then Eqn. 1 reduces to,

$$\mathbf{p}_i \sim \mathcal{N}(\alpha_{it}\mathbf{q}_j + (1 - \alpha_{it})\mathbf{q}_k, \Sigma_t), \quad \alpha_{it} \in (0,1), \ t \equiv \{j,k\}. \tag{2}$$

$\Sigma_t$ is a covariance matrix associated with the atlas patches $\mathbf{q}_j$ and $\mathbf{q}_k$, and $t \in \Psi$, where $\Psi$ is the set of all pairs of atlas patch indices. $\alpha_{it} \in (0,1)$ is the mixing coefficient for the $i^{\text{th}}$ subject patch to the $t^{\text{th}}$ atlas patch-pairs. In essence, each subject patch follows an $\binom{M}{2}$-class Gaussian mixture model (GMM). We assume the patches are i.i.d. and maximize the probability of observing the subject patches $\mathbf{p}_i$ using expectation-maximization (EM) to estimate the $C_2$ contrast patches $\mathbf{u}_i$.

We define $z_{it}$ as the indicator function that $\mathbf{p}_i$ comes from a GMM of the $t = \{j,k\}^{\text{th}}$ atlas pair, $\sum_{t \in \Psi} z_{it} = 1 \ \forall i, \ z_{it} \in \{0,1\}$. Then the probability of observing $\mathbf{p}_i$ can be written as,

$$P(\mathbf{p}_i | z_{it} = 1, \Sigma_t, \alpha_{it}) = \frac{1}{\sqrt{2\pi|\Sigma_t|}} \exp\left\{ -\frac{1}{2}\mathbf{h}_{it}^T \Sigma_t^{-1} \mathbf{h}_{it} \right\}, \tag{3}$$

where $\mathbf{h}_{it} = \mathbf{p}_i - \alpha_{it}\mathbf{q}_j - (1 - \alpha_{it})\mathbf{q}_k, t \equiv \{j,k\}$. The prior probability of having $\mathbf{p}_i$ originating from the distribution of the $t^{\text{th}}$ pair is $P(z_{it} = 1|\Sigma_t, \alpha_{it})$. Without any knowledge of $\mathbf{x}_i$, this prior should ideally depend on a classification of the patch cloud $\mathbf{Q}$. However, we avoid any classification of patches by assuming a uniform prior. Thus the joint probability becomes,

$$P(\mathbf{p}_i, z_{it} = 1|\mathbf{q}_j, \mathbf{q}_k, \Sigma_t, \alpha_{it}) = \frac{1}{|\Psi|} P(\mathbf{p}_i|\mathbf{q}_j, \mathbf{q}_k, z_{it} = 1, \Sigma_t, \alpha_{it}). \tag{4}$$

Writing $\mathbf{Z} = \{z_{it}\}$ and using the i.i.d. assumption on patches, the joint likelihood of all patches can be written as,

$$P(\mathbf{P}, \mathbf{Z}|\Sigma_t, \alpha_{it}) = D \prod_{t \in \Psi} \prod_{i=1}^{N} \left[ \frac{1}{|\Sigma_t|} \exp\left\{ -\frac{1}{2}\mathbf{h}_{it}^T \Sigma_t^{-1} \mathbf{h}_{it} \right\} \right]^{z_{it}}, \tag{5}$$

where $\mathbf{h}_{it}$ is defined in Eqn. 3 and $D$ is a normalization constant. Although it is possible to maximize Eqn. 5 by EM for any $\Sigma_t$, we have experimentally found that an arbitrary positive definite $\Sigma_t$ is often less robust to estimate. Instead, it is assumed to be separable and diagonal,

$$\Sigma_t = \begin{bmatrix} \sigma_{1t}^2 \mathbf{I} & \mathbf{0} \\ \mathbf{0} & \sigma_{2t}^2 \mathbf{I} \end{bmatrix},$$

indicating that the variations of each voxel in a patch are the same around the means, although individual voxels can be of different tissue. Thus, the joint probability becomes,

$$P(\mathbf{P}, \mathbf{Z}|\Theta) = D \prod_{t \in \Psi} \prod_{i=1}^{N} \left[ \frac{1}{\sigma_{1t}\sigma_{2t}} \exp\left\{ -\frac{\|\mathbf{f}_{it}\|^2}{2\sigma_{1t}^2} \right\} \exp\left\{ -\frac{\|\mathbf{g}_{it}\|^2}{2\sigma_{2t}^2} \right\} \right]^{z_{it}},$$

$$\mathbf{f}_{it} = \mathbf{x}_i - \alpha_{it}\mathbf{y}_j - (1 - \alpha_{it})\mathbf{y}_k, \quad \mathbf{g}_{it} = \mathbf{u}_i - \alpha_{it}\mathbf{v}_j - (1 - \alpha_{it})\mathbf{v}_k, \tag{6}$$

The set of parameters is $\Theta = \{\sigma_{1t}, \sigma_{2t}, \alpha_{it}; i = 1, \ldots, N, t \in \Psi\}$. The maximum likelihood estimators of $\Theta$ are found by maximizing Eqn. 6 using EM. The EM algorithm can be outlined as:

1. **E-step:** to find new update $\Theta^{(m+1)}$ at the $m^{\text{th}}$ iteration, compute the expectation $Q(\Theta^{(m+1)}|\Theta^{(m)}) = E[\log P(\mathbf{P}, \mathbf{Z}|\Theta^{(m+1)})|\mathbf{X}, \Theta^{(m)}]$.
2. **M-step:** find new estimates $\Theta^{(m+1)}$ based on the previous estimates using the following equation $\Theta^{(m+1)} = \arg\max_{\Theta^{(m+1)}} Q(\Theta^{(m+1)}|\Theta^{(m)})$.

The **E-step** requires the computation of $E(z_{it}|\mathbf{P}, \Theta^{(m)}) = P(z_{it}|\mathbf{P}, \Theta^{(m)})$. Given that $z_{it}$ is an indicator function, it can be shown that $E(z_{it}|\mathbf{P}, \Theta^{(m)}) = w_{it}^{(m)}$, where,

$$w_{it}^{(m+1)} = \frac{\frac{1}{\sigma_{1t}^{(m)} \sigma_{2t}^{(m)}} \exp\left\{-\frac{\|\mathbf{f}_{it}^{(m)}\|^2}{2\sigma_{1t}^{(m)^2}}\right\} \exp\left\{-\frac{\|\mathbf{g}_{it}^{(m)}\|^2}{2\sigma_{2t}^{(m)^2}}\right\}}{\sum_{\ell \in \Psi} \frac{1}{\sigma_{1\ell}^{(m)} \sigma_{2\ell}^{(m)}} \exp\left\{-\frac{\|\mathbf{f}_{i\ell}^{(m)}\|^2}{2\sigma_{1\ell}^{(m)^2}}\right\} \exp\left\{-\frac{\|\mathbf{g}_{i\ell}^{(m)}\|^2}{2\sigma_{2\ell}^{(m)^2}}\right\}}, \tag{7}$$

$w_{it}^{(m)}$ being the posterior probability of $\mathbf{p}_i$ originating from the Gaussian distribution of the $t^{\text{th}}$ atlas patches $\mathbf{q}_j$ and $\mathbf{q}_k$. $\mathbf{f}_{it}^{(m)}$ and $\mathbf{g}_{it}^{(m)}$ are the expressions defined in Eqn. 6 but with $\alpha_{it}^{(m)}$. $\mathbf{f}_{i\ell}^{(m)}$ and $\mathbf{g}_{i\ell}^{(m)}$ denote the corresponding values with atlas patches belonging to the $\ell^{\text{th}}$ pair, $\ell \in \Psi$, with $\alpha_{i\ell}^{(m)}$. The expected value of the $C_2$ patch is obtained by the following expression,

$$E(\mathbf{u}_i|\Theta^{(m)}) = \sum_{t \in \Psi} w_{it}^{(m)} \left(\alpha_{it}^{(m)} \mathbf{v}_j + (1 - \alpha_{it}^{(m)}) \mathbf{v}_k\right) \tag{8}$$

At each iteration, we replace the value of $\mathbf{u}_i$ with its expectation following the mean-field theory [12]. The **M-step** involves the maximization of the log of the expectation w.r.t. the parameters given the current $w_{it}^{(m)}$. The update equations are given by,

$$\sigma_{1t}^{(m+1)^2} = \frac{\sum_{i=1}^{N} w_{it}^{(m)} \|\mathbf{x}_i - \alpha_{it}^{(m)} \mathbf{y}_j - (1 - \alpha_{it}^{(m)}) \mathbf{y}_k\|^2}{\sum_{i=1}^{N} w_{it}^{(m)}}, \tag{9}$$

$$\sigma_{2t}^{(m+1)^2} = \frac{\sum_{i=1}^{N} w_{it}^{(m)} \|\mathbf{u}_i - \alpha_{it}^{(m)} \mathbf{v}_j - (1 - \alpha_{it}^{(m)}) \mathbf{v}_k\|^2}{\sum_{i=1}^{N} w_{it}^{(m)}}, \tag{10}$$

$\alpha_{it}^{(m+1)} : F\left(\alpha_{it}^{(m+1)}\right) = 0$, where $F(x) = Ax^2(1 - x) - Bx(1 - x) + 2x - 1$, $A = $

$\frac{\|\mathbf{y}_k - \mathbf{y}_j\|^2}{\sigma_{1t}^{(m+1)^2}} + \frac{\|\mathbf{v}_k - \mathbf{v}_j\|^2}{\sigma_{2t}^{(m+1)^2}}$, $B = \frac{(\mathbf{y}_k - \mathbf{x}_i)^T(\mathbf{y}_k - \mathbf{y}_j)}{\sigma_{1t}^{(m+1)^2}} + \frac{(\mathbf{v}_k - \mathbf{u}_i)^T(\mathbf{v}_k - \mathbf{v}_j)}{\sigma_{2t}^{(m+1)^2}}$.

It should be noted that $F(0) = -1, F(1) = 1, \forall A, B$, thus there is always a feasible $\alpha_{it}^{(m)} \in (0, 1)$. Once the EM algorithm converges, the expectation of the final $\mathbf{u}_i$ is considered to be the estimated $C_2$ contrast, and the center voxel of $\mathbf{u}_i$ is used as the $C_2$ replacement of the $i^{\text{th}}$ voxel.

We note that the imaging model (Eqn. 1) is valid for those atlas and subject patches that are close in intensity. Using a non-local type of criteria [13], for every subject patch $\mathbf{x}_i$, we choose a feasible set of $L$ atlas patches such that they are the $L$ nearest neighbors of $\mathbf{x}_i$. Thus the $i^{\text{th}}$ subject patch follows an $\binom{L}{2}$-class GMM and the algorithm becomes $O(NL^2)$. In all our experiments, we choose $3 \times 3 \times 3$ patches with $L = 100$.

## 3   Results

In this section, we describe the applications of intensity transformation on two case-studies, improving segmentation consistency in the presence of scanner and

**Table 1.** Each row shows the Dice coefficient of the hard segmentations between the original MPRAGE acquisition and the listed alternative. The top row is the comparison to segmentation of the original SPGR and represents a baseline for the consistency of the segmentation. The comparisons are based on 20 subjects from the BLSA [1].

|              | CSF               | GM                   | WM                   | Mean              |
|--------------|-------------------|----------------------|----------------------|-------------------|
| **Orig. SPGR**    | $0.815 \pm 0.030$ | $0.703 \pm 0.052$    | $0.854 \pm 0.023$    | $0.793 \pm 0.030$ |
| **Hist. Match**   | $0.784 \pm 0.053$ | $0.751 \pm 0.031$    | $0.859 \pm 0.012$    | $0.804 \pm 0.026$ |
| **Landmark** [4]  | $0.828 \pm 0.027$ | $0.768 \pm 0.026$    | $0.863 \pm 0.013$    | $0.818 \pm 0.016$ |
| **Sparse** [7]    | $0.844 \pm 0.031$ | $0.770 \pm 0.024$    | $0.872 \pm 0.014$    | $0.820 \pm 0.021$ |
| **Probabilistic** | $0.849 \pm 0.030$ | $\mathbf{0.802 \pm 0.023*}$ | $\mathbf{0.870 \pm 0.014}$† | $0.825 \pm 0.021$ |

* Statistically significantly larger than the other four ($p < 0.05$).
† Statistically significantly larger than original, histogram matching and landmark transformation ($p < 0.05$).

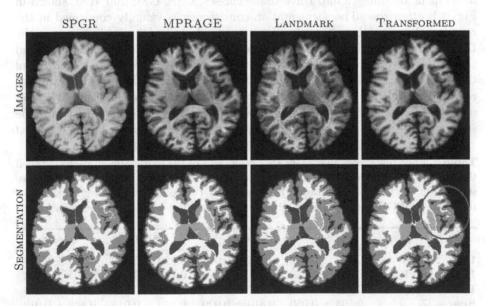

SPGR            MPRAGE            LANDMARK            TRANSFORMED

IMAGES

SEGMENTATION

**Fig. 3.** Top row shows the original SPGR, MPRAGE, the landmark based transformed and the patch based transformed SPGR images of a BLSA subject [1], bottom row shows their segmentations

pulse sequence variations, and improving registration accuracy between $T_1$-w and $b_0$ images in diffusion weighted imaging.

## 3.1 Segmentation Consistency

First we show the effect of the transformation on scans with different pulse sequences. The Baltimore Longitudinal Study of Aging (BLSA) [1] contains subjects having both SPGR and MPRAGE acquisitions from a GE 3T scanner. Each volume is of size $256 \times 256 \times 199$, with $0.94\text{mm}^3$ resolution. All images were first skull-stripped [14], corrected for any intensity inhomogeneity [15] and scaled such that their WM peak intensities are at unity. From our experience, the MPRAGE images usually produces more accurate cortical segmentation than that of the SPGR; thus we transform SPGR images to MPRAGE for 20 subjects, shown in Fig. 3 top row. Assuming MPRAGEs as the target, Dice coefficients between the MPRAGE and the original SPGR and the transformed SPGRs are obtained. Atlases $a_1$ and $a_2$ are chosen as the SPGR and MPRAGE contrast of a randomly chosen subject in the dataset.

Our method is compared with histogram matching, a landmark based intensity transformation [4], and a sparse patch combination method [7]. Histogram matching is usually sensitive to the choice of bin size and landmark based methods are sensitive to the accuracy of the landmarks. We choose three landmarks, namely mean CSF, GM, and WM intensities, each on both $a_2$ and $b_1$ using a 3-class Gaussian mixture model. Once the landmarks are found, the intensities between them are linearly scaled. A fuzzy segmentation [16] method is used to segment the images into three tissue classes, CSF, GM, and WM, shown in Fig. 3 bottom row. The segmentation consistency is visually confirmed in the red circled region (Fig. 3) and quantitatively described in Table 1, where the Dice similarity coefficients between the original MPRAGE segmentation and transformed ones are shown for the three tissue classes. Weighted averages of these three Dice coefficients, weighted by the volume of those tissues, are also reported as the "Mean". Our method significantly improves GM and WM segmentation consistency over other methods. However, it performs statistically the same as to the other methods on CSF segmentation. In general, a landmark based

**Table 2.** Each row shows an average Dice coefficient of the hard segmentations between the MPRAGE acquisition and the listed alternative, averaged over five scans of five subjects in the BIRN [11] dataset. The top row is the comparison to segmentation of the original SPGR and represents a baseline for the consistency of the segmentation.

|  | CSF | GM | WM | Mean |
|---|---|---|---|---|
| **Orig. SPGR** | $0.577 \pm 0.049$ | $0.713 \pm 0.053$ | $0.820 \pm 0.019$ | $0.749 \pm 0.028$ |
| **Hist. Match** | $0.606 \pm 0.052$ | $0.801 \pm 0.025$ | $0.862 \pm 0.018$ | $0.805 \pm 0.014$ |
| **Landmark [4]** | $0.481 \pm 0.066$ | $0.682 \pm 0.067$ | $0.816 \pm 0.059$ | $0.757 \pm 0.078$ |
| **Sparse [7]** | $0.593 \pm 0.050$ | $0.810 \pm 0.020$ | $0.879 \pm 0.015$ | $0.828 \pm 0.012$ |
| **Probabilistic** | $\mathbf{0.733 \pm 0.041}$ | $\mathbf{0.834 \pm 0.015}$ | $\mathbf{0.911 \pm 0.008}$ | $\mathbf{0.871 \pm 0.009}$ |

Bold indicates statistically significantly larger than the other four ($p < 0.05$).

a₁(GE 1.5T)  a₂ (GE 3T)

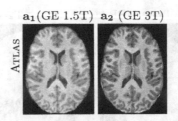

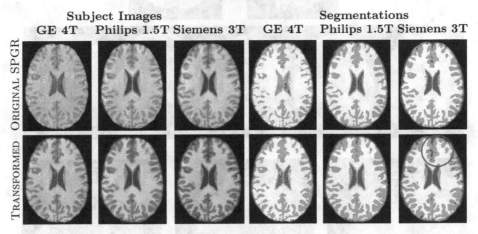

**Fig. 4.** Top row shows atlas SPGR and MPRAGE images from a GE 1.5T and GE 3T scanner. Middle row shows three scans of the same subject from three different scanners and their segmentations. Bottom row shows transformed MPRAGE images, along with the corresponding segmentations.

transformation works well for WM, as a WM landmark can be detected robustly. However, for SPGR images, a GM landmark can be erroneous as the image histograms are often uni or bi-modal [4]. We note that our method is significantly faster ($\sim$ 1 hour) than the sparse patch combination method ($\sim$ 7 hours) to transform a $256 \times 256 \times 199$ volume using $3 \times 3 \times 3$ patches.

Next we experiment on SPGR images on the BIRN [11] traveling subject data to show we can handle the effects of scanner variation. The dataset contains five subjects, each having five SPGRs (one each from a GE 1.5T, GE 4T, Philips 1.5T, and two from a Siemens 3T) and an MPRAGE acquisition (four subjects having GE 3T MPRAGE scans and one having a Siemens 1.5T MPRAGE scan). We transform all the SPGR scans of every subject, using the GE 1.5T SPGR and the GE 3T MPRAGE of the corresponding subject as the atlas images $a_1$ and $a_2$. Three scans and the corresponding transformed images of one subject are shown in Fig. 4 along with their segmentations. Table 2 quantitatively shows that the Dice coefficients between the transformed images and the original MPRAGE segmentation is significantly higher than the other methods, also seen visually in the red circled region in Fig. 4. Both the landmark based method and the histogram matching depend on the shape and range of the histograms of the subject and the target. As the SPGRs are acquired in a variety of scanners, the shape

Atlas T1-w MPRAGE    Atlas T2-w

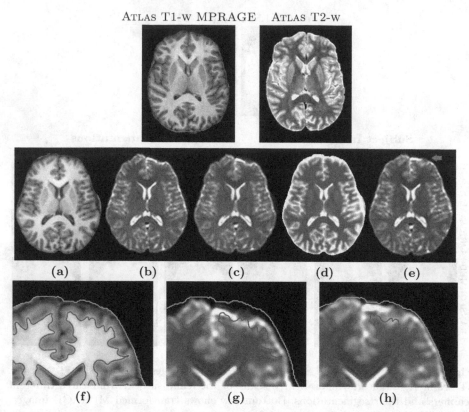

**Fig. 5.** Top row shows MPRAGE and $T_2$-w scans of a normal subject used as atlas. **(a)** and **(b)** shows MPRAGE and a rigidly registered $b_0$ scan of another subject where the $b_0$ scan is distorted near the temporal lobe. A deformable registration [17] of the $b_0$ scan to the MPRAGE is shown in **(c)**. Using the MPRAGE-$T_2$ atlas pair, the MPRAGE image of **(a)** is transformed to $T_2$, shown in **(d)**. The $b_0$ scan in **(b)** is then deformably registered to this $T_2$. The registration result is shown in **(e)**. Zoomed-in versions of **(a)**, **(c)**, and **(e)** are shown in **(f)**- **(g)**. The green contour denotes the CSF-background boundary, while the red contour is the GM-WM boundary.

of the image histograms vary widely [7], resulting in higher standard deviation in the average Dice coefficients for both CSF and GM segmentations. However, our method has consistently low standard deviation, indicating robustness to the variation in scanners.

## 3.2   $b_0$ to $T_1$ Registration

Diffusion MR imaging suffers from geometric distortion due to inhomogeneities in the $b_0$ magnetic field. This distortion is most significant near the boundaries of soft tissues with air or bone. The majority of distortion correction approaches are done by registering the $b_0$ image to a structural image, such as $T_1$-w or $T_2$-w MR images, by non-linear registrations [18]. The $b_0$, in terms of echo times and repetition times used in typical diffusion applications, has image contrast similar to that of a conventional $T_2$-w spin-echo image, thus making $T_2$-w images the preferred target for distortion correction. However, when $T_2$-w images are not acquired, the $T_1$-w image is used, resulting in an inferior correction.

Figs. 5(a)–(b) show an MPRAGE and $b_0$ image acquired in the same imaging session. The $b_0$ image shows significant distortion in the anterior portions of the brain. Fig. 5(c) shows the $b_0$ image after it has been registered to the MPRAGE using the state-of-the-art deformable registration algorithm SyN [17] with mutual information as the similarity metric. The distortion is still visible. For this particular dataset the $T_2$-w image is unavailable. We transform the MPRAGE (Fig. 5(a)) to $T_2$ (Fig. 5(d)), using the atlas images shown at the top of Fig. 5. Here we note that neither histogram matching nor any landmark based method is able to transform an MPRAGE to a $T_2$-w image. Registering the $b_0$ image to this $T_2$ using SyN, with cross-correlation as the similarity metric, yields the $b_0$ distortion corrected image shown in Fig. 5(e). The red arrow in Fig. 5(e) denotes an area of improvement by using the intermediate $T_2$ as the registration target over the MPRAGE. This is reflected quantitatively in the improved mutual information of 0.77 to 0.93, between the MPRAGE and the $b_0$ distortion corrected images from $T_1$-w and $T_2$-w registrations, respectively. Fig. 5(f) shows the GM-WM boundary (red) and the CSF-background contour (green), derived from the MPRAGE, on a zoomed portion of the MPRAGE. The same contours and zoomed portion are shown on the $b_0$ distortion corrected by registering to the $T_1$ and $T_2$ images, Figs. 5(g)–(h) respectively. The contours demonstrate, at least visually, that the $b_0$ after registration to the $T_2$-w image is better spatially aligned to the MPRAGE, than if it had been directly registered to it.

## 4    Discussion and Conclusion

In this paper, we have proposed a probabilistic model to change MR tissue intensities (e.g., from SPGR to MPRAGE or $T_1$ to $T_2$), where the patch selection depends on both contrasts. The transformed images are only used for image processing and not used for any diagnostic purpose. If the atlas does not contain some tissue contrasts, that are present in the atlas, nearby intensities from the subject are used. E.g., if the subject contains lesions, while the atlas does not have any, the lesion intensities will be matched to WM intensities. As our method does not directly rely on any histogram information, it is more robust to scanner variations compared to histogram matching or a landmark based matching technique, as shown on multi-scanner and multi-sequence datasets. Also, unlike the previous transformation method, it can be applied to transform $T_1$-w images to $T_2$-w images, which can be used as a proxy in a registration application, when actual $T_2$ images are not available.

## References

1. Resnick, S.M., Goldszal, A.F., Davatzikos, C., Golski, D., Kraut, M.A., Metter, E.J., Bryan, R.N., Zonderman, A.B.: One-year age changes in MRI brain volumes in older adults. Cerebral Cortex 10(5), 464–472 (2000)

2. Clark, K.A., Woods, R.P., Rottenber, D.A., Toga, A.W., Mazziotta, J.C.: Impact of acquisition protocols and processing streams on tissue segmentation of T1 weighted MR images. NeuroImage 29(1), 185–202 (2006)
3. Fischl, B., Salat, D.H., van der Kouwe, A.J.W., Makris, N., Segonne, F., Quinn, B.T., Dale, A.M.: Sequence-independent segmentation of magnetic resonance images. NeuroImage 23(1), 69–84 (2004)
4. Nyúl, L.G., Udupa, J.K.: On Standardizing the MR Image Intensity Scale. Mag. Reson. Med. 42(6), 1072–1081 (1999)
5. Jäger, F., Hornegger, J.: Nonrigid Registration of Joint Histograms for Intensity Standardization in Magnetic Resonance Imaging. IEEE Trans. Med. Imag. 28(1), 137–150 (2009)
6. Han, X., Fischl, B.: Atlas Renormalization for Improved Brain MR Image Segmentation Across Scanner Platforms. IEEE Trans. Med. Imag. 26(4), 479–486 (2007)
7. Roy, S., Carass, A., Prince, J.: A compressed sensing approach for MR tissue contrast synthesis. In: Székely, G., Hahn, H.K. (eds.) IPMI 2011. LNCS, vol. 6801, pp. 371–383. Springer, Heidelberg (2011)
8. Hertzmann, A., Jacobs, C.E., Oliver, N., Curless, B., Salesin, D.H.: Image analogies. In: Conf. on Comp. Graphics and Interactive Techniques (SIGGRAPH), pp. 327–340 (2001)
9. Cao, T., Zach, C., Modla, S., Powell, D., Czymmek, K., Niethammer, M.: Registration for correlative microscopy using image analogies. In: Dawant, B.M., Christensen, G.E., Fitzpatrick, J.M., Rueckert, D. (eds.) WBIR 2012. LNCS, vol. 7359, pp. 296–306. Springer, Heidelberg (2012)
10. Myronenko, A., Song, X.: Point-Set Registration: Coherent Point Drift. IEEE Trans. Patt. Anal. and Machine Intell. 32(12), 2262–2275 (2010)
11. Friedman, L., Stern, H., Brown, G.G., Mathalon, D.H., Turner, J., Glover, G.H., Gollub, R.L., Lauriello, J., Lim, K.O., Cannon, T., Greve, D.N., Bockholt, H.J., Belger, A., Mueller, B., Doty, M.J., He, J., Wells, W., Smyth, P., Pieper, S., Kim, S., Kubicki, M., Vangel, M., Potkin, S.G.: Test-Retest and Between-Site Reliability in a Multicenter fMRI Study. Human Brain Mapping 29(8), 958–972 (2008)
12. Zhang, J.: The mean field theory in em procedures for markov random fields. IEEE Trans. on Signal Proc. 40(10), 2570–2583 (1992)
13. Mairal, J., Bach, F., Ponce, J., Sapiro, G., Zisserman, A.: Non-local sparse models for image restoration. In: IEEE Intl. Conf. on Comp. Vision, pp. 2272–2279 (2009)
14. Carass, A., Cuzzocreo, J., Wheeler, M.B., Bazin, P.L., Resnick, S.M., Prince, J.L.: Simple paradigm for extra-cerebral tissue removal: Algorithm and analysis. NeuroImage 56(4), 1982–1992 (2011)
15. Sled, J.G., Zijdenbos, A.P., Evans, A.C.: A non-parametric method for automatic correction of intensity non-uniformity in MRI data. IEEE Trans. on Med. Imag. 17(1), 87–97 (1998)
16. Bazin, P.L., Pham, D.L.: Topology-preserving tissue classification of magnetic resonance brain images. IEEE Trans. on Medical Imaging 26(4), 487–496 (2007)
17. Avants, B.B., Epstein, C.L., Grossman, M., Gee, J.C.: Symmetric diffeomorphic image registration with cross-correlation: evaluating automated labeling of elderly and neurodegenerative brain. Medical Image Analysis 12(1), 26–41 (2008)
18. Ardekani, S., Sinha, U.: Geometric distortion correction of high-resolution 3T diffusion tensor brain images. Mag. Reson. Med. 54(5), 1163–1171 (2005)

# Use of Diffusion Tensor Images
# in Glioma Growth Modeling
# for Radiotherapy Target Delineation

Florian Dittmann[1], Björn Menze[2], Ender Konukoglu[1], and Jan Unkelbach[1]

[1] Massachusetts General Hospital, 30 Fruit Street, Boston, MA 02114, USA
[2] Computer Vision Laboratory, ETH Zurich, Switzerland

**Abstract.** In radiotherapy of gliomas, a precise definition of the treatment volume is problematic, because current imaging modalities reveal only the central part of the tumor with a high cellular density, but fail to detect all regions of microscopic tumor cell spread in the adjacent brain parenchyma. Mathematical models can be used to integrate known growth characteristics of gliomas into the target delineation process. In this paper, we demonstrate the use of diffusion tensor imaging (DTI) for simulating anisotropic cell migration in a glioma growth model that is based on the Fisher-Kolmogorov equation. For a clinical application of the model, it is crucial to develop a detailed understanding of its behavior, capabilities, and limitations. For that purpose, we perform a retrospective analysis of glioblastoma patients treated at our institution. We analyze the impact of diffusion anisotropy on model-derived target volumes, and interpret the results in the context of the underlying images. It was found that, depending on the location of the tumor relative to major fiber tracts, DTI can have significant influence on the shape of the radiotherapy target volume.

**Keywords:** glioma, tumor growth model, target delineation, diffusion tensor imaging, radiotherapy.

## 1 Introduction

Gliomas, the most common primary brain tumors, grow infiltratively into the brain parenchyma. Unfortunately, conventional imaging modalities reveal only the central, highly cellular part of the tumor, whereas areas of low tumor cell density appear normal. In standard radiation treatments of high-grade gliomas, the clinical target volume (CTV) is defined by applying an isotropic 1-3 cm margin around the abnormality visible in MRI, to account for potential tumor infiltration in normal appearing brain [1]. However, this process hardly accounts for the growth characteristics of gliomas that are known from histopathological findings [2,3]:

1. preferential spread of tumor cells along the white matter fiber tracts
2. reduced infiltration of gray matter
3. anatomical boundaries that prevent tumor cell migration, e.g. ventricles, falx cerebri, and tentorium cerebelli

L. Shen et al. (Eds.): MBIA 2013, LNCS 8159, pp. 63–73, 2013.
© Springer International Publishing Switzerland 2013

Accounting consistently for these growth patterns can result in a more personalized definition of the CTV, and therefore potentially improve the current treatment procedure. We use a phenomenological tumor growth model, which estimates a spatial tumor cell distribution by formalizing the growth characteristics. The model, which is based on the Fisher-Kolmogorov equation [4,5], is personalized via the patient's MRI imaging data [6]. For radiotherapy planning, the CTV is defined as an isoline of the estimated tumor cell density obtained from the model. For a clinical application, the model is used as a tool that automatically suggests a CTV to the physician, thus making target delineation semi-automatic and more objective. To that end, it is crucial to understand the model's behavior, its capabilities, and its limitations. Previous work has conceptually introduced the Fisher-Kolmogorov model to describe glioma growth [4], including the integration of DTI [7]. However, the specific problems related to radiotherapy planning applications have not been addressed in detail.

In this paper, we evaluate the potential of the Fisher-Kolmogorov model for target delineation. By retrospective analysis of glioblastoma multiforme (GBM) patients treated at our institution, we identify the best clinical use-cases. We determine tumor locations for which the model yields target contours that are more consistent with glioma growth patterns, compared to the manually drawn contours used for treatment. The paper focuses on the use of DTI to model preferential tumor spread along white matter fiber tracts within the glioma growth model. In particular, we characterize anatomical situations in which the additional use of DTI (on top of modeling anatomical barriers and reduced gray matter infiltration) suggests different target volumes.

In section 2, we briefly summarize the underlying tumor growth model and its personalization. Section 3 discusses how DTI is incorporated to model preferential cell migration along white matter fiber tracts. We suggest a new parameterized construction of the cell diffusion tensor from the DTI data, using a single quantitatively interpretable anisotropy parameter. In section 4, we present results for 3 patients. For one case, we present a detailed case study to explain the impact of DTI on CTV delineation. The results are interpreted in the context of the patient anatomy and the imaging data.

## 2 Tumor Growth Model

The glioma growth model formalizes the two processes that describe tumor growth: local *proliferation* of tumor cells and *diffusion* into surrounding brain tissue. It is based on the Fisher-Kolmogorov equation, a reaction-diffusion equation for the normalized tumor cell density $u = u(\boldsymbol{x}, t)$:

$$\frac{\partial u}{\partial t} = \nabla \cdot (D(\boldsymbol{x})\nabla u) + \rho u (1 - u) \tag{1}$$

The proliferation rate $\rho$ is assumed to be spatially constant, but the $3 \times 3$ diffusion tensor $D(\boldsymbol{x})$ depends on the location $\boldsymbol{x}$. The diffusion term $\nabla \cdot (D(\boldsymbol{x})\nabla u)$ represents the migration of tumor cells into the surrounding tissue, and the reaction term $\rho u(1 - u)$ describes the cell proliferation as logistic growth.

**Conversion into a Static Model:** A direct integration of (1) is impractical, because the initial condition that corresponds to the tumor appearance in MRI at the time of treatment planning is unknown. To circumvent this problem, we use the method suggested in [5], which is based on the assumption that the visible tumor is an isoline of the cell density, and the fact that the asymptotic solution of (1) is a traveling wave. Thus, (1) can be approximated by an anisotropic Eikonal equation, which is solved by the anisotropic fast marching algorithm presented in [8]. The result is similar to the geodesic distance model in [9].

**Personalization of the Model:** To apply the model to the patient at hand, an initial segmentation of the brain into tumor, white matter (WM), gray matter (GM), and cerebrospinal fluid (CSF) is performed, using co-registered diagnostic MR images (T1, T2, FLAIR, and T1 post contrast) as input. We utilize Expectation-Maximization-based segmentation similar to the generative tumor segmentation model of [6]. However, the initial segmentation result is enhanced as suggested in [10], in order to reliably incorporate the most prominent anatomical boundaries falx cerebri and tentorium cerebelli. The propagation of infiltration values is restricted to the WM and GM area, and CSF is used to model anatomical boundaries.

## 3 Parameterization of Anisotropic Cell Diffusion

The diffusion tensor $D(x)$ for a voxel $x$ is constructed as

$$D(x) = \begin{cases} D_w T(x), & x \in WM \\ D_g I, & x \in GM \end{cases} \tag{2}$$

where $I$ is the identity matrix, and $D_w$ and $D_g$ are diffusion rates in WM and GM, respectively. By choosing $D_w > D_g$, we model reduced infiltration of GM. In this paper, we set $D_w/D_g = 100$. By constructing $T(x)$ from the water diffusion tensor $DTI(x)$ obtained from DTI, we can describe anisotropic diffusion in WM. The general idea behind the parameterization of $T(x)$ is based on the orthonormal eigenvector matrix $E(x)$ of $DTI(x)$ :

$$T(x) = E(x) \begin{pmatrix} \xi_1 & 0 & 0 \\ 0 & \xi_2 & 0 \\ 0 & 0 & \xi_3 \end{pmatrix} E^T(x) \tag{3}$$

The eigenvectors $e_i$ in $E(x)$ are the eigenvectors of $DTI(x)$ with associated eigenvalues $\lambda_i$. $\xi_1$, $\xi_2$, and $\xi_3$ control the cell diffusion along these eigenvectors, where $\xi_1$ corresponds to the principle eigenvector $e_1$.

### Weighting of Diffusion Anisotropy

Setting $\xi_i = \lambda_i$ leads to $T(x) = DTI(x)$. For this naive construction, one cannot control the degree of anisotropy. Since this paper focuses on the question how diffusion anisotropy can potentially impact target volumes, a parameterization is needed that matches the following criteria: (1) one single parameter controls the amount of anisotropy, (2) the parameter is interpretable quantitatively, (3) the parameterization results in an intuitive behavior of the model.

The main idea of our parameterization is to increase the cell diffusion along the principle diffusion axis, depending on the water diffusion anisotropy and a free constant weighting parameter. To that end, $\xi_2$ and $\xi_3$ are set to $\xi_2 = \xi_3 = 1$, whereas $\xi_1$ is chosen to be larger than 1. To construct $\xi_1$, we first normalize $\lambda_i$ by using the apparent diffusion coefficient (ADC): $\bar{\lambda}_1 = 3\lambda_1 / \sum_i \lambda_i$. With $\bar{\lambda}_1$ being independent from the overall water diffusion at the location $x$, we define $\xi_1$ as:

$$\xi_1 = 1 + \gamma(\bar{\lambda}_1 - 1), \gamma \geq 0 \tag{4}$$

The anisotropy weighting parameter $\gamma$ controls the amount of diffusion that is added to the principal axis. Furthermore, the parameterization has the following desirable properties:

1. For $\gamma = 0$ the diffusion is isotropic and independent from $DTI(x)$.
2. For $\gamma = 1$ the diffusion along the principal axis is equal to the ADC normalized water diffusion.
3. An isotropic water diffusion results in an isotropic $T(x)$.
4. Arbitrary high anisotropy can be introduced through increasing the diffusion along the principal axis via $\gamma$.
5. Because only the cell diffusion along the principal axis is modified, it is easier to trace the influence of anisotropy on the model and on the estimated tumor cell distribution.
6. The diffusion $\xi_1$ along the principal axis scales linearly with $\bar{\lambda}_1$ and $\gamma$, which makes $\gamma$ quantitatively interpretable.

## 4    Model-Based Target Delineation

We performed a retrospective study involving six glioblastoma multiforme patients with varying tumor location treated at our institution. In this section, we report general observations from this group of patients, and illustrate relevant findings. Section 4.1 presents an in-depth analysis of one case to explain the anatomical features (major fiber tracts) that cause difference in model-derived targets when incorporated via DTI. Sections 4.2 and 4.3 show the impact of incorporating DTI data for two additional cases.

### 4.1    Case I

For case I, the tumor is located in the left parietal lobe (right side of the image) close to the corpus callosum (CC). Figure 1a displays the FLAIR image showing peritumoral edema, as well as the segmentation of the contrast enhancing tumor core (green), and the manually delineated CTV (red) from the actually applied treatment plan. The manually delineated CTV covers most of the left hemisphere except for the anterior part of the frontal lobe.

Figure 1c visualizes the principal eigenvector $e_1$ of the diffusion tensor weighted with the normalized first eigenvalue $\overline{\lambda}_1$. As shown, the major fiber tracts adjacent to the tumor core are the CC with a dominant left-right fiber orientation (red), and the tracts with a strong superior-inferior directionality (blue), such as the corticopontine tract and corticospinal tract. The edema surrounding the tumor core leads to a low diffusion anisotropy in this area, visible as low intensity in fig. 1c and in the $\overline{\lambda}_1$ images (fig. 1d to 1f).

## Illustration of the Growth Model without DTI

Figure 1b illustrates the result of the tumor growth model. It shows the isolines of the tumor cell density throughout the brain for isotropic diffusion in WM ($\gamma = 0$). The orange contour in fig. 1a represents the isoline that encompasses the same total volume as the manually drawn CTV (red). The model accounts for the falx cerebri and the ventricles as anatomical barriers, but models tumor cell migration through the CC into the contralateral hemisphere. Here, the growth model suggests an expansion of the target volume into the contralateral hemisphere. This is not accounted for in the manual delineation, which incorporates the falx cerebri as boundary but does not consistently account for the CC. In addition, the model describes the reduced infiltration of gray matter, resulting in a sharp falloff of the tumor cell density within the cortical gray matter surrounding the sulci.

## Influence of DTI on Target Volumes

We now discuss the additional influence of DTI. For that purpose, we calculate the tumor cell densities for $\gamma = 0$, $\gamma = 5$, and $\gamma = 20$. In fig. 1d to 1f, the $\overline{\lambda}_1$ images are overlaid with five selected isolines. For the sake of comparison, the same color of isoline corresponds to the same size of the enclosed volume.[1] In particular, the volume of the orange isolines matches the size of the manually delineated CTV. The red and green contours enclose smaller volumes, which can be used to define radiotherapy boost volumes. The contours in fig. 1d ($\gamma = 0$), serving as reference, are extracted isolines from the cell density distribution shown in fig. 1b.

To show the major differences between targets derived from the isotropic and anisotropic cell diffusion in more detail, figure 2 illustrates the contours, matching the size of the manual CTV, for $\gamma = 0$ (yellow) and $\gamma = 20$ (red) for two axial slices.

---

[1] Instead of isolines with the same infiltration value, it is indicated to compare isolines enclosing a volume of the same size, because the parameterization presented in section 3 introduces higher diffusion rates, resulting in higher infiltration values per se.

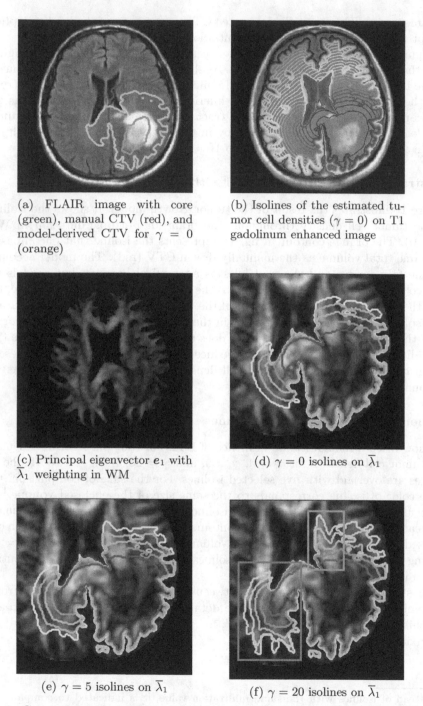

(a) FLAIR image with core (green), manual CTV (red), and model-derived CTV for $\gamma = 0$ (orange)

(b) Isolines of the estimated tumor cell densities ($\gamma = 0$) on T1 gadolinum enhanced image

(c) Principal eigenvector $e_1$ with $\overline{\lambda}_1$ weighting in WM

(d) $\gamma = 0$ isolines on $\overline{\lambda}_1$

(e) $\gamma = 5$ isolines on $\overline{\lambda}_1$

(f) $\gamma = 20$ isolines on $\overline{\lambda}_1$

**Fig. 1.** Comparison of multiple isolines for $\gamma = 0, 5, 20$ ($\gamma = 0$ corresponds to an isotropic growth model without DTI; lines of the same color correspond to the same volume; orange line corresponds to the manual CTV size)

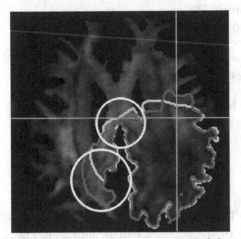
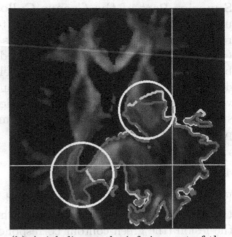

(a) Axial slice at the superior part of the corpus callosum

(b) Axial slice at the inferior part of the corpus callosum

**Fig. 2.** Comparison of the target volumes for $\gamma = 0$ (yellow) and $\gamma = 20$ (red) on visualization of $e_1$ with $\overline{\lambda}_1$ weighting

**Contralateral Hemisphere:** As shown in fig. 1, all contours extend far into the CC due to its close proximity to the tumor core. With increasing anisotropy weighting $\gamma$, the isolines extend further into the contralateral hemisphere (blue box area in fig. 1f). Here, the strong alignment of fibers in the CC results in a high diffusion anisotropy, and therefore in more infiltration of the contralateral side. Especially the blue and the yellow isolines, describing bigger volumes than the manual CTV, are further expanded. For high values of $\gamma$, they reach the smaller peripheral posterior fiber tracts of the contralateral side. The major change of the isolines is visible between the pure isotropic case ($\gamma = 0$) and the case with anisotropy weighting of $\gamma = 5$. Differences between the isolines of $\gamma = 5$ and $\gamma = 20$ are comparatively small.

The tendency that the contralateral side is more likely to be infiltrated in the anisotropic case is also visible in the direct comparison of the contours of $\gamma = 0$ (yellow) and $\gamma = 20$ (red) in fig. 2a (bottom circle) and fig. 2b (left circle).

**Frontal Lobe:** We now consider the region anterior to the tumor core (pink box area in fig. 1f). For the isotropic case ($\gamma = 0$, fig. 1d), the target extension into the frontal lobe is characterized by a smooth contour (mostly defined by the geometric distance in WM from the core). In contrast, in the anisotropic case with high diffusion weighting ($\gamma = 20$, fig. 1f), the isolines have a jagged shape since they incorporate the varying fiber tract orientations in this region. Especially the yellow and the blue lines tend to follow the anterior-posterior oriented fibers, i.e. the anterior part of the internal capsule, and the superior part of the fronto-occipital fascicilus (green fiber tracts in fig. 1c). This effect is also apparent in fig. 2. For a lower anisotropy weighting ($\gamma = 5$, fig. 1e), this effect is less pronounced.

**Superior Part of the Corpus Callosum:** We now compare the target volumes in the superior part of the CC (top circle in fig. 2a). In the anterior direction, the red contour ($\gamma = 20$) does not extend beyond the yellow contour ($\gamma = 0$); the yellow contour is expanded even further than red contour. This is because the dominant fiber direction (left-right) is perpendicular to the primary direction of cell migration. Since we compare contours that encompass the same volume size, and the red contour includes larger areas in the contralateral hemisphere, the target volume is to be trimmed in other regions (e.g. in the superior part of the CC).

## 4.2   Case II

For case II, the tumor core is located in the left temporal lobe adjacent to the brain boundary. Figure 3a shows the FLAIR image in the superior part of the lesion (the green contour corresponds to the contrast enhancing core). The manually delineated CTV (red) covers large areas in the left temporal, occipital, and parietal lobes.

Figure 3b compares the model derived target volumes for the isotropic case (yellow: $\gamma = 0$) and the anisotropic case (red: $\gamma = 20$). Both contours account for the ventricles as anatomical barrier, as well as the effect of reduced gray matter near major sulci. In this case, this becomes most apparent near the lateral sulcus.

The additional impact of DTI on the target volume is visible in the CC and the inferior fronto-occipital fasciculus. Similar to case I, the assumption of preferential spread of tumor cells along major fiber tracts modeled via DTI suggests a further expansion of the target into the CC. However, compared to case I, the effect is reduced because the tumor core is located further away from the CC.

## 4.3   Case III

For case III, the tumor core is located within the left superior frontoparietal region. The FLAIR image shows extensive peritumoral edema around the contrast enhancing core (green contour in fig. 4a). The manually delineated CTV (red) covers most of the left parietal lobe and is partially extended into the left frontal lobe.

Figure 4b shows the location of major fiber tracts and compares of the model-derived target volumes (matching the size of the manual CTV) for $\gamma = 0$ (yellow) and $\gamma = 20$ (red). The findings for this patient are consistent with case I and II: it is illustrated that the integration of anisotropic cell diffusion leads to further extension of the isolines into the CC and the contralateral side. The magnitude of this effect depends on the distance of the tumor from the CC.

Case III also illustrates a limitation of the use of DTI to model preferential tumor cell migration along fiber tracts: within the edematous region the anisotropy signal obtained from DTI is reduced (visible as the hypointense region in fig. 4b). In this region, the information about the dominant fiber orientation is compromised. This reduces the differences between the isotropic and the anisotropic model.

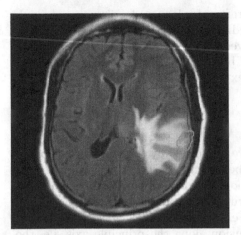

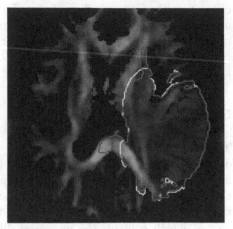

(a) FLAIR image with tumor core (green) and manual CTV (red)

(b) Target volumes for $\gamma = 0$ (yellow) and $\gamma = 20$ (red) overlaid on the visualization of $e_1$ with $\overline{\lambda}_1$ weighting

**Fig. 3.** Case II: Comparison of the target volumes

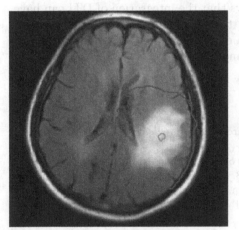

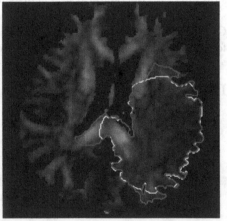

(a) FLAIR image with tumor core (green) and manual CTV (red)

(b) Target volumes for $\gamma = 0$ (yellow) and $\gamma = 20$ (red) overlaid on the visualization of $e_1$ with $\overline{\lambda}_1$ weighting

**Fig. 4.** Case III: Comparison of the target volumes

## 4.4    Application to Low-Grade Gliomas

Model-based CTV definition for low-grade gliomas was not explicitly addressed in this paper. However, the presented methodology would be equally applicable to low-grade gliomas. In current clinical practice, the margin for the manual CTV definition in low-grade cases (1-2 cm, [11]) is smaller than in high-grade cases, resulting in a smaller volume. Therefore, for low grade-gliomas, only high anisotropy of the DTI signal in the immediate neighborhood of the MRI abnormality can have an impact on model-derived CTVs. On the other hand, accurate target delineation and optimal sparing of brain tissue is of particular interest in low-grade gliomas due to the longer life expectancy of patients.

## 5    Conclusion

The spatial growth patterns of gliomas are influenced by the preferential spread of tumor cells along the white matter fiber tracts. This can be formalized via a spatially varying, anisotropic cell diffusion tensor in a reaction-diffusion equation. In this work, we formulated a construction of the cell diffusion tensor from the DTI derived water diffusion tensor. We introduce a single anisotropy parameter $\gamma$, which controls the increased diffusion along the principle axis, i.e. the primary fiber direction.

Based on this comprehensive tensor parameterization, we investigate the influence of DTI on target delineation for radiotherapy. Six patients were analyzed. One of the main findings is that, for tumors located in proximity to the corpus callosum, an anisotropic diffusion parameterization indicates a further expansion into the contralateral side. This shows that the integration of DTI can have significant impact on the model-derived target volume for radiation therapy. Current research addresses the validation of the glioma growth model based on follow-up MR imaging and clinical outcome data.

## References

1. Becker, K.P., Yu, J.: Status quo–standard-of-care medical and radiation therapy for glioblastoma. Cancer J. 18(1), 12–19 (2012)
2. Coons, S.: Anatomy and growth patterns of diffuse gliomas. In: Berger, M., Wilson, C. (eds.) The Gliomas, pp. 210–225. W.B. Saunders Company, Philadelphia (1999)
3. Matsukado, Y., MacCarty, C., Kernohan, J., et al.: The growth of glioblastoma multiforme (astrocytomas, grades 3 and 4) in neurosurgical practice. Journal of Neurosurgery 18, 636 (1961)
4. Harpold, H.L.P., Alvord Jr, E.C., Swanson, K.R.: The evolution of mathematical modeling of glioma proliferation and invasion. J. Neuropathol. Exp. Neurol. 66(1), 1–9 (2007)
5. Konukoglu, E., Clatz, O., Bondiau, P.Y., Delingette, H., Ayache, N.: Extrapolating glioma invasion margin in brain magnetic resonance images: suggesting new irradiation margins. Med. Image Anal. 14(2), 111–125 (2010)
6. Menze, B.H., Van Leemput, K., Lashkari, D., Weber, M.-A., Ayache, N., Golland, P.: A generative model for brain tumor segmentation in multi-modal images. In: Jiang, T., Navab, N., Pluim, J.P.W., Viergever, M.A. (eds.) MICCAI 2010, Part II. LNCS, vol. 6362, pp. 151–159. Springer, Heidelberg (2010)
7. Jbabdi, S., Mandonnet, E., Duffau, H., Capelle, L., Swanson, K.R., Pélégrini-Issac, M., Guillevin, R., Benali, H.: Simulation of anisotropic growth of low-grade gliomas using diffusion tensor imaging. Magn. Reson. Med. 54(3), 616–624 (2005)

8. Konukoglu, E., Sermesant, M., Clatz, O., Peyrat, J.-M., Delingette, H., Ayache, N.: A recursive anisotropic fast marching approach to reaction diffusion equation: application to tumor growth modeling. In: Karssemeijer, N., Lelieveldt, B. (eds.) IPMI 2007. LNCS, vol. 4584, pp. 687–699. Springer, Heidelberg (2007)
9. Cobzas, D., Mosayebi, P., Murtha, A., Jagersand, M.: Tumor invasion margin on the Riemannian space of brain fibers. In: Yang, G.-Z., Hawkes, D., Rueckert, D., Noble, A., Taylor, C. (eds.) MICCAI 2009, Part II. LNCS, vol. 5762, pp. 531–539. Springer, Heidelberg (2009)
10. Unkelbach, J., Menze, B., Motamedi, A., Dittmann, F., Konukoglu, E., Ayache, N., Shih, H.: Glioblastoma growth modeling for radiotherapy target delineation. In: Proc. MICCAI Workshop on IGRT (2012)
11. Grier, J.T., Batchelor, T.: Low-grade gliomas in adults. The Oncologist 11(6), 681–693 (2006)

# Superpixel-Based Segmentation of Glioblastoma Multiforme from Multimodal MR Images

Po Su[1,2], Jianhua Yang[1], Hai Li[2], Linda Chi[3], Zhong Xue[2,*], and Stephen T. Wong[2]

[1] School of Automation, Northwestern Polytechnical University, Xi'an, China
[2] Department of Systems Medicine and Bioengineering, The Methodist Hospital Research Institute, Weill Cornell Medical College, Houston, TX
[3] Department of Diagnostic Radiology, MD Anderson Cancer Center, Houston, TX
zxue@tmhs.org

**Abstract.** Due to complex imaging characteristics such as large diversity in shapes and appearances combining with deformation of surrounding tissues, it is a challenging task to segment glioblastoma multiforme (GBM) from multimodal MR images. In particular, it is important to capture the heterogeneous features of enhanced tumor, necrosis, and non-enhancing T2 hyperintense regions (T2HI) to determine the aggressiveness of the tumor from neuroimaging. In this paper, we propose a superpixel-based graph spectral clustering method to improve the robustness of GBM segmentation. A new graph spectral clustering algorithm is designed to group superpixels to different tissue types. First, a local k-means clustering with weighted distances is employed to segment the MR images into a number of homogeneous regions, called superpixels. Then, the spectral clustering algorithm is utilized to extract the enhanced tumor, necrosis, and T2HI by considering the superpixel map as a graph. Experiment results demonstrate better performance of the proposed method by comparing with pixel-based and the normalized cut segmentation methods.

**Keywords:** GBM, superpixel, spectral clustering, multimodal MR images.

## 1 Introduction

Multimodal magnetic resonance (MR) images have been widely used in diagnosis, treatment planning, and follow-up studies of GBM [1] . In multimodal MR scans, GBM often shows a heterogeneous region including an enhanced tumor region, a necrotic region (necrosis), and a non-enhancing T2HI region that is a combination of active tumor cells and possible edema. Accurate segmentation of different tissues of GBM can help neuroradiologists determine tumor margin and assess its progression and aggressiveness. However, due to the complicated imaging characteristics of GBM, such as large diversity in shapes and appearance combining with deformed surrounding tissue, accurate segmentation of GBM from multimodal MR images is challenging.

In the literature, pixel-based automatic segmentation methods [2-5] are widely used. The basic idea is to assign each voxel to a tissue type by considering its

---

* Corresponding author.

L. Shen et al. (Eds.): MBIA 2013, LNCS 8159, pp. 74–83, 2013.

intensities in multimodal images and the constraints derived from its neighboring pixels or voxels. For example, Clark *et al.* [4] developed a knowledge-based fuzzy clustering algorithm to segment GBM. Prastawa *et al.* [5] considered tumor as outliers of normal tissue, thus the tumor and edema could be isolated by a statistical classification based on learning of intensity distributions for normal brain tissues. Recently, graph cut-based methods [6, 7] have driven more attention. They treat the image as a graph, *i.e.*, pixels as nodes and their similarity as network links or edges. After dividing the graph into sub-networks, the total dissimilarity among different sub-networks and the total similarity within each network are maximized. For example, Corso *et al.* [6] integrated the Bayesian model with graph-based affinities to segment brain tumor from multimodal MR images. However, graph cut-based methods often need to solve a generalized eigenvector problem and may suffer from large computational load when the data set is large. The idea of superpixel [8, 9] can dramatically reduce the number of nodes of the graph and speed up the graph partition while maintaining the image information.

In this paper, we present a superpixel-based graph spectral clustering method for GBM segmentation based on multimodal MR images including T2 weighted (T2), T1 pre-enhanced (T1PRE), T1 post-enhanced (T1POST) and FLAIR. First, a local k-means clustering algorithm with weighted distance is performed to segment the multimodal images into a number of compact and homogeneous superpixels. Then, by considering the brain as a graph of superpixels (*e.g.*, defining nodes as superpixels and links as similarity among superpixels), image segmentation is achieved using spectral clustering of the superpixel network. Compared to the traditional methods, the efficiency and robustness can be improved by using superpixels in the spectral clustering.

In experiments, we first tested the influence of parameters on the segmentation results. Then, we demonstrated the superiority of our method by comparing voxel-based method and standard normalized cut (Ncut) segmentation method.

## 2    Methods

### 2.1    Overview

Fig.1. shows the workflow of the proposed method. The pre-processing step consists of skull stripping and co-registration of multimodal images. The FSL [10] skull stripping (BET) and rigid registration (FLIRT) tools are used. In the next step,

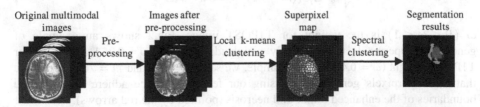

| Original multimodal images | Images after pre-processing | Superpixel map | Segmentation results |

Pre-processing → Local k-means clustering → Spectral clustering

**Fig. 1.** The workflow of the superpixel-based graph spectral clustering method

superpixels are generated using the local k-means clustering algorithm. Finally, the superpixel-based graph is constructed, and the spectral clustering algorithm is performed to classify the superpixels into different groups, including normal brain tissues, enhanced tumor, necrosis and T2HI.

## 2.2    Segmenting Images into Superpixels

We used the local k-means clustering algorithm to segment the image into superpixels. In [8], the algorithm was used to generate superpixels from color images. The CIELAB color $[l\,a\,b]$ and the pixel coordinate $[x\,y]$ were used as the image features. A new distance metric $d$ was introduced by simultaneously considering the image features and the size of superpixel:

$$d = \sqrt{d_f{}^2 + \left(\frac{d_{xy}}{s}\right)^2 m^2}, \tag{1}$$

where

$$d_f = \sqrt{(l_i - l_k)^2 + (a_i - a_k)^2 + (b_i - b_k)^2},$$

$$d_{xy} = \sqrt{(x_i - x_k)^2 + (y_i - y_k)^2}, \tag{2}$$

$$S = \sqrt{N/K}.$$

$N$ is the number of pixels, and $K$ is the desired number of approximately equally-sized superpixels. $(l_i, a_i, b_i, x_i, y_i)^T$ represents the 5-D feature of pixel $i$, and $(l_k, a_k, b_k, x_k, y_k)^T$ is the centroid of the $k$th cluster, $k \in [1, K]$. $d_f$ measures the color proximity, and $d_{xy}$ measures spatial proximity. $m$ is a parameter that controls the compactness of superpixels, and larger $m$ will induce more compact superpixels. The searching region of the local k-means algorithm is limited to local neighboring region with the size $2S \times 2S$. This results in a significant reduction of computational load over the standard k-means algorithm.

In order to generate superpixels adhering more tightly to the tissue boundaries, we use different weights on T1 post-enhanced image that captures enhanced tumor and necrosis well. Let $[f_{1i}\,f_{2i}\,f_{3i}\,f_{4i}\,x_i\,y_i]$ represents the 6-D feature vector of pixel $i$, where $f_{1i}, f_{2i}, f_{3i},$ and $f_{4i}$ represent the image intensities of pixel $i$ located at $(x_i, y_i)$ in T2, T1PRE, FLAIR, and T1POST images, the feature distance between pixel $i$ and the $k$th cluster center is defined as,

$$d_f = \sqrt{\frac{1-\omega}{3}\sum_{j=1}^{3}\left(f_{ji} - f_{jk}\right)^2 + \omega(f_{4i} - f_{4k})^2}, \tag{3}$$

$\omega$ ($0 < \omega < 1$) is the weight for T1POST image. Fig.2 shows an example of generating superpixels using equally weighted distance ($\omega = 0.25$) and a higher T1POST weight ($\omega = 0.4$). In this example, we set $K = 600$, and $m = 70$. We can see that the superpixels generated by using our feature distance adhere better to the boundaries of the enhanced tumor and necrosis (pointed by the red arrows).

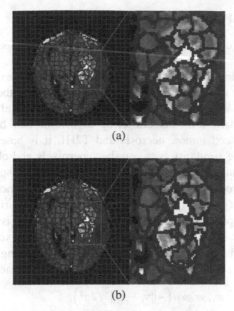

(a)

(b)

**Fig. 2.** Superpixels generated using standard local k-means clustering and our method. (a) Standard equally weighted; (b) with more weights on T1POST.

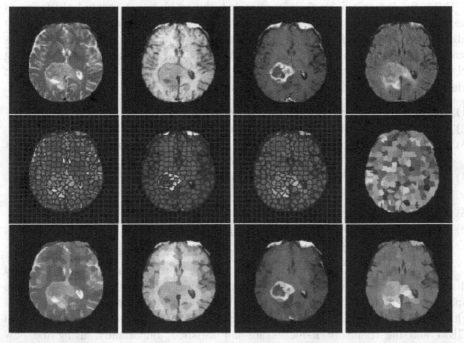

**Fig. 3.** Examples of superpixel segmentation. Top: original multimodal images (T2, T1PRE, T1POST, and FLAIR); middle: superpixels generated by our method; bottom: superpixels in each modality, from left to right: T2, T1PRE, T1POST, FLAIR.

## 2.3    Graph Spectral Clustering of Superpixels

After brain pixels are classified into superpixels, with each superpixel consisting of the adjacent pixels with similar multimodal image intensities, we need to further classify them into several major tissue groups. Fig. 3 shows an example of generating superpixels. In the last row, each superpixel is represented by the average intensities in four modalities, and we will use them as features for superpixel classification.

Although the standard k-means clustering algorithm can be used to segment superpixels into enhanced tumor, necrosis and T2HI, it is based on the Euclidean distance to measure the similarity between the superpixels and cluster centroids, and the algorithm is only suitable when data manifold in the feature space is convex. If the data manifold is curved or not convex, the Euclidean distance is inadequate for distinguishing different tissue types. To better handle the similarity and classification of superpixels, the graph partition-based segmentation method is used for superpixel classification. Specifically, for a graph $G = \{V, E\}$ with vertexes $V = \{v_1, v_2, \cdots, v_K\}$ representing superpixels, and edge $E$ representing affinity among the superpixels, the affinity of superpixels $i$ and $j$, $w_{ij}$, is defined as a Gaussian kernel with width $\sigma$,

$$w_{ij} = \exp\left(-\|\mathbf{v}_i - \mathbf{v}_j\|^2 / 2\sigma^2\right). \tag{4}$$

$\mathbf{v}_i$ and $\mathbf{v}_j$ are the average intensity vectors in the four modalities of the vertexes $v_i$ and $v_j$.

After the superpixel graph is constructed, the graph-based spectral clustering is applied to classify the superpixels into different tissue types. The spectral clustering algorithm [11, 12] reflects the intrinsic data manifolds in the feature space and is suitable for classification of no-convex data. Herein, the normlized spectral clusering algorithm [11] is used. Given the affinity matrix $W = [w_{ij}]$ and the number of the clusters $C$ ($\sigma = 20$, $C=6$), the following six steps are performed:

1) Define $D$ to be a diagonal matrix with $D_{ii} = \sum_{j=1}^{K} w_{ij}$.
2) Compute the normalized Laplacian matrix $L = D^{-1/2}(D - W)D^{-1/2}$.
3) Compute top $C$ eigenvectors $z_1, z_2, \cdots, z_C$ of $L$ and form the matrix $Z = [z_1\, z_2\, \cdots\, z_C] \in R^{K \times C}$ by stacking the eigenvectors in columns.
4) Form matrix $Y \in R^{K \times C}$ from $Z$ by normalizing the rows to have unit length, i.e., $y_{ij} = z_{ij} / \left(\sum_{c=1}^{C} z_{ic}^2\right)^{1/2}$.
5) Run the k-means clustering to group the row vector $Y$.
6) Assign the original point $v_i$ to cluster $j$ if and only if row $i$ of the matrix $Y$ is assigned to cluster $j$.

Finally, the GBM tissue segmentation can be obtained based on the intensity distribution of each group. Fig. 4 shows the sample segmentation results using the spectral clustering algorithm and k-means. For both methods, we set the number of clusters to $C= 6$. We can see that spectral clustering succeeds to segment all parts of GBM and the results of k-means are not satisfied. Importantly, using the new algorithm, it is much easier to distinguish necrosis with grey matter, as well as T2HI with other white matters.

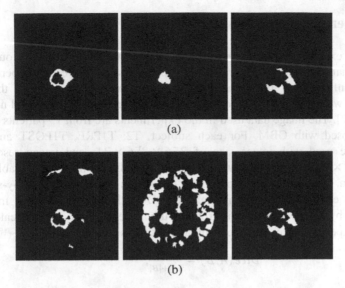

(a)

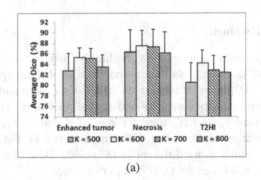

(b)

**Fig. 4.** Results using spectral clustering and k-means. (a) Results of spectral clustering. From left to right are enhanced tumor, necrosis, and T2HI; (b) results of k-means clustering.

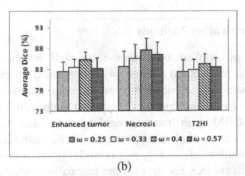

(a)

(b)

**Fig. 5.** The influence of parameter $K$ and $\omega$ on GBM tissue segmentation. (a) Segmentation results using different $K$ ($\omega = 0.4$); (b) segmentation results using different $\omega$ ($K = 600$).

# 3        Experiments and Results

Two sets of experiments were conducted to evaluate the performance of our method. The performance of our method relies on superpixels. So in the first experiment, we tested the influence of the parameters on superpixels generation. In the second experiment, we compared our algorithm with voxel-based method [4] and normalized cut (Ncut) [7]. The image data used in the experiments are from 15 patients who have been diagnosed with GBM. For each subject, T2, T1PRE, T1POST and FLAIR images were used with image size of $256 \times 256 \times 21$, and image resolution of $0.78 \times 0.78 \times 6.5$ mm$^3$. The low resolution in $z$-direction is not suitable for 3D segmentation, so we adopted superpixels to process the images slice-by-slice. The algorithm is extendable for supervoxels for 3D MRI data. The manual marking of GBM tissue by an expert is used as ground truth. Dice similarity score is calculated to evaluate the performance. The Dice similarity score is defined as:

$$Dice(A, B) = \frac{2|A \cap B|}{|A| + |B|}, \tag{5}$$

$A$ represents the pixel sets of GBM tissue of ground truth, $B$ represents the pixel sets of GBM tissue using proposed method or other methods.

## 3.1        Selection of Parameter

The quality of superpixel segmentation is highly dependent on the choice of parameters: $K$, $m$ and $\omega$. $m$ controls the compactness of the superpixels and is often set in the range [10,100]. $m = 70$ is adopted in all our experiments, and it offers a good balance between intensity similarity and spatial proximity. To achieve the best segmentation performance, we have tried a range of $K$ and $\omega$. Fig. 5 (a) shows the GBM tissue segmentation results using different $K$ ($\omega = 0.4$). Fig. 5 (b) shows the GBM segmentation results using different $\omega$ ($K = 600$). Based on our experiments, we found $K = 600, \omega = 0.4$ can the yield best performance.

## 3.2        Comparison with other Methods

In the experiment, we applied our method as well as the other two classic segmentation methods, pixel-based method [4] and normalized cut (Ncut) [7] to our image data and compared the segmentation results, both qualitative and quantitative. We found that pixel-based method and Ncut are vulnerable when dealing with complicated cases (GBM with more irregular shape and more heterogeneous intensity). Fig. 6 shows an example of applying the three methods to one subject with complicated GBM characteristics. Fig. 6 (a) and Fig. 6 (b) are the FLAIR and T1POST images of this subject. Fig. 6 (c) is the manually labeled ground truth. Fig. 6 (d) is the result of pixel-based method. Fig. 6 (e) is the result of Ncut. Fig. 6  (f) is the result of our algorithm. From Fig. 6, we can see our method outperform voxel-based method and Ncut on this complicated case.

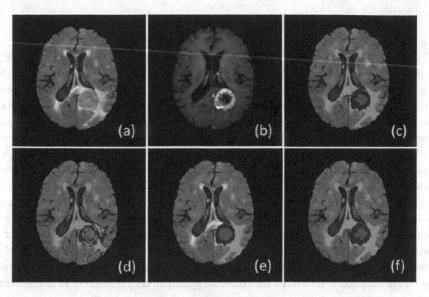

**Fig. 6.** Comparison of segmentation results on a complicated GBM sample. (a)(b): original FLAIR and T1POST images; (c) groundtruth; (d) pixel-based method; (e) normalized cut; (f) our algorithm. (enhanced tumor: blue region, necrosis: red region, T2HI: green region).

The quantitative results are shown in Fig. 7. We can see that our algorithm is more accurate. Pixel-based segmentation method does not take local or global spatial information into account and easily generate unsatisfied segmentations when the intensity of GBM tissues overlaps each other. For Ncut, it can yield good results when the shape of GBM tumors are compact and regular, when the shape of GBM is irregular and complicated, this method is limited (see Fig. 6 (e)). Furthermore, Ncut needs to solve a generalized eigenvector problem, when the image size is large, it suffers high computational load. Compared with other two methods, our algorithm combines the advantages of superpixel and spectral clustering is more suitable for GBM segmentation.

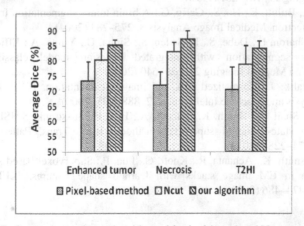

**Fig. 7.** Comparison of our algorithm with pixel-based and Ncut methods

# 4    Conclusion

We developed a superpixel-based graph spectral clustering algorithm that combines superpixel and graph spectral clustering to segment GBM from multimodal MR images. The basic idea is that the superpixel method groups spatially relate pixels with similar intensities together, and the graph spectral clustering on superpixels reduces the computational load and improves the accuracy of the segmentation. Comparative study showed the proposed method can achieve more accurate results. Because the $z$-direction resolution of our image data is very low, we used superpixel instead of supervoxel. It can be easily extended to use supervoxel for 3D scans. Quantitative segmentation of GBM from multimodal images provides detailed diagnostic information. For example, the shape and size of the enhanced tumor, necrosis, the region of T2 hyperintensity (T2HI), the intensity distribution within each region, as well as the transition from enhanced tumor to T2HI may provide important information about the aggressiveness of GBM. In the future, we plan to extract these features and correlate with the pathological finding aiming at providing more quantitative diagnostic measures for GBM subtyping and aggressiveness assessment.

# References

1. Petrella, J.R., Provenzale, J.M.: MR perfusion imaging of the brain: techniques and applications. American Journal of Roentgenology, 207–219 (2000)
2. Constantin, A.A., Bajcsy, B.R., Nelson, C.S.: Unsupervised segmentation of brain tissue in multivariate MRI. In: 2010 IEEE International Symposium on Biomedical Imaging: From Nano to Macro, pp. 89–92. IEEE (2010)
3. Fletcher-Heath, L.M., Hall, L.O., Goldgof, D.B., Murtagh, F.R.: Automatic segmentation of non-enhancing brain tumors in magnetic resonance images. Artificial Intelligence in Medicine 21, 43–63 (2001)
4. Clark, M.C., Hall, L.O., Goldgof, D.B., Velthuizen, R., Murtagh, F.R., Silbiger, M.S.: Automatic tumor segmentation using knowledge-based techniques. IEEE Transactions on Medical Imaging 17, 187–201 (1998)
5. Prastawa, M., Bullitt, E., Ho, S., Gerig, G.: A brain tumor segmentation framework based on outlier detection. Medical Image Analysis 8, 275–283 (2004)
6. Corso, J.J., Sharon, E., Dube, S., El-Saden, S., Sinha, U., Yuille, A.: Efficient multilevel brain tumor segmentation with integrated bayesian model classification. IEEE Transactions on Medical Imaging 27, 629–640 (2008)
7. Shi, J.B., Malik, J.: Normalized cuts and image segmentation. IEEE Transactions on Pattern Analysis and Machine Intelligence 22, 888–905 (2000)
8. Achanta, R., Shaji, A., Smith, K., Lucchi, A., Fua, P., Susstrunk, S.: SLIC superpixels compared to state-of-the-art superpixel methods. IEEE Trans. Pattern Anal. Mach. Intell. 34, 2274–2282 (2012)
9. Lucchi, A., Smith, K., Achanta, R., Knott, G., Fua, P.: Supervoxel-based segmentation of mitochondria in EM image stacks with learned shape features. IEEE Trans. Med. Imaging 31, 474–486 (2012)

10. Smith, S.M., Jenkinson, M., Woolrich, M.W., Beckmann, C.F., Behrens, T., Johansen-Berg, H., Bannister, P.R., De Luca, M., Drobnjak, I., Flitney, D.E.: Advances in functional and structural MR image analysis and implementation as FSL. Neuroimage 23, 208 (2004)
11. Ng, A.Y., Jordan, M.I., Weiss, Y.: On spectral clustering: Analysis and an algorithm. In: Advances in Neural Information Processing Systems, pp. 849–856 (2001)
12. Von Luxburg, U.: A tutorial on spectral clustering. Statistics and Computing 17, 395–416 (2007)

# Mapping Dynamic Changes in Ventricular Volume onto Baseline Cortical Surfaces in Normal Aging, MCI, and Alzheimer's Disease

Sarah K. Madsen[1], Boris A. Gutman[1], Shantanu H. Joshi[2], Arthur W. Toga[1], Clifford R. Jack, Jr.[3], Michael W. Weiner[4,5], and Paul M. Thompson[1] for the Alzheimer's Disease Neuroimaging Initiative (ADNI)

[1] Imaging Genetics Center, Laboratory of Neuro Imaging, UCLA School of Medicine, Los Angeles, CA 90095, USA
[2] Laboratory of Neuro Imaging, UCLA School of Medicine, Los Angeles, CA 90095, USA
[3] Mayo Clinic, Rochester, MN, USA
[4] Departments of Radiology, Medicine, Psychiatry, UC San Francisco, San Francisco, CA, USA
[5] Department of Veterans Affairs Medical Center, San Francisco, CA, USA

**Abstract.** Ventricular volume (VV) is a powerful global indicator of brain tissue loss on MRI in normal aging and dementia. VV is used by radiologists in clinical practice and has one of the highest obtainable effect sizes for tracking brain change in clinical trials, but it is crucial to relate VV to structural alterations underlying clinical symptoms. Here we identify patterns of thinner cortical gray matter (GM) associated with dynamic changes in lateral VV at 1-year (N=677) and 2-year (N=536) intervals, in the ADNI cohort. People with faster VV loss had thinner baseline cortical GM in temporal, inferior frontal, inferior parietal, and occipital regions (controlling for age, sex, diagnosis). These findings show the patterns of relative cortical atrophy that predict later ventricular enlargement, further validating the use of ventricular segmentations as biomarkers. We may also infer specific patterns of regional cortical degeneration (and perhaps functional changes) that relate to VV expansion.

**Keywords:** imaging biomarkers, brain imaging, magnetic resonance imaging, quantitative image analysis, statistical analysis, temporal/longitudinal image series analysis.

# 1    Introduction

The lateral ventricles are a fluid-filled region within the brain that expands to fill space formerly occupied by degenerating brain tissue inside the fixed volume of the skull. Ventricular volume (VV) is a widely-used biomarker of Alzheimer's disease (AD) progression; it offers one of the highest effect sizes for tracking brain change over time, and for detecting disease effects, making it highly advantageous in clinical trials.

Clinically, VV is commonly used by radiologists to help diagnose neurodegeneration, more so than many of the more complex brain MRI measures analyzed in research. Even

L. Shen et al. (Eds.): MBIA 2013, LNCS 8159, pp. 84–94, 2013.
© Springer International Publishing Switzerland 2013

so, information is sorely needed on what VV changes imply in terms of alterations in regions underlying cognitive functions, such as the cortex. Cross-structure correlations linking changes in VV to differences in other brain tissues have been largely ignored in univariate analyses of single structures or maps.

Reductions in gray/white matter contrast with age make it challenging to detect longitudinal change in many brain structures - such as the hippocampus and cortex - usually requiring time-consuming manual edits even with the most widely-used segmentation packages. In contrast, the boundary demarcating the lateral ventricles (cerebrospinal fluid (CSF)/brain tissue) is easier to detect, making ventricular segmentation reliable and robust [1]. As brain atrophy progresses, changes in cortical structure become even more extreme, along with further reductions in contrast at the gray/white interface. Segmentation of cortical structures, which tend to have greater functional significance, becomes even more difficult in the aging population.

The lateral ventricles can be measured in brain MRI scans using several different techniques. VV [7], shape [2], and boundary shift integral [8] have been validated as highly sensitive biomarkers of AD and mild cognitive impairment (MCI), offering high classification accuracy and greater consistency than some cognitive tests [9], [10]. Longitudinal studies show that VV is a very sensitive biomarker of ongoing atrophy in elderly populations. In elderly non-demented adults, VV changes at a markedly faster rate (2.80-4.4% per year) than hippocampal volumes (0.68-0.84% per year) [7,8]. Changes in VV may be faster in MCI and early AD than in later AD or normal aging [5], but accumulated VV differences are most extreme in later stages of AD [2].

Prior methods for VV segmentation have used semi-automated, automated [4], and single-atlas or multi-atlas methods [5]. In this analysis, we segmented the ventricles with a modified multi-atlas approach. Our segmentation method makes use of group-wise surface registration of existing templates, and applies surface-based template blending for more accurate results [5]. For cortical segmentation, we use the standard FreeSurfer tools (v5.0.0) [6].

Most studies of VV have been univariate, looking at the ventricles alone as a single structure, which does not allow more detailed interpretations of how changes in VV relate to other brain regions. Two groups have related VV to shape and volume differences in periventricular brain structures (including the hippocampus) [12], [3]; however, as far as we know, ours is the first study to use VV to infer cortical brain structure differences. By inferring cortical alterations from ventricular changes, we can better interpret results of clinical trials that show a deceleration in the rate of VV loss.

## 2    Methods

### 2.1    Cohort Studied

We analyzed 677 individuals who had received a high-resolution, T1-weighted structural MRI brain scan as part of phase 1 of the Alzheimer's Disease Neuroimaging Initiative

(ADNI1) and whose scans passed quality control for both ventricular and cortical segmentations. Segmentations were assessed visually from multiple views for defects. All subjects passed quality control (QC) for ventricle segmentations and six subjects were excluded during QC of cortical GM surfaces.

ADNI is a multi-site, longitudinal study of patients with Alzheimer's disease (AD), individuals with mild cognitive impairment (MCI) and healthy elderly controls (HC). Standardized protocols maximize consistency across sites.

## 2.2    Scan Acquisition and Processing

For VV segmentation, we analyzed baseline, 1-year (N=677), and 2-year (N=536) follow-up brain MRI scans (1.5-Tesla, T1-weighted 3D MP-RAGE, TR/TE = 2400/1000 ms, flip angle = 8°, slice thickness = 1.2 mm, final voxel resolution = 0.9375 x 0.9375 x 1.2 mm$^3$). Raw MRI scans were pre-processed to reduce signal inhomogeneity and were linearly registered to a template (using 9 parameters).

For cortical GM segmentation, we analyzed 677 baseline brain MRI scans (1.5-Tesla, T1-weighted 3D MP-RAGE, TR/TE = 2400/1000 ms, flip angle = 8°, slice thickness = 1.2 mm, 24-cm field of view, a 192×192×166 acquisition matrix, final voxel resolution = 1.25×1.25×1.2 mm$^3$, later reconstructed to 1 mm isotropic voxels). To simplify the presentation, we did not perform cortical segmentation at later time points, as the baseline differences tend to reflect the overall level of atrophy, and to some extent they also reflect the rate of atrophy.

Bias field correction (N3) was applied as part of the standard ADNI dataset pre-processing before scans were downloaded. We used a registration with 9 parameters as it corrects for scanner voxel size variation and arguably outperforms 6 parameter registration in multi-site studies such as ADNI [13], [14]. Independent alignment procedures were used for the ventricles and for the cortex, as described below (**Sections 2.3 and 2.4**), using methods optimized for each structure.

## 2.3    Ventricular Segmentation

Ventricular segmentation was performed using a validated method [15]. Ventricular surfaces were extracted using an inverse-consistent fluid registration with a mutual information fidelity term to align a set of hand-labeled ventricular templates to each scan. The template surfaces were registered as a group following a medial-spherical registration method [15]. To improve upon the standard multi-atlas segmentation, which generally involves a direct, or a weighted average of the warped binary masks, we selected an individual template that best fits the new boundary at each boundary point. A naïve formulation of this synthesis can be written as below:

$$S(p) = \sum_i W^i(p)T_i(p), \quad W^i(p) = \begin{cases} 1 & if\ s(I,I_i)[p] > s(I,I_j)[p]\ \forall j \neq i \\ 0 & otherwise \end{cases} \quad (1)$$

Here, $I, S$ are the new image and boundary surface, $\{I_i, T_i\}_i$ are template surfaces and images warped to the new image, and $s(I,I_i)[p]$ is some local normalized similarity measure at point $p$. Normalized mutual information around a neighborhood of each point was used as similarity. This approach allows for more flexible segmentation, in particular for outlier cases. Even a weighted average, with a single weight applied to each individual template, often distorts geometric aspects of the boundary that are captured in only a few templates, perhaps only in one. However, to enforce smoothness of the resulting surface, care must be taken around the boundaries of the surface masks $W^i$. An effective approach is to smooth the masks with a spherical heat kernel, so that our final weights are $W_\sigma^i(q) = \int_{\mathbb{S}^2} K_\sigma(p,q)W^i(p)dp$.

## 2.4    Cortical Segmentation

Cortical reconstruction and volumetric segmentation were performed with the FreeSurfer (v5.0.0) image analysis suite, which is freely available online (http://surfer.nmr.mgh.harvard.edu/). Details of these procedures have been described previously [6]. Briefly, the processing includes removal of non-brain tissue, intensity normalization, tessellation of the cortical gray/white matter boundary, automated topology correction and surface deformation along intensity gradients to optimally define cortical surface borders, registration to a spherical atlas using individual cortical folding patterns to align cortical anatomy across individuals, and creation of 3D maps of GM (as measured with thickness, volume, and surface area) at each cortical surface point. After processing, images are in an isotropic space of 256 voxels along each axis (x, y, and z) with a final voxel size of 1 mm$^3$.

## 2.5    Statistical Analysis: Mapping Ventricular Change onto the Cortical Surface

Statistical tests were conducted at each point on the cortical surface separately for 1-year and 2-year change in VV after applying cortical smoothing (kernel radius=25 mm, full width at half maximum). We tested a series of general linear models (GLM) of change in VV on cortical GM thickness after: (1) controlling for effects of sex, age, and diagnosis (AD, MCI, or healthy elderly controls) in all individuals (1-year change: N=677; 2-year change: N=536), (2) controlling for sex and age in AD, MCI and control groups, separately (1-year: AD N=142, MCI N=335, Control N=200; 2-year: AD N=109, MCI N=251, Control N=176), and (3) controlling for sex and age in matched groups of N=100 AD, MCI and controls. Analyses were run separately for associations within each hemisphere (i.e., for change in left VV with left cortical GM thickness and for change in right VV with right cortical GM thickness). To control the rate of false positives, we enforced a standard false discovery rate (FDR) correction for multiple statistical comparisons across voxels in the entire left and right brain surfaces, using the conventionally accepted false positive rate of 5% ($q$=0.05) [16] .

## 2.6    *Post Hoc* Statistical Analysis: Linear Relationships between Regional Cortical Thickness and Ventricular Change

We identified clusters that passed FDR in the 3D cortical surface maps for the matched groups of N=100 AD, MCI, and controls for the GLM of 2-year change in

VV on cortical GM thickness after controlling for sex and age. Within each statistically significant cluster on the cortical surface, we calculated mean cortical GM thickness for each subject. We then plotted each subject's mean cortical GM thickness and raw 2-year change in VV for each group (AD, MCI, and controls for N=100), to understand the characteristics (i.e., magnitude and shape) of the significant associations we found in our surface GLM between the two measures.

## 3     Results

In the full sample, we found that (Figure 1) 1-year (N=677) and 2-year (N=536) changes in VV were significantly associated with baseline cortical GM thickness in temporal, inferior and anterior frontal, inferior parietal, and some occipital regions, after controlling for age, sex, and diagnosis. The significant regions were somewhat more expansive, in the same areas, for the 2-year change compared to the 1-year change in VV. If ventricular change is linear, these two maps should be the same, but the 2-year map may show more extensive or stronger associations because the 2-year measures have greater SNR. All results presented pass a hemispheric FDR correction at $q=0.05$.

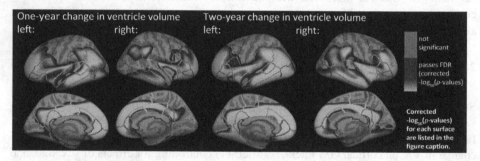

**Fig. 1.** Hemispheric 3D maps show significant negative associations in the entire sample between 1-year ($N=677$) and 2-year ($N=536$) change in VV and baseline cortical GM thickness in all individuals, after controlling for age, sex, and diagnosis (AD, MCI, or healthy elderly) (1-year change, *left*: $-\log_{10}(p\text{-values})=1.53\text{-}3.76$, right: $-\log_{10}(p\text{-values})=1.70\text{-}3.96$; 2-year change, left: $-\log_{10}(p\text{-values})=1.51\text{-}3.77$, right: $-\log_{10}(p\text{-values})=1.55\text{-}3.80$, corrected). Results are corrected for multiple comparisons by thresholding at a $q=0.05$ false discovery rate (FDR) threshold across the entire brain surface. Blue represents areas where $p$-values passed the corrected significance threshold for a negative relationship between progressive ventricular enlargement and baseline cortical thickness values (greater VV enlargement associated with lower cortical GM thickness at baseline).

Looking separately at diagnosis (Figure 2), 1-year and 2-year changes in VV were most strongly associated with baseline cortical GM thickness in MCI, with maps similar to those for the full cohort. In MCI, left inferior and anterior frontal, temporal, inferior parietal, and inferior occipital regions were significantly negatively associated with 1-year change in VV (left: $-\log_{10}(p\text{-values})=1.58\text{-}3.84$, right:

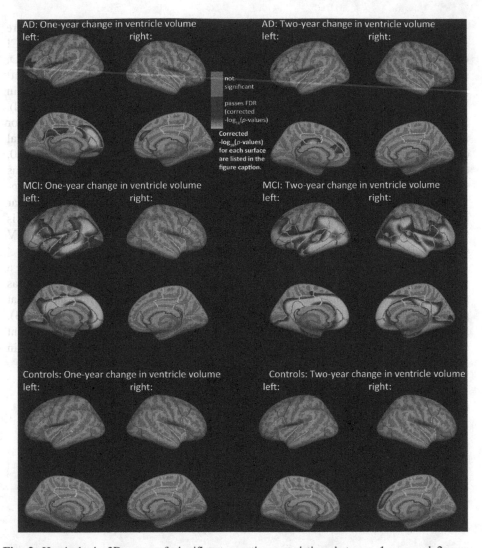

**Fig. 2.** Hemispheric 3D maps of significant negative associations between 1-year and 2-year change in VV and baseline cortical gray matter thickness in AD (1-year: N=142; 2-year N: 109), MCI (1-year: N=335; 2-year N: 251), and healthy elderly individuals (1-year: N=200; 2-year N: 176), after controlling for age and sex (AD: 1-year change, left: $-\log_{10}(p\text{-values})$=2.39-4.64, right: $-\log_{10}(p\text{-values})$=3.04-5.03, 2-year change, left: $-\log_{10}(p\text{-values})$=2.95-5.20, right: $-\log_{10}(p\text{-values})$=3.64-5.90; MCI: 1-year change, left: $-\log_{10}(p\text{-values})$=1.58-3.84, right: $-\log_{10}(p\text{-values})$=3.28-5.54, 2-year change, left: $-\log_{10}(p\text{-values})$=1.55-3.81, right: $-\log_{10}(p\text{-values})$=1.55-3.80; Controls: 1-year change, left: $-\log_{10}(p\text{-values})$=1.98-4.24, right: $-\log_{10}(p\text{-values})$=2.36-4.62, 2-year change, left: $-\log_{10}(p\text{-values})$=3.42-5.68, right: $-\log_{10}(p\text{-values})$=3.32-5.58, corrected). Results were corrected for multiple comparisons by thresholding at a $q$=0.05 false discovery rate (FDR) threshold across the entire brain surface. Blue represents areas where $p$-values passed the corrected significance threshold for a negative relationship between ventricular enlargement and cortical thickness values (greater VV enlargement associated with lower cortical GM thickness at baseline).

-$\log_{10}(p$-values)=3.28-5.54, corrected). Somewhat larger regions, bilaterally, were significantly negatively associated with 2-year change in ventricular volume in MCI (left: -$\log_{10}(p$-values)=1.55-3.81, right-$\log_{10}(p$-values)=1.55-3.80, corrected). In AD, significant negative associations were found in the bilateral superior frontal, left middle frontal, and left anterior and posterior cingulate cortex for 1-year change in VV (left: -$\log_{10}(p$-values)=2.39-4.64, right: -$\log_{10}(p$-values)=3.04-5.30, corrected). Significant negative associations for 2-year change in VV were found in left anterior and posterior cingulate cortex and small clusters in the left superior and middle frontal cortex for AD (left: -$\log_{10}(p$-values)=2.95-5.20, right: -$\log_{10}(p$-values)=3.64-5.90, corrected). In elderly controls, right superior frontal GM thickness at baseline was significantly negatively associated with 2-year change in VV (right: -$\log_{10}(p$-values)=3.32-5.582, corrected); no significant associations were detected for 1-year change, perhaps because SNR for tracking change is poorer when the interval is shorter, especially in this group which is expected to have slower rates of VV expansion.

In MCI, longitudinal changes in VV are associated with cortical GM thickness in a well-known pattern of areas vulnerable to AD pathology [17], [18], such as progressive accumulation of beta-amyloid that precedes cognitive decline and tau that parallels cognitive decline, as measured by F18-FDDNP PET brain scans (Figure 3). Primary sensorimotor areas that are spared in AD, which are also difficult to segment due to very thin GM and overabundance of myelin creating poor tissue contrast in MRI, were not significant in our maps.

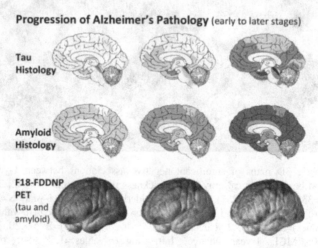

**Fig. 3.** Canonical progression of AD pathology (adapted from [17], [18]) as has been mapped previously in non-overlapping elderly samples. These patterns agree well with those seen in our cortical mapping of changes in VV, with significant associations in areas known to be susceptible to AD pathology and no detected relationship in areas that do not have a significant disease burden (primary sensorimotor cortex).

To examine if insufficient power contributed to differences in results for groups with smaller sample size, we re-analyzed subsets of N=100 matched by age and sex in the AD, MCI, and control groups at 1-year and 2-years. In the equally-sized subsets, 1-year change in VV was negatively associated with right superior frontal cortex thickness in AD (left: not significant, right: $-\log_{10}(p$-values$)=3.66$-$5.92$). No other significant results were found for 1-year change in VV for MCI or elderly controls with N=100. Two-year change in VV (Figure 4, top panel) was negatively associated with GM thickness in left posterior and rostral anterior cingulate, lateral orbitofrontal, and rostral middle frontal cortex in AD (left: $-\log_{10}(p$-values$)=2.15$-$4.41$, right: not significant) and left pars orbitalis, fusiform, the isthmus and posterior cingulate, and superior frontal cortex in MCI (left: $-\log_{10}(p$-values$)=2.15$-$4.41$, right: not significant). In elderly controls, 1-year change in VV was negatively associated with GM thickness in the right insula, superior frontal, precuneus, supramarginal, transverse temporal, inferior parietal, and isthmus of the cingulate cortex (left: not significant, right: $-\log_{10}(p$-values$)=2.28$-$4.54$).

After limiting the sample size of all groups to N=100 (the approximate size of the smallest group), the extent of significant regions appears roughly similar across groups, supporting the interpretation that the more prominent effects seen in the full-sized MCI sample (twice as large as the other groups) may be attributed to increased power rather than specific to this diagnostic category.

To better understand the characteristics of the relationship we found between VV and GM thickness in the surface GLMs (Figure 4, top panel), we plotted raw 2-year change in VV against mean GM thickness at baseline (averaged across all surface points within distinct statistically significant regions from the surface GLMs) in each subject from the N=100 subsets for AD, MCI, and CON (Figure 4, bottom panel). As expected, all plots show negative relationships (greater VV expansion over time is associated with thinner baseline GM). Plots for AD (top row of plots) and MCI (second and third rows of plots) show greater variance and higher rates of expansion in 2-year VV compared to healthy elderly controls (bottom two rows of plots) for all statistical regions of interest. The plots also show that elderly controls have higher baseline GM thickness in several regions compared to AD and MCI groups. Steeper slopes for the healthy elderly control group may be explained by greater variance in baseline GM thickness compared to AD and MCI groups.

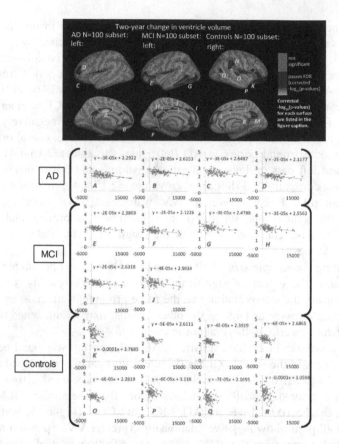

**Fig. 4.** *Top Panel:* Hemispheric 3D maps of significant negative associations between 2-year change in VV and cortical GM thickness in matched N=100 sub-samples for AD, MCI, and healthy elderly individuals, after controlling for age and sex (AD: 2-year change, left: $-\log_{10}(p\text{-}$ values$)$=2.58-4.84, right: not significant; MCI: 2-year change, left: $-\log_{10}(p\text{-}$values$)$=2.15-4.41, right: not significant; Controls: 2-year change, left: not significant, right: $-\log_{10}(p\text{-}$values$)$=2.28-4.54, corrected). Results are corrected for multiple comparisons by thresholding at a $q$=0.05 false discovery rate (FDR) threshold across the entire brain surface. Blue represents areas where $p$-values passed the corrected significance threshold for a negative relationship between ventricular enlargement and cortical thickness values (greater VV enlargement associated with lower cortical GM thickness at baseline).

*Bottom Panel:* Plots of 2-year VV change against mean baseline GM thickness (x-axis: raw 2-year VV change in mm$^3$, y-axis: mean baseline GM thickness for statistically significant regions in mm). Each data point represents one subject within the matched N=100 subsets for AD, MCI, and healthy elderly control groups (AD: first row, MCI: second and third rows, Controls: last two rows). Each plot represents a distinct and continuous cortical region that passed correction with FDR in the surface GLM maps shown in the top panel of this figure. Within each statistically significant cortical region, GM thickness was averaged across all significant surface vertices. Letters correspond to labels on the cortical surface maps in the top panel and are ordered first by group (AD: A-D; MCI: E-J, controls: K-R) and then by cortical region (from highest to lowest corrected p-value, all passed FDR in GLMs).

# 4    Discussion

Our results complement the current literature on change in ventricular enlargement as a robust clinical biomarker of disease progression in the early stages of AD. We also make a novel contribution to the field, which has largely ignored cross-structural correlations with VV, by showing how changes in VV relate to cortical GM thickness in normal aging and in varying stages of Alzheimer's dementia. These results allow us to make stronger inferences about functionally important areas of the cortex, based on ventricular segmentations.

The cortical regions significantly associated with dynamic changes in VV are among those that are regarded as most susceptible to AD-related pathologies in multiple domains, including accumulation of amyloid plaques and tau neurofibrillary tangles, metabolic disruption, functional and connectivity alterations, and structural GM loss. The lateralization of our findings (left in AD and MCI, right in controls) may not hold up in larger samples with higher statistical power. In equally-sized samples the extent of significant associations was similar across groups.

Ventricular measures on MRI are among the most reliable and robust, but have been previously limited as it has been hard to make inferences about specific alterations in cortical structure and their clinical or functional consequences. Cortical regions can be difficult to segment in elderly brains, so relating cortical changes to a highly reliable measure such as VV has great clinical advantages. Combining information from cortical architecture and ventricular enlargement may allow us to better understand factors affecting normal aging and different stages of neurodegeneration in disease. Future work will also apply the reverse approach, to map summary measures from the cortex (average and change in GM thickness in regions of interest) onto 3D ventricular shapes, to see which ventricular changes are most strongly associated with longitudinal changes in cortical thickness.

# References

1. Ferrarini, L., et al.: Ventricular shape biomarkers for Alzheimer's disease in clinical MR images. Magnetic Resonance in Medicine: Official Journal of the Society of Magnetic Resonance in Medicine 59(2), 260–267 (2008)
2. Apostolova, L.G., et al.: Hippocampal atrophy and ventricular enlargement in normal aging, mild cognitive impairment (MCI), and Alzheimer Disease. Alzheimer Disease and Associated Disorders 26(1), 17–27 (2012)
3. Qiu, A., et al.: Regional shape abnormalities in mild cognitive impairment and Alzheimer's disease. Neuroimage 45(3), 656–661 (2009)
4. Cardenas, V.A., et al.: Comparison of methods for measuring longitudinal brain change in cognitive impairment and dementia. Neurobiology of Aging 24(4), 537–544 (2003)
5. Nestor, S.M., et al.: Ventricular enlargement as a possible measure of Alzheimer's disease progression validated using the Alzheimer's Disease Neuroimaging Initiative database. Brain 131, 2443–2454 (2008)
6. Jack Jr., C.R., et al.: Comparison of different MRI brain atrophy rate measures with clinical disease progression in AD. Neurology 62(4), 591–600 (2004)

7. Fjell, A.M., et al.: One-year brain atrophy evident in healthy aging. The Journal of Neuroscience 29(48), 15223–15231 (2009)
8. Zhang, Y., et al.: Acceleration of hippocampal atrophy in a non-demented elderly population: the SNAC-K study. International Psychogeriatrics 22(1), 14–25 (2010)
9. Chou, Y.Y., et al.: Automated ventricular mapping with multi-atlas fluid image alignment reveals genetic effects in Alzheimer's disease. Neuroimage 40(2), 615–630 (2008)
10. Chou, Y.Y., et al.: Mapping correlations between ventricular expansion and CSF amyloid and tau biomarkers in 240 subjects with Alzheimer's disease, mild cognitive impairment and elderly controls. Neuroimage 46(2), 394–410 (2009)
11. Fischl, B., Dale, A.M.: Measuring the thickness of the human cerebral cortex from magnetic resonance images. PNAS 97(20), 11050–11055 (2000)
12. Ferrarini, L., et al.: Shape differences of the brain ventricles in Alzheimer's disease. Neuroimage 32(3), 1060–1069 (2006)
13. Hua, X., et al.: Optimizing power to track brain degeneration in Alzheimer's disease and mild cognitive impairment with tensor-based morphometry: An ADNI study of 515 subjects. Neuroimage 48(4), 668–681 (2009)
14. Paling, S.M., et al.: The application of serial MRI analysis techniques to the study of cerebral atrophy in late-onset dementia. Medical Image Analysis 8(1), 69–79 (2004)
15. Gutman, B.A., et al.: Shape matching with medial curves and 1-D group-wise registration. 2012 9th IEEE International Symposium on Biomedical Imaging, 716–719 (2012)
16. Benjamini, Y., Hochberg, Y.: Controlling the False Discovery Rate - a Practical and Powerful Approach to Multiple Testing. Journal of the Royal Statistical Society. Series B (Methodological) 57(1), 289–300 (1995)
17. Braak, H., Braak, E.: Neuropathological stageing of Alzheimer-related changes. Acta Neuropathologica 82(4), 239–259 (1991)
18. Braskie, M.N., et al.: Plaque and tangle imaging and cognition in normal aging and Alzheimer's disease. Neurobiology of Aging 31(10), 1669–1678 (2010)

# Unsupervised Fiber Bundles Registration Using Weighted Measures Geometric Demons

Viviana Siless[1,2], Sergio Medina[1,2], Pierre Fillard[1], and Bertrand Thirion[1,2]

[1] Parietal Team, Inria Saclay-Île-de-France, Saclay, France,
viviana.siless@inria.fr
http://parietal.saclay.inria.fr
[2] CEA, DSV, I²BM, Neurospin bât 145, 91191 Gif-Sur-Yvette, France

**Abstract.** Brain image registration aims at reducing anatomical variability across subjects to create a common space for group analysis. Multi-modal approaches intend to minimize cortex shape variations along with internal structures, such as fiber bundles. A difficulty is that it requires a prior identification of these structures, which remains a challenging task in the absence of a complete reference atlas. We propose an extension of the log-Geometric Demons for jointly registering images and fiber bundles without the need of point or fiber correspondences. By representing fiber bundles as Weighted Measures we can register subjects with different numbers of fiber bundles. The efficacy of our algorithm is demonstrated by registering simultaneously $T_1$ images and between 37 and 88 fiber bundles depending on each of the ten subject used. We compare results with a multi-modal $T_1$ + Fractional Anisotropy (FA) and a tensor-based registration algorithms and obtain superior performance with our approach.

**Keywords:** Registration, neural fibers, diffeomorphism, Demons Algorithm, multi-modal registration, image, geometry, log-domain.

## 1 Introduction

In medical image analysis, non-linear image registration intends to reduce anatomical variability across subjects in order to ease subsequent subjects or population comparisons. Over the last decades the availability of different image modalities has increased, bringing hope for more accurate registration procedures. $T_1$ weighted image ($T_1$ image in the sequel) registration is mainly driven by the contrast of the the grey matter and ventricles. In these images, the white matter appears uniform, giving no relevant information about its internal structures, which are composed of neural fibers connecting cortical areas. However Diffusion Tensor Imaging (DTI) can be used to reveal the microscopic structure of the white matter. Aligning white matter structures can help to increase the sensitivity of fMRI activation detection as shown in [1], and in [4] a group analysis on DWI was performed for early detection of schizophrenia. Tensor-based registration has recently been proposed to improve white matter alignment [14,13].

L. Shen et al. (Eds.): MBIA 2013, LNCS 8159, pp. 95–106, 2013.
© Springer International Publishing Switzerland 2013

Nevertheless, mis-registration may persist in regions where the tensor field appears uniform [5].

Multi-modal registration combines information from different image modalities to provide more anatomical details. For instance, the registration algorithm in [3] uses $T_1$ images and FA from DTI to better align grey and white matter. Geometric registration specifically targets the alignment of Structures of Interest (SOIs), such as in [12] for cortical surfaces, or [5] for fiber bundles. While those clearly improve SOI registration, they may not be suitable for aligning other structures than those used specifically during registration.

Hybrid techniques propose to jointly consider SOIs and images during registration. For instance, in [2,7] the mathematical framework of Measures and Currents respectively, were used to simultaneously register images and geometric descriptors such as sulcal lines or surfaces, while [9] proposed a Markovian solution to the same problem.

In the log-Geometric Demons with Currents (CGD) [8] an hybrid multi-modal registration of iconic and geometric descriptors has been proposed that uses Currents to model fibers but relies on a one-to-one fiber bundles correspondences across subjects. Correspondences across subjects are hard or even impossible to obtain. Individual fiber bundles show important differences in compactness, length and density. These characteristics might depend on the subject, tractography parameters and on the quality of the images. Furthermore, in some cases bundles may be cut, fused or absent in some subjects.

We propose to represent our geometric descriptors of fiber bundles as Weighted Measures to relax the hypothesis of explicit fiber correspondences across subjects. We define a flexible framework in which subjects can have different number of bundles, and no assumption is made about the bundle size.

The rest of the paper is organized as follows. First, we propose a mathematically sound extension of the log-Geometric Demons, the Weighted Measures Geometric Demons (WMGD), that relies on the log-domain daemons framework for computation purposes and handles geometric constraints as Weighted Measures. Then, we evaluate the WMGD $T1$ + bundles constraints registration on a dataset of 10 subjects and compare them with a tensor-based [13], and ANTS [3] a $T_1$ + FA multi-modal registration. We also study the sensitivity of the results with respect to the various parameters.

## 2    Weighted Measures Geometric Demons (WMGD)

WMGD is a multi-modal algorithm that jointly registers image and geometric descriptors. We shortly describe in Section 2.1 the $T_1$ diffeomorphic demons registration, for then explain in Section 2.2 the extension to the geometric registration and the modeling of our constraints as Weighted Measures.

### 2.1    Image Registration: The Diffeomorphic Demons

The goal of image registration is to find the displacement field $s$ that aligns as accurately as possible the corresponding structures from a moving image $M$, to the structures in the fixed image $F$. Ideally the displacement field $s$ minimizes a distance between the fixed and the moving image, while holding some properties such as being diffeomorphic.

In the Demons framework[10] a correspondence field $c$ was introduced to make the minimization of the functional energy tractable: $E(c,s) = \frac{1}{\sigma_i^2}\text{Sim}(F, M \circ c) + \frac{1}{\sigma_x^2}\text{dist}(s,c)^2 + \frac{1}{\sigma_T^2}\text{Reg}(s)$, where Sim is a similarity measure between images defined by the sum of square differences (SSD) and $\text{Reg}(s)$ a regularization term chosen to be the harmonic energy $\|\nabla s\|^2$. The amount of regularization is controlled with $\sigma_T$ while $\sigma_i$ accounts for the image noise.

The term $\text{dist}(s,c)^2$ imposes the displacement field $s$ to be close to the correspondence field $c$. And $\sigma_x$ weights the spatial uncertainty on the deformation. The energy minimization is performed by alternating minimization w.r.t. $c$ and $s$. In [11], small deformations are parametrized by a dense displacement field $u$: $c \leftarrow s \circ \exp(u)$, $\exp()$ being the exponential map in the Lie group sense, which ensures that the result is diffeomorphic. In the log-domain demons $s$ is encoded with the exponential map as $s = \exp(v)$ and the inverse of $s$ can be easily computed as $s^{-1} = exp(-v)$; then $dist(s,c) = \|log(s^{-1} \circ c)\|$ and $\text{Reg}(s) = \|\nabla log(s)\|^2$ where $log = \exp^{-1}$.

## 2.2  $T_1+$ Geometric Registration

We build on the extension of the Demons framework proposed in [8], that includes geometric descriptors into the variational formulation. The definition of $c$ carries information coming from both image and geometry. Let $\mathcal{G}^F$ be the fixed geometric descriptors and $\mathcal{G}^M$ the moving one, we aim at minimizing the following energy:

$$E(c,s) = \frac{1}{\sigma_i^2}\left[\text{Sim}_I(F, M \circ c) + \text{Sim}_G(c \star \mathcal{G}^F, \mathcal{G}^M)\right] +$$
$$\frac{1}{\sigma_x^2}\text{dist}(s,c)^2 + \frac{1}{\sigma_T}\text{Reg}(s), \tag{1}$$

where $\text{Sim}_I$ is the image similarity criterion, $\text{Sim}_G$ the geometric similarity criterion, and $c \star \mathcal{G}^F$ denotes the action of $c$ on the geometry. Then $c$ is parametrized by an update field of image and geometry which is described at the end of this section. Note that $s$ goes from $F$ to $M$, thus the inverse of $s$ gives the geometric deformation.

## 2.3  Fiber Bundles Representation

In the Currents GD fiber bundles were represented in the space of currents as it provides a pose and shape-sensitive measure, independent of the number of fibers per bundle. The main issue with this metric is the need for corresponding bundles, hence requiring prior identification. Currents could in theory be used to represent a set of geometric objects without explicit correspondences, but they require an orientation to be chosen for each fiber: given a curve $L$ and a sequence of points $L = x_1, ..., x_n$ a current is defined as $\sum_i \tau_i \delta_{c_i}$, where $c_i = \frac{x_i + x_{i+1}}{2}$, $\tau_i = x_i - x_{i+1}$, in other words, a set of positions and tangent vectors. A current can thus be seen as a sum of oriented segments. Therefore it is important to find a consistent orientation, otherwise the same fiber with the opposite orientation cannot be registered properly. It is extremely hard to find a consistent orientation on a large number of one-dimensional objects in 3D without a prior segmentation and labeling in each subject. As subject variability is high and –in the absence of complete fiber atlas– correspondence mistakes can lead to poor solutions, we propose to relax this hypothesis and represent the geometry using Weighted Measures.

## 2.4   Compression of the Tractography Output

Depending on the resolution of the diffusion images the number of fibers can go from few thousands to few millions, generally leading to high computational cost. For this reason we want to reduce the fibers to a set of few representatives, and give these representatives a weight corresponding to the number of fibers that they represent. For registration purposes we need bundles to be highly homogeneous so that each representative summarizes the bundle accurately. To obtain low variance bundles we require many of them (typically 500) among which the small ones are considered as outliers and discarded.

For registration we take the largest (i.e. more than 50 fibers) and the longest ones (i.e. more than 50mm) as we believe they can better lead the alignment of the white matter. Ideally this yields to 50-100 fiber bundles. Large bundles have higher probability of being well defined, hence detected across subjects. Short fibers, specifically U-shape fibers are accumulated around the cortex and it is hard to distinguish one from the others because of their resemblance on position and shape. In consequence, they can easily mislead the registration close to the cortical foldings.

## 2.5   Weighted Measures

Having a set of bundles from the fixed fibers $C^F$ (and moving $C^M$), we define the set of points in $\mathcal{G}^F$ as $x_{i,j}, i \in [1..|C^F|], j \in [1..|C_i^F|]$, where $x_{i,j}$ the j-th point of the representative from the i-th bundle in $C^F$. We can associate with this sequence a specific measure as a sum of weighted Dirac Measures: $\mu_{\mathcal{G}}^F = \sum_{i=1}^{|C^F|} \sum_{j=1}^{|C_i^F|} w_{i,j} \delta_{x_i}$ where $w_{i,j} = \frac{|C_i^F|}{\sum_{i=0}^{|C^F|} |C_i^F|}$, which weights measures according to the number of fibers that the bundle of $C_i^F$ represents. From now on, to simplify notations, we refer to points from the geometry in $\mathcal{G}^F$ as $x_i$ and to points from $\mathcal{G}^M$ as $y_i$, and we assume that $w_i^x$ (resp. $w_i^y$) is the weight of the $x_i$ (resp. $y_i$) given by the corresponding bundle size. We define the geometry in the fixed subject as $\mathcal{G}^F = \sum_{i=0}^{N} w_i^x \delta_{x_i}$ and for the moving subject as $\mathcal{G}^M = \sum_{j=0}^{M} w_j^y \delta_{y_j}$.

Let $\mathcal{G}^F = (x_1, ..., x_N)$ and $\mathcal{G}^M = (y_1, ..., y_M)$ be the fixed and a moving geometric descriptor and $N, M$ being the number of objects. Let $K_\beta$ be a Gaussian kernel of size $\beta$. Then the scalar product between two sums of Weighed Measures can be expressed conveniently with a pre-defined kernel $K_\beta$:

$$\langle \mathcal{G}^F, \mathcal{G}^M \rangle_\beta = \langle \sum_{i=1}^{N} w_i^x \delta_{x_i}, \sum_{j=1}^{M} w_j^y \delta_{y_j} \rangle_\beta = \sum_{i=1}^{N} \sum_{j=1}^{M} K_\beta(x_i, y_j) w_i^x . w_j^y \quad (2)$$

Then the distance between Weighted Measures is defined as follows:

$$d_\beta^2(\mathcal{G}^F, \mathcal{G}^M) = ||\mathcal{G}^F||^2 + ||\mathcal{G}^M||^2 - 2\langle \mathcal{G}^F, \mathcal{G}^M \rangle_\beta \quad (3)$$

The distance captures misalignment and shape dissimilarities at the resolution $\beta$. Distances much larger than $\beta$ do not influence the metric, while smaller ones are considered as noise and thanks to the smoothing effect of the kernel they are not taken into account.

Given the current deformation $s$, we define the action of the correspondence field $c$ on $\mathcal{G}$ as: $c \star \mathcal{G} = \{s \circ \exp(u_G)(x_i)\}_{i \in [1,N]} \approx s(x_i) + u_G(s(x_i))\}_{i \in [1,N]}$.

Since we deal with a discrete set of points, we choose to parametrize the dense update field $u_G$ by a finite set of vectors $u_{G,i}$ using radial basis function extrapolation: $u_G(x) = \sum_{i=1}^{N} h(||x - x_i||)\lambda_i$, where $h(x) = e^{-\frac{x^2}{\gamma^2}}$, $\lambda_i$ are the interpolation coefficients and $\gamma > 0$ is the interpolation scale. $\lambda_i$ are calculated such that $u_G(x_i) = u_{G,i} \forall i$. Let us define the matrix $A$ such that $[A]_{i,j} = h(||x_i - x_j||)$ ($[A]_{i,j}$ denotes the $(i,j)$ entry of $A$), $\Lambda = [\lambda_1, ..., \lambda_N]$ the vector of $\lambda$s, $H(x)$ the vector such that $[H(x)]_i = h(||x - x_i||)$ and $U = [u_{G,1}, ..., u_{G,N}]$. We can write: $u_G(x) = H(x)A^{-1}U$. Minimizing $\nabla E_G(s, u_G) = 0$ w.r.t. $u_G$ via gradient descent yields to the following update field equation:

$$u_{G,i} = -\epsilon[-\frac{2}{\beta^2} \sum_{l=0}^{N} w_l^x w_i^x K_\beta(s(x_i), s(x_l))(s(x_i) - s(x_l))$$

$$+ \frac{2}{\beta^2} \sum_{j=0}^{M} w_i^x w_j^y K_\beta(s(x_i), y_j)(s(x_i) - y_j)], \quad (4)$$

where $\epsilon \in [0, 1]$, and $\gamma \in [1, 4]$mm.

Finally, a new update field is defined by the additive combination of the image update field $u_I$ described in [11], and the geometric update field $u_G$ in eq. (4): $u = u_I + u_G$. The algorithm follows as in [11] where a regularization is applied and the transformation $s$ is updated. In [8] non-intersecting domains where assumed between the image and the geometry of the fibers. However, this contradicts the minimization procedure, thus we do not use such a splitting here.

## 3    Joint $T_1$ MRI and Brain Bundle Registration

In this section we describe the experiments of the extended joint $T_1$ MRI and brain fibers bundles registration. We first analyse the behaviour of the method itself, and we later compare it against other methods.

## 3.1  Data Description

We used ten healthy volunteers from the Imagen database scanned with a 3T Siemens Tim Trio scanner. Acquisitions were MPRAGE for $T_1$ weighted ( $240 \times 256 \times 160, 1.09375 \times 1.09375 \times 1.1mm^3$) and DW-MRI ($128 \times 128 \times 60, 2.4 \times 2.4 \times 2.4mm^3$) with TR $=$ 15000 ms, TE $=$ 104 ms, flip angle $= 90^o$, 36 gradient directions, and b-value $= 1300s/mm^2$.

For each subject we obtained the linear transformation from the non-weighted image $B = 0$ to $T_1$ to align bundles with $T_1$ images. Eddy currents correction were applied to DTI data, and skull and neck were removed from $T_1$ images using the FSL software.

We used MedInria for fiber tractography, and splines to extrapolate for uniformly distributed points. Fibers shorter than $50mm$ were discarded in order to discard U-shape fibers. Within U-shape brain fibers variability is high and mismatch across subjects can be easily introduced during registration. We rather trust the image for those regions around the cortex.

As discussed in section 2.4 we are not interested in using the whole fiber tracktography output, but rather the bundles representatives. We use QuickBundles algorithm [6] to obtain a clustering of the fibers, and used the representatives given by the algorithm for registration. The threshold value for the bundles spread width was set to $10mm$, which gives a trade-off between low cluster variability and number of fibers per cluster. This yielded an average of 600 bundles per subject (range: $[323, 927]$), where a bundle contains at least one fiber. Selecting bundles with more than 50 fibers leads to an average of 63 bundles (range: $[37, 88]$). In the sequel we refer to this subset as the Training Set, and bundles with less than 50 fibers as the Test Set.

Before registering with WMGD we apply a $T_1$ affine transformation using the MedInria software to take subjects to the target space, and apply the inverse to the fibers.

After running WMGD we obtained a deformation field that we applied to the moving $T_1$ and the inverse of the deformation to the fibers.

The rest of this section explains the experiments performed. To assess the sensitivity to parameters we arbitrary choose a subject as target to register the rest of the dataset. Then, for performance comparison with other algorithms, we register the subjects to one another, and average the pairwise distances.

## 3.2  Weighted Measures Kernel Size

To analyze the impact the $\beta$ parameter we register the whole dataset to an arbitrary subject chosen as target by using the Training Set of bundles. Typically large kernels would be able to capture large misalignment and handle details as noise.

We run Weighted Measures Geometric Demons with the following parameters fixed $\epsilon = 0.3, \gamma = 3mm, \sigma_T = 2, \sigma_i = 1, \sigma_x = 1$ with a 3-steps multi-scale approach with $15, 10$ and $5$ iterations at each scale (from small to large).

We vary $\beta$ from 0 to 30mm and show results in Figure 1 for fibers (a) and for image (b). However, we believe that decreasing $\beta$ through iterations might avoid local minima for fiber registration and improve the accuracy of image registration. We decrease it 0.5% at each iteration and results are shown in Figure 1 for fibers (c) and for image (d).

### 3.3   Regularization

To analyze the smoothness of the deformation field, we run experiments with values of $\sigma_T$ varying from 0 to 3.0 and analyze the impact over the results. Analogous to Section 3.2 we register the dataset to an arbitrary subject chosen as target, and we use the Training Set of fibers for registration. We use the same parameter setting with $\beta = 20mm$. In Figure 2 results are shown for fibers (a), image (b) and the regularization term (c).

### 3.4   Performance Comparison

We conducted a cross-validation experiment by performing registration on the Training Set, and validating results over the Test Set (bundles left out for containing less than 50 fibers). To validate the robustness of the results we register subjects dataset to one another and plot the average pairwise distance.

We run Weighted Measures Geometric Demons with the following parameters $\epsilon = 0.3, \gamma = 3mm, \beta = 10mm, \sigma_T = 2, \sigma_i = 1, \sigma_x = 1$. $\beta$ was decreased by 0.5% at each iteration of the algorithm. Symmetric Tensor Demons (STD) was run with its defaults parameters. For ANTS we used recommended parameters from documentation except for the weight of $T_1$ and $FA$ where different combinations were tested. We finally show results with both equal to 1, which we found to be a fair trade-off. Each algorithm was tested on the 3-steps multi-scale approach with $15, 10$ and 5 iterations at each scale (from small to large).

We recall that for WMGD we first apply a $T_1$ affine transformation using the MedInria software to take subjects to the target space, and apply the inverse to the fibers. After running WMGD we obtained a deformation field that we applied to the moving $T_1$ and the inverse of the deformation to the fibers. We compare our results to those of ANTS, a multi-modal image registration combining $T_1$ image and FA, and Symmetric Tensor Demons, a tensor-based registration algorithm. Before running ANTS, corresponding FA and $T_1$ were aligned using a linear transformation. The resulting affine transformation and deformation field were applied to the moving $T_1$ image, and their inverse to the fibers. For tensor-based registration, tensor images were taken to the target $T_1$ space using an affine transformation for the moving subjects, but preserving original resolution. The resulting deformation field was up-sampled to the $T_1$ resolution for application to the image and then inverted for application to the geometry.

## 4   Results and Discussion

### 4.1   Weighted Measure: $\beta$ Value

As expected, Figure 1 shows that higher $\beta$ values give better scores for fiber registration, while loosing accuracy on the image registration. Each curve in

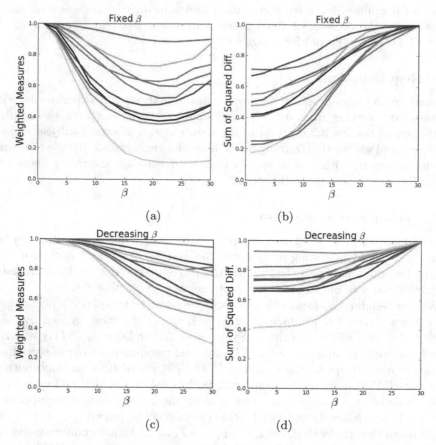

(a)                                        (b)

(c)                                        (d)

**Fig. 1.** Registration of the dataset to an arbitrary subject chosen as target. Each curve encodes one subject registration to the target. $\beta$ varies in the x-axis. Figures (a) and (b) show the metric for fiber and image respectively at each $\beta$ value fixed through iterations. Figures (c) and (d) show respectively the metric for fibers and image at each initial value of $\beta$, and with a 0.5% decrease at each iteration. Curves were normalized by their maximal value.

Figure 1 has been normalized by its maximum value in order to analyze the impact of the parameter in each subject. However minimum values across figures are not comparable as they depend on the maximum value achieved. When defining a fixed $\beta$ though the iteration we quickly lose accuracy for the image registration. When decreasing iteratively $\beta$, we can see that with an initial values between 10 and 15, we improve fiber alignment while still holding the image one.

## 4.2   Regularization

In Figure 2 we see that as we increase the regularization, the image accuracy decreases. However, low regularization will result in sharp deformations, which

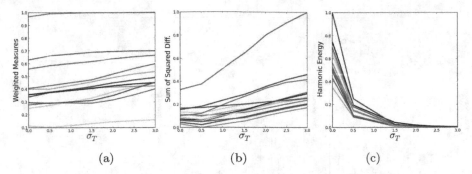

**Fig. 2.** Registration of the dataset to an arbitrary chosen as target with varying $\sigma_T$. Each curve encodes one subject registration to the target. Weighted Measures metric is shown in (a) for increasing $\sigma_T$, Sum of Squared Diff. of the image in (b) and in (c) we show the harmonic energy results. Curves were scaled using min-max normalization.

are often undesirable for the purposes of registration. As for the fiber accuracy we find the impact is low, nevertheless, a fair compromise with the harmonic energy can be found for $\sigma_T$ between 1.5 and 2. The difference of regularization impact over the image and the fibers are related to the resolution differences.

### 4.3   Performance Comparison

The aim of WMGD is to align $T_1$ images and neural fibers simultaneously by only using a set of bundles that represent well the white matter structure. We compare our results to a tensor-based registration (Symmetric Tensor Demons) and a multi-modal registration of $T_1 + $ FA (ANTS).

Average results for registering the individual datasets to each other are shown in Fig. 3 for training set (a), test set (b) and image (c). The WMGD method outperforms the others on the bundles used in the registration as shown in (a), which is expected, given that the minimized energy considered those specific bundles. For a fair comparison we tested our metric on the remaining bundles; the corresponding results are shown in (b). For the left aside bundles, results are similar but generally improved by our method. These results suggest that a sparse bundle selection according to their importance can be sufficient and that there is no need to require datasets to have the same number of bundles. Last, in (c) we compare the methods with respect to image registration accuracy. It is important to mention that diffusion images had a lower resolution than the $T_1$ images, giving advantage to ANTS and our algorithm in accuracy. WMGD yields better performance than ANTS, proving that improvements on bundles registration was not obtained at the expense of image accuracy.

In Fig. 4 we can see the result of registering the dataset to an arbitrary chosen as target. In (d) we see the fibers even before applying an affine registration, and in (g) we can see some improvements with respect to (e) and (f) regarding the borders of the image, and a better alignment of the corpus callosum.

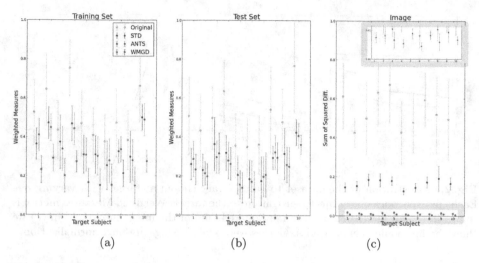

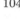

(a)    (b)    (c)

**Fig. 3.** Registration of the dataset to each subject. STD, ANTS, and WMGD show the average accuracy of the registration to each subject for the corresponding method. Original corresponds to the original distances between the dataset and the chosen target subject. Values were scaled using min-max normalization.

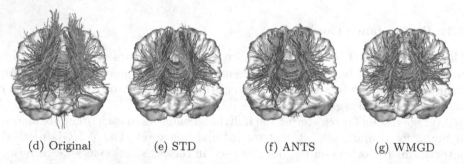

(d) Original    (e) STD    (f) ANTS    (g) WMGD

**Fig. 4.** Overlapping of fiber bundle representatives from all subjects registered to an arbitrary one chosen as target. Colors encode the different subjects. Behind we see the 3D $T_1$ image of the target subject.

We time all algorithms with an Intel Xeon 8proc. 2.53GHz, 11.8Gb and obtained: STD=5.11min, Ants=29.43min, WMGD=44.0min.

## 5    Conclusion

We presented a novel approach of hybrid multi-modal registration based on $T_1$ images and representative fiber bundles. Our algorithm does not require to have the same number of fiber bundles per subject, neither does it require them to be oriented, which makes it usable in much more general and realistic situations than previous approaches.

We have compared our algorithm to other well-known available registration algorithms with different modalities ($T_1$ + FA and Tensors) to show the benefits of using geometric descriptors. We obtain very good results for training fiber bundles, and improvements on test fibers and image alignment can be seen.

We also show that using fiber bundles instead of tensor information or FA adds relevant features, which amounts to include some priors: Tractography algorithms have to deal with uncertain regions on DTI images and use prior knowledge to overcome this difficulties. We strongly believe that this information should not be discarded. Also, keeping only long fibers introduces prior knowledge into the registration process.

Future extensions of the present work could include a joint labeling/registration framework. One can expect that including fiber classification across the iterations of the registration will improve accuracy and also give relevant information for posterior analyses of groups of subjects.

In addition, the high performance of the algorithm makes it worthwhile for validating results on diseases where the white matter is degenerated.

Since neural fibers contains information about connected regions, we also conjecture that this methodology will increase sensitivity in fMRI activation detection experiments.

**Acknowledgments.** This work was supported by ANR grant (ANR-10-BLAN-0128). The data were acquired within the Imagen project.

# References

1. Ardekani, B.A., Bachman, A.H., Strother, S.C., Fujibayashi, Y., Yonekura, Y.: Impact of inter-subject image registration on group analysis of fmri data. ICS 1265, 49–59 (2004)
2. Auzias, G., Colliot, O., Glaunes, J., Perrot, M., Mangin, J.F., Trouve, A., Baillet, S.: Diffeomorphic brain registration under exhaustive sulcal constraints. IEEE Trans. Med. Imaging (2011)
3. Avants, B.B., Tustison, N.J., Song, G., Cook, P.A., Klein, A., Gee, J.C.: A reproducible evaluation of ants similarity metric performance in brain image registration. NeuroImage 54(3), 2033–2044 (2011)
4. DeLisi, L.E., Szulc, K.U., Bertisch, H., Majcher, M., Brown, K., Bappal, A., Branch, C.A., Ardekani, B.A.: Early detection of schizophrenia by diffusion weighted imaging. Psychiatry Research: Neuroimaging 148(1), 61–66 (2006)
5. Durrleman, S., Fillard, P., Pennec, X., Trouvé, A., Ayache, N.: Registration, atlas estimation and variability analysis of white matter fiber bundles modeled as currents. NeuroImage 55(3), 1073–1090 (2011)
6. Garyfallidis, E., Brett, M., Correia, M.M., Williams, G.B., Nimmo-Smith, I.: Quickbundles, a method for tractography simplification. Frontiers in Neuroscience 6(175) (2012)
7. Ha, L., Prastawa, M., Gerig, G., Gilmore, J.H., Silva, C.T., Joshi, S.: Image registration driven by combined probabilistic and geometric descriptors. In: Jiang, T., Navab, N., Pluim, J.P.W., Viergever, M.A. (eds.) MICCAI 2010, Part II. LNCS, vol. 6362, pp. 602–609. Springer, Heidelberg (2010)

8. Siless, V., Glaunès, J., Guevara, P., Mangin, J.-F., Poupon, C., Le Bihan, D., Thirion, B., Fillard, P.: Joint T1 and brain fiber log-demons registration using currents to model geometry. In: Ayache, N., Delingette, H., Golland, P., Mori, K. (eds.) MICCAI 2012, Part II. LNCS, vol. 7511, pp. 57–65. Springer, Heidelberg (2012)

9. Sotiras, A., Ou, Y., Glocker, B., Davatzikos, C., Paragios, N.: Simultaneous geometric - iconic registration. In: Jiang, T., Navab, N., Pluim, J.P.W., Viergever, M.A. (eds.) MICCAI 2010, Part II. LNCS, vol. 6362, pp. 676–683. Springer, Heidelberg (2010)

10. Thirion, J.P.: Image matching as a diffusion process: an analogy with Maxwell's demons. Medical Image Analysis 2(3), 243–260 (1998)

11. Vercauteren, T., Pennec, X., Perchant, A., Ayache, N.: Symmetric Log-Domain Diffeomorphic Registration: A Demons-Based Approach. In: Metaxas, D., Axel, L., Fichtinger, G., Székely, G. (eds.) MICCAI 2008, Part I. LNCS, vol. 5241, pp. 754–761. Springer, Heidelberg (2008)

12. Yeo, B., Sabuncu, M., Vercauteren, T., Ayache, N., Fischl, B., Golland, P.: Spherical demons: Fast diffeomorphic landmark-free surface registration. IEEE Trans. Med. Imaging 29(3), 650–668 (2010)

13. Yeo, B., Vercauteren, T., Fillard, P., Peyrat, J.M., Pennec, X., Golland, P., Ayache, N., Clatz, O.: Dt-refind: Diffusion tensor registration with exact finite-strain differential. IEEE Trans. Med. Imaging 28(12), 1914–1928 (2009)

14. Zhang, H., Yushkevich, P.A., Alexander, D.C., Gee, J.C.: Deformable registration of diffusion tensor mr images with explicit orientation optimization. Medical Image Analysis 10(5), 764–785 (2006)

# Classification Forests and Markov Random Field to Segment Chronic Ischemic Infarcts from Multimodal MRI*

Jhimli Mitra[1], Pierrick Bourgeat[1], Jurgen Fripp[1], Soumya Ghose[1],
Stephen Rose[1], Olivier Salvado[1], Alan Connelly[2], Bruce Campbell[3],
Susan Palmer[2], Gagan Sharma[3], Soren Christensen[3], and Leeanne Carey[2]

[1] Australian e-Health Research Centre, CSIRO, Australia
[2] The Florey Institute of Neuroscience and Mental Health, Australia
[3] Royal Melbourne Hospital, Australia
www.START.csiro.au

**Abstract.** Accurate identification of ischemic lesions and brain atrophy is critical in the management of stroke patients and may serve as an important biomarker in studying post-stroke depression. In this paper we present an automated method to identify chronic ischemic infarcts in gray matter and gray/white matter partial volume areas that may be used to measure the amount of tissue loss due to atrophy in the area. The measure of tissue loss may then be used as a potential biomarker in analyzing the relation between stroke and post-stroke depression. The automated segmentation method relies on Markov random field (MRF) and random forest based classifications. The MRF classification identifies the possible lesion areas from the fluid attenuated inversion recovery (FLAIR) magnetic resonance (MR) images. Thereafter, the multimodal (T1-, T2-weighted, FLAIR, and apparent diffusion coefficient (ADC)) MR images of the possible lesion areas are fed into the classification forests along with other context-aware features and probability maps of the gray and white matter regions. The results of classification from the MRF and the classification forests are finally combined using connected component analysis to identify the final lesion area. The accuracy of the method in identifying infarcted regions from multimodal MR images has been validated on 17 patient datasets with a mean accuracy of 99%, a mean positive predictive value (PPV) of 75% and a mean negative predictive value (NPV) of 99% and a volume correlation of $r = 0.98$.

**Keywords:** Ischemic lesion segmentation, classification forest, MRF, MRI.

## 1 Introduction

The magnetic resonance imaging (MRI) parameters within an ischemic lesion are time dependent and are heterogeneous; i.e., they vary between acute (less than

---

\* The START Research Team.

L. Shen et al. (Eds.): MBIA 2013, LNCS 8159, pp. 107–118, 2013.

7 days) and chronic (3 months) stages. Therefore, it is unlikely that a single MR parameter can characterize the complexity of the cerebral tissue [1]. In clinical practice, diffusion-, T1-, T2-weighted (DWI, T1W, T2W) and fluid attenuated inversion recovery (FLAIR) images are acquired during the progression of stroke. Chronic ischemic lesions appear as hyperintense regions in FLAIR with heterogeneities around the lesions. In comparison, in T1W images the ischemic lesion intensities are hypointense compared to the normal tissue areas.

The fate of some cells in the ischemic area is normally death at the chronic stage while others are salvageable early. The dead cells are usually removed in the process of phagocytosis by the macrophages [2]. These areas are in turn filled with the cerebrospinal fluid (CSF). Figure 1(a) shows a stroke lesion at the chronic stage where parts within the stroke are filled with CSF and hence are hypointense compared to the remaining lesion. Therefore, the CSF areas around the ischemic lesions are usually enlarged compared to the normal part of the cortex. Measuring the CSF volume difference between the ipsilesional volume-of-interest (VOI) around the ischemic area and the contralesional VOI would provide an estimate of the tissue lost due to stroke. The measure of tissue loss associated with the index stroke, as well evidence of atrophy in putative depression regions may be used as a useful biomarker in the study of post-stroke depression [3]. In most cases, ischemic strokes appear in partial volume areas between the gray matter (GM) and the white matter (WM). Therefore, the macrophagic action and hence, filling of CSF is mostly observed in these areas. Although, CSF filling can also occur for pure WM strokes, in this paper we have limited our automatic detection method to the GM areas and considered the WM strokes only if they are connected to the GM strokes. This is beacuse detection of pure WM strokes in FLAIR images becomes extremely difficult in the presence of WM diseases or hyperintensities around the peri-ventricular regions [4], especially when WM strokes have an increased tendency to fuse with the periventricular region WM hyperintensities. Therefore, DWI images of the acute/sub-acute stages are necessary to isolate the stroke area from other areas of WM hyperintensities. Figure 1(b) shows a stroke region and other similar hyperintensities on a FLAIR image. In the available literature, ischemic lesion detection at the acute and sub-acute stages is predominant, rather than detection at the chronic stage. Dastidar et al. [5] proposed a semi-automatic method for segmenting ischemic lesions at the sub-acute stage from T1W and T2W MRI. The method involved amplitude segmentation of intensity histograms followed by region growing and decision trees [6], but required extensive manual intervention at each step to refine the segmentation. High correlation was reported between the extracted lesion volumes using this method and that by an expert. Jacobs et al. [7] applied the ISODATA (Iterative Self-organizing Data) algorithm [8] on integrated images comprising of T1W, T2W and DWI MR images to segment ischemic lesions at 3 time-points. The lesion volume extracted by the automated method showed high correlation with either the T2W or DWI volume across different time-points. Kabir et al. [9] suggested an automatic segmentation method based on MRF from multimodal MRI images comprising of DWI, T2W and FLAIR. The primary objective of the

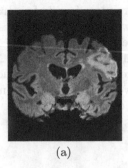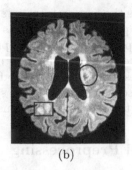

(a)                                    (b)

**Fig. 1.** Intensity heterogeneities in stroke lesions at the chronic stage and white matter hyperintensities in FLAIR. (a) Heterogenous intensities inside chronic stage stroke lesion due to CSF filling. The light red mask denotes the entire stroke area as marked by an expert, (b) anomalous FLAIR hyperintensities. The circular region in the image depicts a stroke region while the square area contains other white matter hyperintensities.

method was to categorize the stroke sub-types at the acute, sub-acute and later stages by registering with the blood supply territories atlas, therefore no quantitative results were presented related to the accuracy of the stroke detection. Mean-shift procedure on edge-confidence maps was proposed by Hevia-Montiel et al. [10] with subsequent region adjacency analysis and pruning to segment acute ischemic lesions from DWI images. The method showed a high average volume correlation with a high variance when compared to the manually segmented lesion volumes. Shen et al. [11] used extended fuzzy C-means to include the prior GM, WM, and CSF probability maps in the objective function. Finally Bray Curtis distance [12] between the fuzzy membership and prior probability of each voxel was used to isolate lesions from normal voxels. Qualitative results on T1W images showed good agreement of the method with an expert observation.

The methods in the literature show good accuracy in terms of volume correlation and visual agreement, although some methods required manual intervention and some required threshold values to be set at some stages. Most of the available methods deal with DWI images of the acute stage showing hyperintense stroke regions and can be easily targeted to isolate the ischemic stroke from other brain diseases. It appears that the methods in the literature also do not deal with the challenges of ischemic stroke segmentation in the presence of WM hyperintensities in FLAIR. We have designed our automated segmentation method, motivated by some of the works in literature and Zikic et al. [13] to: a) identify the location of the lesion with high confidence (without DWI and avoiding known WM hyperintensities); b) extract the extent of the ischemic lesion and c) find out possible focal atrophies other than known WM hyperintensities that may have significant impact on post-stroke impairment and recovery. These are achieved by: 1) a two-stage MRF classification of the probable lesion areas; 2) using random forests on the intensities of the probable lesion areas; and finally 3) applying an ad-hoc rule to refine the results iterating between random forests and MRF classifications using connected component analysis. To the best of our knowledge this is the first attempt to apply random forests for stroke lesion segmentation. The paper is organized as follows: Section 2 provides the detail of the multimodal patient data and the preprocessing steps, Section 3 provides the description of the MRF classification using Iterated Conditional Modes (ICM), the random forests method with the feature-space and the ad-hoc rule for refinement of the segmentation in its respective subsections, and finally Section 4 and 5 deal with the results, discussions and conclusions.

## 2    Data and Preprocessing

A total of 20 patient datasets of size $181 \times 217 \times 181$ voxels are used in our experiments. All patients have stroke lesions and T1W, T2W, FLAIR and ADC (apparent diffusion coefficient) maps of the chronic stage are available. The T1W images are acquired with TE=2.55ms, TR=1900ms, flip angle=9°, voxel spacing=$(1 \times 1 \times 1)$mm; the T2/FLAIR volumes are acquired with TE=388ms, TR=6000ms, T1=2100ms, flip angle=120° with isotropic 1mm voxels. The ADC maps are generated from the diffusion weighted images with B=1000 in 25 directions with isotropic voxel spacing of 2.5mm. The voxels sizes for all the modalities are converted to 1mm isotropic voxels for our experiment. All patient data are rigidly registered to the (Montreal Neurological Institute) MNI atlas. Bias correction for the patient MRIs is done using the method of Van Leemput et al. [14] that also provides the segmented masks of GM, WM and CSF. Skull stripping is done by applying the GM, WM, CSF segmented masks to remove the remaining part of the brain. The probabilistic GM and WM estimates for each patient are obtained by non-rigidly aligning [15] the GM/WM masks of other patients to the target patient and then averaging the aligned masks. This method ensures that the effect of atrophies that are likely to be present in the individual patient tissue masks is minimized.

## 3    The Proposed Method

This section explains the different steps involved in our method. Figure 2 shows the schematic diagram of our method. The MRF classification from the FLAIR image provides the possible lesion areas. The multimodal MRI images of these areas are then used as inputs to the random forests training and classification, and finally connected component analysis with ad-hoc rules are applied on the random-forests and MRF classifications to refine the segmentation results. The rationale behind using a part of the brain i.e. possible lesion areas as input to the random forest as opposed to the sub-sampled entire brain is to reduce the overhead of computational complexity and to avoid missing smaller lesions in the random forests training phase. Sections 3.1 and 3.2 provide terse theoretical backgrounds of MRF and random forests and how each classification method is applied in our experiment. Finally, Section 3.3 describes the connected component analysis rules used to refine the segmentation results.

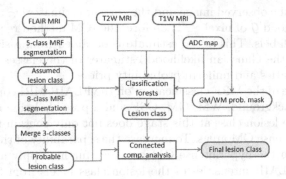

**Fig. 2.** A schematic diagram of the proposed method for ischemic stroke lesion segmentation

## 3.1   Markov Random Field (MRF) Segmentation

Given $\mathcal{F} = \{f_s\}_{s \in S}$ a set of image data where $f_s$ denotes the gray value at pixel $s$. A segmentation problem is to find the labeling $\hat{\omega}$ which maximizes $P(\omega|\mathcal{F})$. Bayes theorem suggests that $P(\omega|\mathcal{F}) = \frac{P(\mathcal{F}|\omega)P(\omega)}{P(\mathcal{F})}$. Actually $P(\mathcal{F})$ does not depend on the labeling $\omega$ and we have the assumption from conditional probability that $P(\mathcal{F}|\omega) = \prod_{s \in S} P(f_s|\omega_s)$. The MRF on each of the pixel $s$ is defined by the clique potentials and by a neighborhood-system $\mathcal{G}$. Let $C$ denote a clique of $\mathcal{G}$, and $\mathcal{C}$ the set of all cliques. The restriction of the label $\omega$ to the site of a given clique $C$ is denoted by $\omega_C$. The clique potentials $E_C(\omega_C)$ for every $C$ in $\mathcal{C}$ and every $\omega \in \Omega$, where $\Omega$ is the set of all possible discrete labellings. Following the definition of MRF and the Bayes theorem, the global labeling which we are trying to find is given by:

$$\hat{\omega} = \max_{\omega \in \Omega} \prod_{s \in S} P(f_s|\omega_s) \prod_{C \in \mathcal{C}} \exp(-E_C(\omega_C)). \tag{1}$$

The energies of cliques of order 2 and more reflect the probabilistic modelings of labels taking the neighborhood-system into account, i.e. the pixels would be labeled considering the neighborhood labels. Let us assume that $P(f_s|\omega_s)$ is Gaussian, the discrete class $\lambda$ is represented by its mean value $\mu_\lambda$ and its deviation $\sigma_\lambda$. We get:

$$\hat{\omega} = \min_{\omega \in \Omega} \left( \sum_{s \in S} \left( \log(\sqrt{2\pi}\sigma_{\omega_s}) + \frac{(f_s - \mu_{\omega_s})^2}{2\sigma_{\omega_s}^2} \right) + \sum_{C \in \mathcal{C}} E_C(\omega_C) \right) \tag{2}$$

Using the above equation, the local energy of any labeling $\omega$ at site $s$ would be:

$$\varepsilon_s(\omega) = \log(\sqrt{2\pi}\sigma_{\omega_s}) + \frac{(f_s - \mu_{\omega_s})^2}{2\sigma_{\omega_s}^2} + \sum_{C_s \in \mathcal{C}} E_{C_s}(\omega_{C_s}). \tag{3}$$

The estimation of $\hat{\omega}$ is done through the energy minimization using the ICM algorithm [16]. The key to the ICM method is that the probability of the label at pixel $s$ given the observed image and the current estimates $\omega_C$ of all the labels in the neighborhood $\mathcal{G}$ of pixel $S$. Therefore, the ICM method requires an initial estimate of the labels. This initial estimate is obtained from a simple Bayesian classification of the Gaussian likelihood estimates of the classes based only on the image intensities and uniform probability priors.

The first stage of the MRF classification on the FLAIR MRI considers 5 tissue classes as the background, WM, GM, CSF and a possible lesion class. The segmentation of the lesion class at this stage does not only contain the lesion area but also hyperintense GM areas. To increase the separability of the hyperintense lesion areas from the hyperintense GM areas we further apply a MRF classification on the FLAIR intensities of the lesion class labels from the first stage. This second stage of classification attempts to separate the possible lesion class into 8 classes to maximize the separation between the Gaussian density functions. As mentioned in the introduction, ischemic stroke lesions have intensities dropping around the edges, therefore a merging of the labeled components from the 3 classes with highest mean values ensures that a maximum of the lesion area is included in the segmentation. Nevertheless, hyperintensities in the periventricular regions, basal ganglia and the hippocampal regions similar to the stroke areas, still incorporate errors in the MRF segmentation process. Therefore, the intensities of the merged possible lesion class are further passed into classification forests described in the following section.

## 3.2   Random Forests (RF) Classification

In this method, standard classification forests based on spatially non-local features combined with probabilistic tissue estimates of GM $(P_{GM})$ and WM$(P_{WM})$ are used. The MRI input channels used in the classification are FLAIR, T1W, T2W and ADC maps. Additionally, the labeled probable tissue class $(L_{les})$ is also used as a channel input. Therefore an input channel comprises of $C_j = (I_{FLAIR}, I_{T1}, I_{T2}, I_{ADC}, P_{GM}, P_{WM}, L_{les})$.

In our method we use 3 spatial and context-aware features [13] along with the voxel position and its respective intensity set. Let us consider $x \in \mathcal{X}$ is a spatial point, to be assigned a class (lesion/background) and $I_j$ is an input channel. $N_j^s(x)$ denotes a 3D neighborhood with edge lengths $s = (s_x, s_y, s_z)$, $v \in \mathbb{R}^3$ is an offset vector. The contextual features are as follows: 1) $I_{j1}(x) - I_{j2}(x + v)$, where $I_{j1} = I_{j2}$ is allowed; 2) difference of cuboid means, i.e. $\mu(N_{j1}^{s1}(x)) - \mu(N_{j2}^{s2}(x + v))$, where $j1 \neq j2$; and 3) this feature assumes that lesions usually appear as partial volumes of GM and WM areas and CSF borders the other side of the lesion, therefore the difference of intensity along a 3D line as $\max_\lambda(I_j(x + \lambda v)) - \min_\lambda(I_j(x + \lambda v))$ with $\lambda \in [0, 1]$.

In classification forests training, each tree $t$ in the forest receives the full training set $V$, along with the label at the root node and selects a test along randomly chosen dimensions of the feature space to split $V$ into two subsets in order to maximize the information gain. The left and the right child nodes receive their respective subsets $V_i$ and the process is repeated at each child node to grow the next level of the tree. Each node in a decision tree also contains a class predictor

$p_t^i(c|x)$, which is the probability corresponding to the fraction of points with class $c$ in $V_i$. Growth is terminated when either information gain is minimum or the tree has grown to maximum depth. At testing, a point to be classified is pushed through each tree $t$ by applying the learned split functions. When reaching a leaf node $l$, posterior probabilities $p_t^l(c|x))$ are gathered in order to compute the final posterior probability of the voxel defined by $p(c|x) = \frac{1}{n}\sum_{t=1}^n p_t^l(c|x)$. The actual class estimate is chosen as the most probable class by $\arg\max_c p(c|x)$.

### 3.3  Ad-hoc Connected Component Analysis

In this step, we firstly remove the periventricular areas and the WM areas from the MRF classification results by applying a non-rigidly registered [15] mask of the automated anatomical labeling (AAL) atlas [17] that models the GM. This means that the lesion areas falling under the zero labels (WM) and the labels 71/72 (periventricular regions) of the registered atlas are ignored. Since the lesion areas are much smaller compared to the whole brain, the input to the RF are probable lesion areas from the MRF classification to avoid unbalanced data. Nonetheless, the probable lesion areas are much larger than the actual lesion area. Therefore, RF provides sparse classification of the true positive areas while managing to eliminate the false positives in most of the cases. Therefore, we applied a pruning step to remove more than 10 connected voxels (analyzing 8-connectivity) and then a morphological closing operator with a circular mask of radius 3. Isolated lesion components from RF may be parts of the same lesion which may be verified from the MRF classification. The components of the RF classification that have more than $\epsilon$ percent overlap with the corresponding components in MRF are retained and the others are removed as outliers. In the final output, the component from MRF classification is replaced for these lesions. It may be the case, when the resulting component is less than $\epsilon$ percent of the volume of the corresponding RF component, then the larger component from the RF is replaced in the final output. This step further ensures that the WM lesion areas that are connected with the GM areas are also included in the final lesion volume and only the pure WM strokes are eliminated. In summary, the iterative approach ensures that maximum lesion areas either from the MRF or RF are included. Finally, a morphological closing operation of radius 2 ensures that some of the hypointense regions embedded inside the hyperintense regions are mostly included in the lesion volume.

## 4   Evaluation and Discussions

A total of 20 patient datasets are used in the training and validation procedure. Three patients have pure WM strokes; although we have included these data in the MRF and RF classification stages, they are automatically removed in the connected component analysis step when the WM areas and periventricular areas are removed from the MRF classification using the AAL atlas. Therefore, the final lesion results are evaluated only on 17 patients. The RF training/testing

**Table 1.** Quantitative results for ischemic lesion detection using MRF and RF. DSC (Dice similarity coefficient) is in fraction, PPV (positive predictive value), NPV (negative predictive value) and ACC (accuracy) are in %. $\mu$ is the average and $\sigma$ is the standard deviation.

| Patient# | DSC | PPV | NPV | ACC |
|---|---|---|---|---|
| 1 | 0.71 | 87.46 | 99.92 | 99.90 |
| 2 | 0.75 | 97.78 | 99.90 | 99.89 |
| 3 | 0.55 | 51.32 | 99.98 | 99.96 |
| 4 | 0.33 | 31.23 | 99.99 | 99.97 |
| 5 | 0.81 | 94.35 | 99.86 | 99.84 |
| 6 | 0.44 | 73.37 | 99.98 | 99.98 |
| 7 | 0.73 | 88.40 | 99.89 | 99.87 |
| 8 | 0.44 | 40.66 | 99.99 | 99.97 |
| 9 | 0.65 | 79.38 | 99.83 | 99.77 |
| 10 | 0.78 | 88.38 | 100.00 | 100.00 |
| 11 | 0.34 | 35.15 | 99.99 | 99.98 |
| 12 | 0.46 | 93.76 | 99.97 | 99.97 |
| 13 | 0.73 | 94.14 | 99.76 | 99.74 |
| 14 | 0.36 | 53.90 | 99.93 | 99.91 |
| 15 | 0.58 | 81.77 | 99.96 | 99.96 |
| 16 | 0.62 | 85.97 | 99.98 | 99.98 |
| 17 | 0.70 | 95.57 | 99.88 | 99.87 |
| $\mu$ | 0.59 | 74.86 | 99.93 | 99.92 |
| $\sigma$ | 0.16 | 22.95 | 0.07 | 0.08 |

are carried out with 100 full-grown trees in a leave-one-patient-out manner. The offset vector $v$ in Section 3.2 is empirically chosen as 8mm and the 3D neighborhood is restricted to $3 \times 3 \times 3$ voxels. The value of $\epsilon$ for the connected component analysis of Section 3.3 is empirically learned from the datasets as 20. An expert neurologist segmented the ischemic lesions on the FLAIR images. Table 1 shows the quantitative results in terms of Dice similarity coefficient (DSC)= $2 \times TP/(FP + 2 \times TP + FN)$, i.e. the fraction of overlap between the manual segmentation and the automated segmentation method showing a mean of $0.59 \pm 0.16$; positive predictive value or the precision rate (PPV)=$TP/(TP + FP)$ denotes the proportion of true positives i.e. a high PPV would indicate that a patient identified with a lesion does actually have the lesion. Negative predictive value (NPV)=$TN/(TN + FN)$ denotes the proportion of negative results in the test, i.e. a high NPV indicates that the method rarely misses the lesion; while accuracy (ACC)=$(TP + TN)/(TP + TN + FP + FN)$ measures the degree of closeness to the actual measurements. Here $TP$ ='true positives', $TN$ ='true negatives', $FP$ ='false positives' and $FN$ ='false negatives'. The volume correlation between the manually segmented volume and that by the automated method is $r = 0.98$. The DSC values show a maximum high value of 0.81 and a low value of 0.33. This variation is due to several reasons, for e.g., the expert neurologist marked the lesions which were deemed to be stroke,

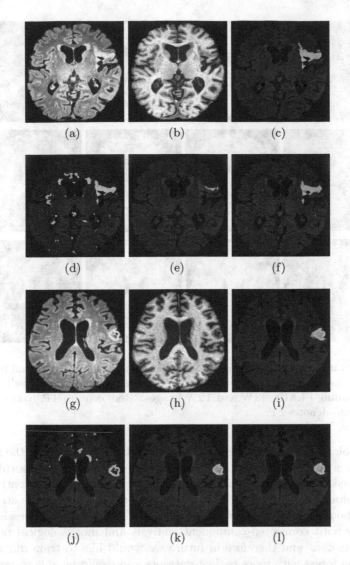

**Fig. 3.** Classification results from MRF, RF and connected component analysis. (a) to (f) are the results corresponding to patient 1 and (g) to (l) are the results corresponding to patient 2. (a) & (g) are the FLAIR images that show hyperintensities for stroke lesions and (b) & (h) are the T1W images showing hypointense regions of stroke. The manual segmentations by the expert radiologist are shown in (c) & (i); segmentations from MRF (merged 3-classes) are shown in (d) & (j); segmentations from RF classifications are shown in (e) & (k) and the final lesions after ad-hoc connected component analysis are shown in (f) & (l) for patients 1 and 2 respectively.

but the patients might actually contain other hyperintense areas other than WM diseases which are extracted by our algorithm and may eventually cause atrophies that are important for the study of post-stroke recovery and depression.

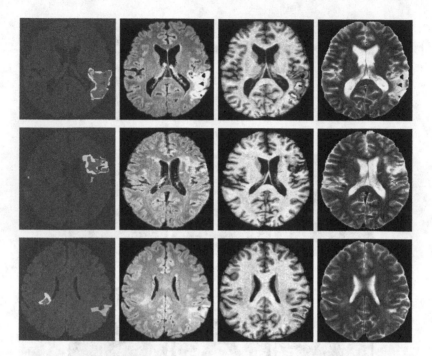

**Fig. 4.** Qualitative results of ischemic lesion segmentation. Rows correspond to patients 5, 9 and 14. The $1^{st}$ column shows the overlap image and the $2^{nd}$, $3^{rd}$ and $4^{th}$ represent the corresponding FLAIR, T1W and T2W images. 'Red' denotes TP, 'yellow' denotes FN and 'green' denotes FP.

The morphological operation helps to fill-up the CSF areas within the stroke in most cases, while if the areas are too large then the uniform morphological operator mask radius used is not good enough to approximate the entire stroke area. Therefore, our algorithm provides an underestimation of the stroke area and hence poor overlap measures for those patients. The post-processing of the lesion areas with connected-component analysis and morphological processing is data dependant and therefore in future we would like to train our model of classification forest with more patient datasets and would be able to remove the ad-hoc step. Nevertheless, at this stage with a limited number of datasets, the ad-hoc step is required to obtain clinically meaningful results.

Figure 3 shows the classification results for patients 1 and 2 at each stage of the proposed method. Figures 3(d) shows the result after 3-classes with highest means are merged from the 8-class MRF classification, while 3(e) shows the results from the classification forest. It is observed that a significant part of the lesion is missing from the RF classification while in the final output (Figure 3(f)), the connected component analysis manages to extract a larger part of the lesion that is similar to the manual segmentation as in Figure 3(c). In the case of patient 2, Figure 3(j) shows a missing part of the lesion from MRF classification (being hypointense in FLAIR), while Figure 3(k) shows the complete lesion after

RF classification followed by morphological closing operation, therefore the final output in Figure 3(l) from connected component analysis shows a lesion area conforming to the manual segmentation of Figure 3(i).

Figure 4 shows the qualitative results of patients 5, 9 and 14 which show very high, medium and low overlap areas with the manual segmentation. The TP areas are shown in red, the FN areas are shown in yellow and the FP areas are shown in green. Observing Figure 4 it is evident that the results of our method show high overlap for patient 5 (row 1). The last row in the figure shows false positive areas in green which are hyperintense in FLAIR and T2W MRI and hypointense in T1W MRI. This suggests that our method is capable of extracting ischemic stroke lesions and some added lesions which might have been caused by some other disease but may have significant structural and functional impact on the patient brain. Therefore identifying such lesions is also important for the post-stroke depression study.

All our implementations are done in C++ and ITK platform on a 6-core CPU of 3.2GHz with 23.5GB of memory. The MRF classification requires 6min−7min on an average for each patient, the RF training requires an average of 2 hours to train in leave-one-patient-out manner, while each testing requires 5min. The connected component analysis also takes 10s−15s on average.

## 5   Conclusions

The method described in this paper deals with a two-stage classification based on MRF and classification forests to identify chronic ischemic stroke lesions in the human brain. The first stage results from the MRF are used as inputs to the classification forests as well as help reduce misclassified and missing lesion areas obtained from the classification forests. The method shows good accuracy in identifying the lesion areas which is useful for the post-stroke depression study. Since, our method is also capable of identifying most of the hyperintense areas on FLAIR images, we would like to use the DWI images of the acute/sub-acute stages to discriminate between strokes (both GM and WM lesions) and other WM hyperintensities which would provide additional biomarkers consistent with the hypotheses in the post-stroke depression study [3]. We would like to validate our method with more stroke patients in future and would probably not require the ad-hoc connected component analysis step if the RF is trained with more patients which would increase the generalization power of classification forests.

**Acknowledgments.** We would like to acknowledge the Stroke Imaging Prevention and Treatment (START) program of research which is supported in part by the CSIRO of Australia through the Preventative Health Flagship Cluster, the National Health and Medical Reserch Council of Australia, and a Victorian Government Operational Infrastructure Support Grant. In particular, we wish to acknowledge the stroke patients, radiologists and START researchers who contributed to the data collected for this study. Leeanne Carey is supported by an Australian Research Council Future Fellowship [number FT0992299]. The funding sources had no role in conduct of the study or writing of the report.

# References

1. Baird, A.E., Warach, S.: Magnetic resonance imaging of acute stroke. J. Cereb. Blood Flow Metab. 18, 583–609 (1998)
2. Mosser, D.M., Edwards, J.P.: Exploring the full spectrum of macrophage activation. Nature Reviews Immunology 8, 958–969 (2008)
3. Carey, L., et al.: START-PrePARE PREdiction and Prevention to Achieve Optimal Recovery Endpoints after stroke: Study rationale and protocol. In: 7th World Cong. of Neurorehab. (2012)
4. Campbell, B.C., et al.: Assessing response to stroke thrombolysis: validation of 24-hour multimodal magnetic resonance imaging. Arch. Neurol. 69(1), 46–50 (2012)
5. Dastidar, P., et al.: Volumetric measurements of right cerebral hemisphere infarction: use of a semiautomatic MRI segmentation technique. Comput. in Biol. & Med. 30, 41–54 (2000)
6. Heinonen, T., et al.: Semiautomatic tool for segmentation and volumetric analysis of medical images. Med. Biol. Eng. Comput. 36, 291–296 (1998)
7. Jacobs, M.A., et al.: Multiparametric MRI tissue characterization in clinical stroke with correlation to clinical outcome: Part 2. Stroke 30, 950–957 (2001)
8. Jacobs, M.A., et al.: A model for multiparametric MRI tissue characterization in experimental cerebral ischemia with histological validation in rat: Part 1. Stroke 32, 943–949 (2001)
9. Kabir, Y., et al.: Multimodal MRI segmentation of ischemic stroke lesions. In: IEEE EMBS, pp. 1595–1598 (2007)
10. Hevia-Montiel, N., et al.: Robust nonparametric segmentation of infarct lesion from diffusion-weighted MR images. In: IEEE EMBS, pp. 2102–2105 (August 2007)
11. Shen, S., et al.: An improved lesion detection approach based on similarity measurement between fuzzy intensity segmentation and spatial probability maps. Mag. Reson. Imag. 28, 245–254 (2010)
12. Bray, J.R., Curtis, J.T.: An ordination of the upland forest communities of southern wisconsin. Ecol. Monogr. 27, 325–349 (1957)
13. Zikic, D., et al.: Decision forests for tissue-specific segmentation of high-grade gliomas in multi-channel MR. In: Ayache, N., Delingette, H., Golland, P., Mori, K. (eds.) MICCAI 2012, Part III. LNCS, vol. 7512, pp. 369–376. Springer, Heidelberg (2012)
14. Van Leemput, K., et al.: Automated model-based tissue classification of MR images of the brain. IEEE Trans. in Med. Imag. 18(10), 897–908 (1999)
15. Modat, M., et al.: Fast free-form deformation using graphics processing units. Comput. Meth. Prog. Biomed. 98(3), 278–284 (2010)
16. Besag, J.: On the statistical analysis of dirty pictures. J. R. Statist. Soc. Ser. B 48, 259–302 (1986)
17. Tzourio-Mazoyer, N., et al.: Automated anatomical labeling of activations in SPM using a macroscopic anatomical parcellation of the MNI MRI single-subject brains. NeuroImage 15(1), 273–289 (2002)

# Registration of Brain CT Images to an MRI Template for the Purpose of Lesion-Symptom Mapping

Hugo J. Kuijf, J. Matthijs Biesbroek, Max A. Viergever,
Geert Jan Biessels, and Koen L. Vincken

University Medical Center Utrecht, The Netherlands

**Abstract.** Lesion-symptom mapping is a valuable tool for exploring the relation between brain structure and function. In order to perform lesion-symptom mapping, lesion delineations made on different brain CT images need to be transformed to a standardized coordinate system. The preferred choice for this is the MNI152 template image that is based on T1-weighted MR images. This requires a multi-modal registration procedure to transform lesion delineations for each CT image to the MNI152 template image. A two-step registration procedure was implemented, using lesion-masking and contrast stretching to correctly align the soft tissue of the CT image to the MNI152 template image. The results were used to transform the lesion delineations to the template. The quality of the registration was assessed by an expert human observer. Of the 86 CT images, the registration was highly successful in 71 cases (83%). Slight manual adjustments of the lesion delineations in the standard coordinate system were required to make unsuccessful cases suitable for a lesion-symptom mapping study.

## 1 Introduction

Acute ischemic stroke frequently causes cognitive deficits. [1] Besides the volume of lesions, the exact location of lesions is an important factor in explaining the variance in post-stroke cognitive performance. [1] The study of these patients with acquired brain damage is a valuable tool for exploring the relationship between brain structure and function. Lesion-symptom mapping studies have provided valuable insights in neuroanatomical correlates of various cognitive functions. [2]

Traditional approaches to lesion-symptom mapping include comparing the performance of groups of patients with and without lesions at one or more predefined locations. [2, 3] Recently, more sophisticated methods have emerged, such as voxel-based lesion-symptom mapping (VLSM). [3, 4] A major advantage of VLSM over traditional approaches is that it allows for assumption-free calculation of associations between brain injury and behavioral performance at each individual location (i.e. voxel) in the image.

A prerequisite for performing voxel-wise analyses is that the lesions have to be segmented and registered to a standard space. Segmentation of the lesions is

L. Shen et al. (Eds.): MBIA 2013, LNCS 8159, pp. 119–128, 2013.

done by delineating the location of lesions manually or (semi-)automatically on structural imaging (usually CT or MRI T1- or T2-weighted sequences), resulting in a lesion mask for each subject. Next, all lesion masks are transformed into a standardized coordinate system. Each voxel in this standardized coordinate system contains information regarding the presence or absence of a lesion at that specific location for each subject. Finally, a VLSM approach is used to investigate the relation between the occurrence of a lesion at a specific location and cognitive performance.

The MNI152 standard-space MRI T1-weighted average structural template image (shortened as: MNI152 template) is often used as the standardized coordinate system that all lesion masks are transformed to. [5, 6] This MNI152 template is derived from 152 individual images, as described by Fonov et al. For this template, a number of anatomical atlases are available, making it a popular choice when performing lesion-symptom mapping. [7]

Ischemic brain lesions are often imaged using CT—because of higher availability and shorter acquisition time—whereas the MNI152 template is based on MR images. This complicates the registration procedure. A common solution is to acquire a T1-weighted MR image of each subject and perform a two-step registration. Hereby the CT image is registered to the T1-weighted image and the T1-weighted image to the MNI152 template. Both transformations are combined to transform the CT image directly to the standard coordinate space. If T1-weighted images are not available, which is the case by imaging of acute ischemic lesions, the CT image has to be registered to the MNI152 template directly. This is more complicated, because the registration procedure has to deal with both the difference in modality and shape of the head.

In literature, some methods are described to perform this inter-subject registration between CT and MR (template) images. [8, 9] The general consensus is that a deformable registration optimizing a mutual information metric is required. However, details of the practical implementation of this approach are not always described. Especially for the purpose of lesion-symptom mapping studies, where the presence of brain lesions and the low soft tissue contrast in the CT images complicates the registration. A recent publication by Gao et al. describes a procedure for registering brain CT images to an MRI template, by including the mid-sagittal plane to constrain the deformable registration. [10] However, the presence of brain lesions is not reported and the results were only evaluated for the total brain volume, disregarding the difficulties of registering the soft tissue within the brain.

The goal of the present study is to develop a method to transform lesion masks to a standardized space for the purpose of lesion-symptom mapping, by registration of CT images directly to the MNI152 template. The proposed method consists of two steps: an affine registration to globally align the CT image with the MNI152 template and a deformable registration to locally match the template. The resulting transform is applied to the delineated lesions and the quality of the transformed lesion masks is assessed.

# 2 Methods and Materials

## 2.1 Participants and CT

From a prospectively collected database of patients who were admitted between November 2005 and December 2012 with ischemic stroke to the University Medical Center Utrecht, we included 86 patients. Patients fulfilled the following inclusion criteria: (1) first-ever ischemic stroke; (2) an infarction on follow-up CT; (3) no infarcts from earlier date. Because the data were gathered in order to study the relation between lesion location and cognitive performance, patients with known pre-existent impaired cognition were also excluded.

All CT scans were performed in the setting of standard clinical care and were acquired using a Philips Mx8000 16, Brilliance 64, or Brilliance iCT 256 CT scanner.

Lesion locations were manually delineated on the CT images by an experienced observer, with an in-house developed tool based on MeVisLab (MeVis Medical Solutions AG, Bremen, Germany [11]).

## 2.2 Affine Registration

All registrations, both affine and deformable, were performed with the `elastix` toolbox. [12] The used MNI152 template has a voxel size of 1.0 mm$^3$. To globally align the CT image with the MNI152 template, an affine registration considering only the bone was performed.

The bone was extracted from the CT images: intensity values below 500 HU were set to zero, intensity values equal to or above 500 HU were untouched. The MNI152 template was modified to extract the bone. First, the template image intensities were inverted to produce high intensity values at the location of the bone. Next, the image was thresholded to extract the bone and a mask was applied to suppress the background. An example is shown in Figure 1. Note that the ventricles are visible in the bone-extracted MNI152 template image, because of their low intensities. This does not influence the registration, since there are no intensities to match in the bone-extracted CT image.

An affine registration was used to transform the bone-extracted CT image to the bone-extracted MNI152 template, following the recommended settings of `elastix`: a multi-resolution approach with four resolutions, the Advanced Mattes Mutual Information metric, and the Adaptive Stochastic Gradient Descent optimizer. [13–15]

## 2.3 Deformable Registration

Following the affine registration to align the bone-extracted CT and MNI152 images, a deformable registration was used to align the soft tissue of the brain with the template. A B-spline with its control points placed in a regular 3D grid, spaced 10 mm apart, was used to deform the CT image. [16, 17] The Advanced Mattes Mutual Information metric was optimized with a standard gradient descent optimizer. [18] The previously computed affine transform and

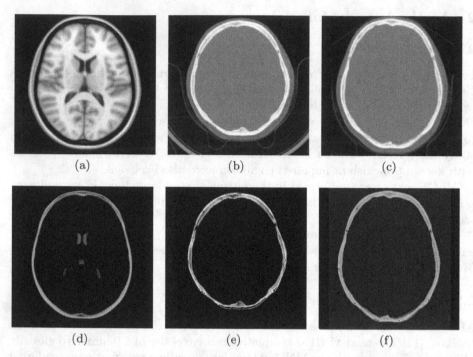

**Fig. 1.** Left: (a) the MNI152 template image and (d) the bone-extracted image. Middle: (b) an example CT image and (e) the bone-extracted image. The image in (e) was transformed to (d) with an affine registration. Right: transformed CT image after registration.

the B-spline transform were composed together, to avoid repeated interpolations. A lesion-masking approach was used to prevent a bias in the transformation caused by the presence of the lesion, by ignoring the manually delineated lesion area in the computation of the metric. [19]

However, the lack of sufficient contrast in soft tissue of the brain on CT images makes it challenging to directly transform such images to the MNI152 template. The features that need to be aligned with the MNI152 template— the gray matter, white matter, and cerebrospinal fluid—all have intensity values between 0 HU and 50 HU. The used Advanced Mattes Mutual Information metric computes a joint histogram of the intensity values of the CT image and MNI152 template. The number of bins of this joint histogram is set to 32 bins (`elastix` default value). This results in a bin size of approximately 90 HU, rendering it impossible to make a meaningful deformation of the CT image: the little contrast that was present in the soft tissue vanished into a single bin. This is illustrated in the top row of Figure 2. The effect of this can be seen in Figure 3(c), where the soft tissue after deformable registration is identical to the soft tissue after affine registration in Figure 3(b).

To overcome this, contrast stretching by means of histogram equalization and the removal of (outlier) intensities below the 5th and above the 95th percentile was

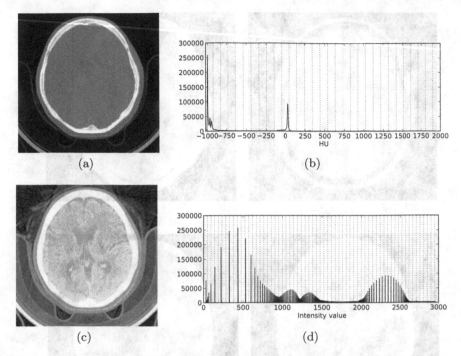

Fig. 2. Top row: original CT image with its histogram of intensities. The peak around 25 HU represents the soft tissue; the dotted vertical lines are the histogram bins used by the metric. Bottom row: contrast enhanced CT image with its histogram. The soft tissue now has intensity values between 2000 and 2500, which are spread over more bins in the histogram. The number of histogram bins has been increased as well (dotted lines).

applied. Furthermore, the number of bins of the joint histogram was increased to 64 bins. By doing this, the intensities of the gray matter, white matter, and cerebrospinal fluid were distributed over approximately 15 bins in the joint histogram, as can be seen in Figure 2. This enabled the registration procedure to compute a meaningful deformation of the CT image to the MNI152 template, as can be seen in Figure 3.

## 2.4   Experiments

The described procedure was used to transform the CT images and the lesion delineations of the 86 participants to the MNI152 template. Since the proposed method was developed for the purpose of lesion-symptom mapping, a correct positioning of the lesions was the main goal. An experienced human observer visually assessed the quality of the transformation of the lesion delineations and determined if the quality was sufficient for VLSM.

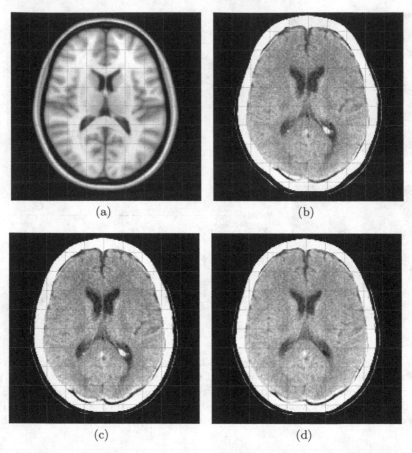

**Fig. 3.** The effect of contrast stretching on the deformable registration. Note that for viewing purposes only, the contrast settings have been altered to highlight the soft tissue and a reference grid is included. (a) The MNI152 template. (b) The CT image after affine registration. (c) The CT image after deformable registration without contrast stretching. (d) The CT image after deformable registration with contrast stretching.

## 3    Results

Of the 86 CT images, the registration was successful in 71 cases (83%). Some example results are shown in Figure 4.

In eight of the unsuccessful cases there was a misalignment of the tentorium cerebelli (separates cerebellum from cerebral hemispheres). An example is shown in the top row of Figure 5. In six unsuccessful cases there was a misalignment of the ventricles, caused by either edema with midline shift (four cases, example in bottom row of Figure 5) or atrophy with enlargement of the ventricular system (two cases). In one unsuccessful case there was no evident cause. All misalignments were resolved by slight manual adjustments of the lesion delineations in the standard space, as can be seen in Figures 5(c) and (f).

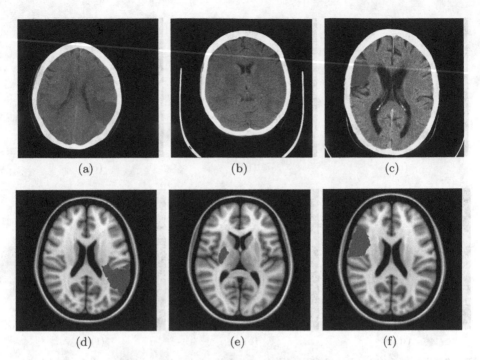

(a)                    (b)                    (c)

(d)                    (e)                    (f)

**Fig. 4.** Top row: original CT images with the lesion delineation overlaid in red. Note that the viewing settings have been altered to highlight the soft tissue. Bottom row: lesion delineations transformed to the MNI152 template image.

## 4  Discussion

The proposed registration procedure to transform lesion delineations from CT images to the MNI152 template image proved to be highly successful. In 83% of the cases, the lesion delineations were correctly transformed and suitable for usage in a lesion-symptom mapping study. Slight manual adjustments of the transformed lesion delineations were needed in the remaining cases.

Performing an initial affine registration with bone-extracted images was required in order to correctly align the CT image with the MNI152 template. Otherwise, there is a risk that the optimization procedure will converge into a local optimum when only using a deformable registration. The bone of the CT image might then be aligned with the gray matter on the MNI152 template, as there are strong edges at those locations. The presence of the ventricles in the bone-extracted MNI152 template (see Figure 1(d)) did not influence the affine registration, since there are no corresponding intensities at that location in the bone-extracted CT image.

The deformable registration used a contrast stretched CT image to perform the registration with the MNI152 template. By applying a simple contrast stretching, the CT image intensities were spread over multiple bins in the joint histogram of the used metric. This allowed the registration procedure to correctly align the gray matter, white matter, and cerebrospinal fluid.

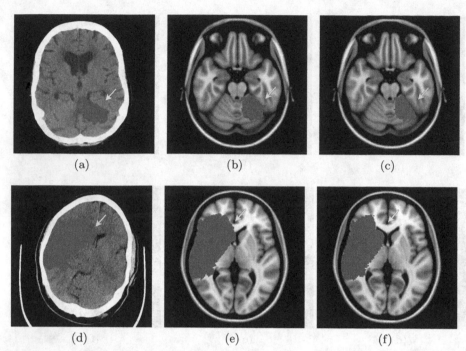

(a)                    (b)                    (c)

(d)                    (e)                    (f)

**Fig. 5.** Top row: (a) original CT with lesion delineation in red, (b) transformed lesion delineation on MNI152 template image is incorrect around the tentorium cerebelli, (c) manually adjusted lesion delineation. Bottom row: (d) original CT with lesion delineation in red, (e) transformed lesion delineation on MNI152 template image is incorrect because of edema with midline shift, (f) manually adjusted lesion delineation.

Unfortunately, this issue is not addressed by the publication of Gao *et al.* [10] In this publication, Dice's coefficient and the Hausdorff distance are reported in the results, but only for the total brain volume. The accuracy of the alignment of structures within the brain tissue (for example cortical gray matter, white matter, basal ganglia, and thalamus) are not evaluated. When performing lesion-symptom mapping, accurate alignment of these structures is essential.

The final goal of the proposed registration procedure was to transform lesion delineations, in order to perform VLSM. Therefore, the quality of the resulting transformations was assessed by an experienced observer with this goal in mind. Lesion delineations on the original CT images were visually compared to the transformed lesion delineations on the MNI152 template image. In the case that slight manual adjustments were needed to correct misalignments, the registration was deemed unsuccessful. However, as can be seen in Figure 5, large portions of the lesion delineations were correctly transformed in all the unsuccessful cases. In eight unsuccessful cases there was a misalignment of the tentorium cerebelli, a structure that is hardly visible on the CT images and therefore difficult to transform correctly. However, lesions generally do not cross the tentorium cerebelli. Manual adjustments in the standard coordinate space are thus easily made by erasing the inaccurate parts. In the unsuccessful cases caused by edema with midline shift, one of the lateral ventricles is suppressed by the lesion. Because of the lesion masking approach and the absence of a lateral ventricle, the deformation field is interpolated at these areas, since there are no features to compute the metric. This results in an enlarged lesion in the standard coordinate space, which is easily corrected by erasing the parts that overlap the lateral ventricles. Inclusion of the mid-sagittal plane, as proposed by Gao *et al.*, is unlikely to solve this problem, because computation of the mid-sagittal plane is inaccurate in the case of midline shift. The inclusion of a (curved) mid-sagittal surface [20] constraint might prevent the lesion from being transformed into the wrong hemisphere, but the absence of a lateral ventricle is the largest problem in these cases.

## 5   Conclusion

In this work, we proposed a procedure for the registration of CT images to the MNI152 template image for the purpose of lesion-symptom mapping. Lesion delineations on the CT images were successfully transformed to the MNI152 template image. Slight manual adjustments of the transformed lesion delineations were needed in a limited number of cases.

## References

1. Gorelick, P.B., Scuteri, A., Black, S.E., DeCarli, C., Greenberg, S.M., Iadecola, C., Launer, L.J., Laurent, S., Lopez, O.L., Nyenhuis, D., Petersen, R.C., Schneider, J.A., Tzourio, C., Arnett, D.K., Bennett, D.A., Chui, H.C., Higashida, R.T., Lindquist, R., Nilsson, P.M., Roman, G.C., Sellke, F.W., Seshadri, S.: Vascular contributions to cognitive impairment and dementia: A statement for healthcare professionals from the american heart association/american stroke association. Stroke 42(9), 2672–2713 (2011)
2. Rorden, C., Karnath, H.O.: Using human brain lesions to infer function: a relic from a past era in the fmri age? Nature Reviews Neuroscience 5(10), 812–819 (2004)
3. Biesbroek, J.M., Kuijf, H.J., van der Graaf, Y., Vincken, K.L., Postma, A., Mali, W.P.T.M., Biessels, G.J., Geerlings, M.I., on behalf of the SMART Study Group: Association between subcortical vascular lesion location and cognition: A voxel-based and tract-based lesion-symptom mapping study. The smart-mr study. PLoS ONE 8(4), e60541 (2013)
4. Rorden, C., Karnath, H.O., Bonilha, L.: Improving lesion-symptom mapping. Journal of Cognitive Neuroscience 19(7), 1081–1088 (2007)
5. Fonov, V., Evans, A., McKinstry, R., Almli, C., Collins, D.: Unbiased nonlinear average age-appropriate brain templates from birth to adulthood. NeuroImage 47(supp.1) (2009), S102; Organization for Human Brain Mapping 2009 Annual Meeting
6. Fonov, V., Evans, A.C., Botteron, K., Almli, C.R., McKinstry, R.C., Collins, D.L.: Unbiased average age-appropriate atlases for pediatric studies. NeuroImage 54(1), 313–327 (2011)

7. Evans, A.C., Janke, A.L., Collins, D.L., Baillet, S.: Brain templates and atlases. NeuroImage 62(2), 911–922 (2012)
8. Maintz, J.B.A., Viergever, M.A.: A survey of medical image registration. Medical Image Analysis 2(1), 1–36 (1998)
9. Pluim, J.P.W., Maintz, J.B.A., Viergever, M.A.: Mutual-information-based registration of medical images: a survey. IEEE Transactions on Medical Imaging 22(8), 986–1004 (2003)
10. Gao, A., Chen, M., Hu, Q.: Non-rigid registration between brain ct images and mri brain atlas by combining grayscale information, point correspondence on the midsaggital plane and brain surface matching. In: Proceedings of the 2nd International Conference on Computer Science and Electronics Engineering. Advances in Intelligent Systems Research, pp. 222–225 (2013)
11. Ritter, F., Boskamp, T., Homeyer, A., Laue, H., Schwier, M., Link, F., Peitgen, H.O.: Medical image analysis: A visual approach. IEEE Pulse 2(6), 60–70 (2011)
12. Klein, S., Staring, M., Murphy, K., Viergever, M.A., Pluim, J.P.W.: elastix: A toolbox for intensity-based medical image registration. IEEE Transactions on Medical Imaging 29(1), 196–205 (2010)
13. Thevenaz, P., Unser, M.: Optimization of mutual information for multiresolution image registration. IEEE Transactions on Image Processing 9(12), 2083–2099 (2000)
14. Klein, S., Pluim, J.P.W., Staring, M., Viergever, M.A.: Adaptive stochastic gradient descent optimisation for image registration. International Journal of Computer Vision 81(3), 227–239 (2009)
15. Klein, S., Staring, M.: elastix: the manual, 4.6 edn. (2012)
16. Rueckert, D., Sonoda, L.I., Hayes, C., Hill, D.L.G., Leach, M.O., Hawkes, D.: Non-rigid registration using free-form deformations: application to breast mr images. IEEE Transactions on Medical Imaging 18(8), 712–721 (1999)
17. Unser, M.: Splines: a perfect fit for signal and image processing. IEEE Signal Processing Magazine 16(6), 22–38 (1999)
18. Klein, S., Staring, M., Pluim, J.P.W.: Evaluation of optimization methods for nonrigid medical image registration using mutual information and b-splines. IEEE Transactions on Image Processing 16(12), 2879–2890 (2007)
19. Brett, M., Leff, A.P., Rorden, C., Ashburner, J.: Spatial normalization of brain images with focal lesions using cost function masking. NeuroImage 14(2), 486–500 (2001)
20. Kuijf, H.J., Viergever, M.A., Vincken, K.L.: Automatic extraction of the curved midsagittal brain surface on MR images. In: Menze, B.H., Langs, G., Lu, L., Montillo, A., Tu, Z., Criminisi, A. (eds.) MCV 2012. LNCS, vol. 7766, pp. 225–232. Springer, Heidelberg (2013)

# A Dynamical Clustering Model of Brain Connectivity Inspired by the $N$-Body Problem

Gautam Prasad[1], Josh Burkart[2], Shantanu H. Joshi[1], Talia M. Nir[1], Arthur W. Toga[1], and Paul M. Thompson[1]

[1] Imaging Genetics Center, Laboratory of Neuro Imaging, UCLA School of Medicine, Los Angeles, CA, USA
[2] Department of Physics, UC Berkeley, Berkeley, CA, USA

**Abstract.** We present a method for studying brain connectivity by simulating a dynamical evolution of the nodes of the network. The nodes are treated as particles, and evolved under a simulated force analogous to gravitational acceleration in the well-known $N$-body problem. The particle nodes correspond to regions of the cortex. The locations of particles are defined as the centers of the respective regions on the cortex and their masses are proportional to each region's volume. The force of attraction is modeled on the gravitational force, and explicitly made proportional to the elements of a connectivity matrix derived from diffusion imaging data. We present experimental results of the simulation on a population of 110 subjects from the Alzheimer's Disease Neuroimaging Initiative (ADNI), consisting of healthy elderly controls, early mild cognitively impaired (eMCI), late MCI (LMCI), and Alzheimer's disease (AD) patients. Results show significant differences in the dynamic properties of connectivity networks in healthy controls, compared to eMCI as well as AD patients.

**Keywords:** gravity, n-body simulation, diffusion, connectivity, MRI.

## 1 Introduction

Modeling human brain connectivity is essential for understanding the higher level network organization of the brain [1]. Because the underlying neuronal interconnections cannot be directly observed, constructing the brain connectivity map is an inference problem. Further, there are different approaches for constructing brain networks based upon the imaging modality and the type of connectivity. For example, the neuronal fiber tracts manifest in structural anatomical connectivity [2] that is observed using diffusion-weighted imaging. Sporns et al. [1] referred to the comprehensive map of these connections as the *connectome*. However, to understand the functional organization of the brain, we can model the correlations of task activations [3] and the BOLD response from functional magnetic resonance image (fMRI). A different approach by He and Evans et al. [4] observes statistical inter-dependencies of pertinent signals in the brain. This approach is general and can also be applied to cortical thickness measures from

L. Shen et al. (Eds.): MBIA 2013, LNCS 8159, pp. 129–137, 2013.

the brain. These types of networks also known as inference networks are useful in highlighting the compensatory processes that modulate structural measures (morphology, volume, thickness) in the brain.

At an abstract level, brain connectivity is often characterized using a connectivity matrix [5]. This connectivity matrix is an adjacency matrix that quantifies and organizes information on the connectivity between different regions of the brain. In white matter connectivity, tractography methods can assist in computing either the number or the density of extracted fibers that intersect any pair of brain regions, and provide a measure of their anatomical connectivity. The matrix of these connectivity values can also be understood as a network, which can be described using a variety of graph measures. By statistically analyzing connectivity measures from multiple subjects - of different ages or with different clinical diagnoses - it is possible to discover factors that affect the brain's connectivity network with aging and disease, and even how it is affected by our genes. Despite this, the final network representation is a topological structure, and usually does not include information on the location or size of the regions being analyzed. The size of the regions may even be regressed out using normalization to study connection density, and the relative locations of the regions are usually ignored if only the network topology is examined.

Most methods study brain connectivity as a static problem and use several sophisticated models for estimating the underlying structure. We take a different approach here and aim to model the nodal interconnectivity as a dynamical problem. This approach adapts a well known physics-based problem, the $N$-body simulation for dynamic modeling of particles under physical forces, imposing a dynamic structure on the nodes of the brain network. This conveniently allows one to model the nature of the interconnections by using forces proportional to the edge strengths. Traditionally, $N$-body simulations are used to understand dynamic systems of particles/objects under the influence of gravity. These simulations have been used by astrophysicists to understand the nonlinear formation of galaxies and related structures.

In our work, we design an $N$-body simulation that embodies the connectivity information of the brain to create a dynamic system of particles representing regions in the brain that interact depending on their volume and connectivity with other regions. The use of a gravitational force was motivated by the fact that, often, subnetworks with local connectivity integrate information first, and their hubs then communicate this information to other more distant centers of communication. This transfer strongly resembles the way in which $N$-body systems have submodules that interact and coalesce locally before interacting with other parts of the system. As such, the dynamics of the system incorporates constraints on information flow that depend on the physical proximity of the regions as well as the strength of their interaction.

Our goal is to create new measures of brain connectivity that may be useful for distinguishing disease. Our solution is a dynamic system of the locations, volumes, and fiber connectivity of a cortical segmentation, and contrasts the traditional fiber connectivity matrix with only pairwise connectivity information. Another source for our motivation is evidence of hierarchical brain organization [6].

To this end, we encoded brain measures into a gravitational $N$-body simulation. We used the simulation as a dynamical clustering algorithm able to produce 3D configurations of cortical segments based on connectivity rather than true physical location. We exploited similarities between information flow in brain networks and hierarchical structures formed by gravitationally interacting systems.

We present a detailed description of our connectivity based $N$-body simulation, outline a method for incorporating empirical connectivity data into the simulation, and describe time-dependent statistics. Additionally, we present methods for using the simulation statistics to discriminate between Alzheimer's disease and healthy control subjects in a large elderly cohort. Overall, we aim to define and simulate new models of network interaction, and observe if their properties can reveal biological differences between diagnostic groups.

## 2   Methods

Before designing the simulation, we assume that each subject has precomputed connectivity information that includes a parcellation of the cortex (and sometimes subcortical regions) into a set of regions with an accompanying $N \times N$ matrix characterizing their connectivity. Additionally, we also expect to know the location, size, and relationship of each region to every other region. There are several well-known approaches for partitioning the brain into a set of nodes, and for the purpose of representing the initial connectivity, our method allows any such connectivity matrix to be incorporated into our analysis.

In the following simulation design the various terms and forces are designed to restrict particle movement and bring them to a steady state reasonably quickly. We designed the particles so that their initial locations are the centroids of cortical regions and their masses are the corresponding volumes, but those initial locations are not enforced in the simulation and are quickly washed away in the early timesteps.

### 2.1   Gravitational $N$-Body Simulation

We now describe how we adapt the gravitational $N$-body simulation problem to brain networks. Each connectivity node corresponding to one of $N$ regions in the cortex, is treated as a particle whose mass is proportional to the region's volume. The equations of motions for each particle $i$, in the traditional $N$-body problem are

$$\ddot{r}_i = -G \sum_{j=1;j \neq i}^{N} \frac{m_j(r_i - r_j)}{|r_i - r_j|^3}. \tag{1}$$

where $\ddot{r}_i$, $m_i$, and $r_i$ are the acceleration, mass, and position of particle $i$, with $G$ as a gravitational constant; in astrophysics, this is simply a fixed universal constant. To allow for stronger interactions between some pairs of network nodes (particles), we set the gravitational term to be the value of the connectivity matrix indexed by $i$ and $j$ and modified the expression so that $G$ is replaced by

$G_{ij}$, which is the connectivity value for regions $i$ and $j$. Intuitively, this induces a force on each particle that depends on its connectivity strength with each of the others.

In addition to the gravitational force, we include an additional attraction term, a repulsion force, and a damping force. We also include an additional attraction term to deal with "evaporation", when particles acquire too much energy and become unbound. This prevents drifting of the centroid of the $N$-body system. We choose the attraction term to increase as the particle separation becomes greater, as

$$-G_{ij}m_j\hat{r}_{ij}\frac{(|r_{ij}|/R)^b}{r_0^2},\tag{2}$$

where $\hat{r}_{ij}$ is the unit direction of the vector from $i$ to $j$ and $|r_{ij}|$ is its norm. $R$ is the overall size of the space and (in our neuroimaging application) is set to the largest dimension of the T1-weighted brain image and $r_0 = RN^{-1/3}$ is the inter-particle spacing. If volume of the image space is $R^3$, the per-particle volume is $R^3/N$, making $((R^3)/N)^{(1/3)} = RN^{(-1/3)}$ the initial interparticle distance. The repulsion force keeps the particles from getting too close together and prevents Equation 1 from blowing up and decreasing the timestep of the numerical solver. It is also critical for bonding of the particles in an equilibrium state. Formally, the force is

$$G_{ij}m_j\hat{r}_{ij}\frac{d^{2a-2}}{|r_{ij}|^{2a}},\tag{3}$$

where $d = r_0/10$ and $a = 3$. Parameter $d$ specifies the typical distance between particles in the equilibrium state. We chose $d = r_0/10$ to give particles sufficient initial energy to allow randomization prior to the equilibrium state's development; however, this choice is somewhat arbitrary so long as $d << r_0$. The damping force moves the system into equilibrium over time and is

$$\frac{-v_i}{t_d},\tag{4}$$

where $t_d = 10$ and controls the strength of the damping and time till equilibrium.

The virial theorem [7] of gravitational dynamics is

$$2\langle T\rangle + \langle V\rangle = 0,\tag{5}$$

where $T$ is the kinetic energy of the system and $V$ is the potential energy. It ensures that the system reaches equilibrium over time. Given this we set the typical collision time to be $t_0 = 1$ so that $r_0/v_0 = 1$ and scaled the gravity, masses, and velocity accordingly.

When combined, our modified gravity force, the attraction term, repulsion force, and damping force, specify the equations of motion for a particle as

$$\ddot{r}_i = \sum_{j=1;j\neq i}^{N} G_{ij}\hat{r}_{ij}m_j\left(\frac{-1}{|r_i-r_j|^2} + \frac{d^{2a-2}}{|r_i-r_j|^{2a}} - \frac{(|r_i-r_j|/R)^b}{r_0^2}\right) - \frac{v_i}{t_d},\tag{6}$$

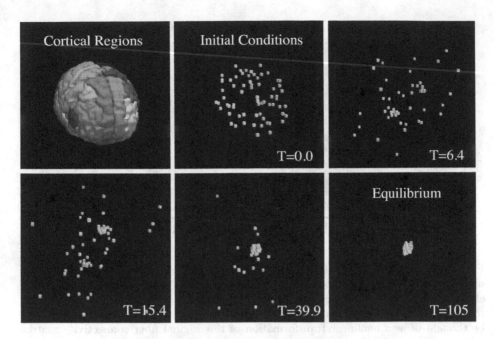

**Fig. 1.** We show a summary of states in our dynamical simulation of connectivity in the brain for a single subject. Each particle represents a region of the cortex and our initial conditions place a particle at the centroid of the corresponding region and assign it a mass proportional to the volume of the region. At time zero (T=0.0), we show the initial positions of all the particles coloring those in the right hemisphere green and those in the left hemisphere orange. The particles interact with each other depending on $G_{ij}$, which is proportional to their connectivity value and at T=6.4 and T=15.4 we can see two distinct clusters of particles in their respective hemispheres. At T=39.9 the kinetic energy of the system reduces as the system begins to reach equilibrium shown at T=105. We presented the cortical segmentation as a reminder of the initial configuration of the particles, but those locations are not enforced in the simulation and are quickly washed away in the early timesteps.

where the parameters could still be adjusted if we wanted to change how the simulation evolves. This set of equations are solved through numerical integration using the explicit Runge-Kutta (4,5) formula [8] with adaptive time steps. The simulation proceeds with the particles in each hemisphere forming clusters and ends by reaching an equilibrium configuration of the particles.

## 2.2 Simulation Features

We computed an $N$-body connectivity matrix derived from the equilibrium state. Each connectivity value represents the Euclidean distance between two particles in the final configuration with a comparison to the standard fiber connectivity matrix shown in Figure 2.

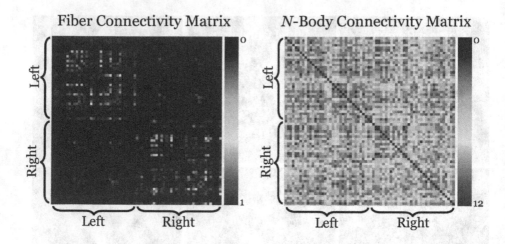

**Fig. 2.** We show the standard fiber connectivity matrix and our $N$-body connectivity matrix. The standard fiber connectivity matrix is an adjacency matrix where each element represents the connectivity strength between two region that is quantified by the number of fibers intersecting both regions. Our $N$-body connectivity matrix can be thought of as a nonlinear transformation of the original fiber connectivity matrix by incorporating the size and locations of the cortical regions into a dynamic system of particles.

The connectivity features we used from our method are the network measures derived from the $N$-body connectivity matrix, the time for the system to first reach equilibrium, the average speed for the centroid of the particles in addition to each particle, the total displacement of the centroid and the individual particles, and the change of distance from the initial and equilibrium states of the centroid and individual particles.

We tested the features from the simulation using two-sample $t$-tests to understand their ability to discriminate disease states in our data.

## 3   Experimental Results

We used a collection of 110 subjects scanned as part of the ADNI-2 [9], an extension of the ADNI project where diffusion imaging was added to the standard MRI protocol. The dataset was composed of 28 cognitively normal elderly controls (C), 56 early- and 11 late-stage MCI subjects (eMCI, LMCI), and 15 with Alzheimer's disease (AD). These subjects were scanned with a 3-Tesla GE Medical Systems scanner, which acquired both T1-weighted 3D anatomical spoiled gradient echo (SPGR) sequences ($256 \times 256$ matrix; voxel size = $1.2 \times 1.0 \times 1.0$ mm$^3$; TI=400 ms; TR = 6.98 ms; TE = 2.85 ms; flip angle = $11°$), and diffusion weighted images (DWI; $256 \times 256$ matrix; voxel size: $2.7 \times 2.7 \times 2.7$ mm$^3$; scan time = 9 min). The DWIs consisted of 41 diffusion images with $b = 1000$ s/mm$^2$ and 5 T2-weighted

$b_0$ images. To process the T1-weighted images, we automatically removed extra-cerebral tissues from the images, corrected for intensity inhomogeneities using the MNI N3 tool [10], and aligned to the Colin27 template [11] with FSL FLIRT [12]. We segmented the resulting images into 34 cortical regions (in each hemisphere) using FreeSurfer [13]. These labels were then dilated with an isotropic box kernel of $5 \times 5 \times 5$ voxels to ensure they overlapped the white matter for connectivity analysis. These images were corrected for head motion and eddy current distortion in each subject by aligning the DWI images to the average $b_0$ image with FSL's eddy correct tool. We skull-stripped the brain using FSL and EPI-corrected with an elastic mutual information registration algorithm that aligned the DWI images to the T1-weighted scans. We generated close to 5,000 tractography fibers for each subject using a probabilistic tractography algorithm [14] and used them to compute a corresponding connectivity matrix where the connectivity value was the number of fibers that intersected a pair of regions from our dilated cortical labels.

We ran the $N$-body simulation for 200 timesteps (T=0-200), which provided enough time for the system to reach equilibrium, usually after 100 timesteps. In Figure 1, we step through a simulation for one subject from our experimental dataset, and visually describe the positions of the particles and their relationship to the cortical regions of our connectivity analysis. Additionally, we compared this $N$-body connectivity matrix to the fiber connectivity matrix that we used to define $G_{ij}$ by computing ten different network measures [15]. These measures included mean eccentricity (ECC), global efficiency (GE), mean local efficiency (LE), mean degree (MD), transitivity, small world (SW), path length (PL), density, modularity, and the mean connectivity matrix (CM) value. We normalized the fiber connectivity matrix by the total number of fibers computed. We tested the features we computed during the simulation in two-sample $t$-tests comparing disease states in controls vs. AD, controls vs. LMCI, controls vs. e-MCI, and e-MCI vs. LMCI. We found the total displacement of the centroid over the simulation to be significant in discriminating controls vs. AD with a $p$-value of .012. We found the total displacement for one of the particles in the simulation was also significantly different comparing controls vs. AD with a $p$-value of

**Table 1.** We show the $p$-values from two-sample $t$-tests comparing features derived from the standard connectivity matrix versus our $N$-body connectivity matrix across a set of disease states that include 20 normal elderly controls, 56 early mild cognitively impaired (e-MCI) patients, 11 late MCI (LMCI) patients, and 15 Alzheimer's disease patients. We list the features with the lowest $p$-values. The features in the table are mean eccentricity (ECC), global efficiency (GE), mean connectivity matrix (CM) value, mean local efficiency (LE), and mean degree.

| Test | Fiber Connectivity | | $N$-Body Connectivity | |
|---|---|---|---|---|
| | Measure | $p$-value | Measure | $p$-value |
| Control vs. AD | Mean ECC | $8.73 \times 10^{-4}$ | Mean Degree | $1.29 \times 10^{-6}$ |
| Control vs. eMCI | GE | $3.10 \times 10^{-2}$ | Mean Degree | $8.40 \times 10^{-14}$ |
| Control vs. late-MCI | Mean CM | $1.44 \times 10^{-2}$ | Mean Degree | $1.55 \times 10^{-5}$ |
| eMCI vs. late-MCI | Mean LE | $1.69 \times 10^{-1}$ | Mean CM | $1.34 \times 10^{-4}$ |

$3.54 \times 10^{-4}$ which passes the multiple comparison correction threshold at .05. In addition, one of the mean particles speeds was significant in the controls vs. AD comparison with a $p$-value of $1.43 \times 10^{-5}$.

## 4  Discussion

We presented a novel approach that simulates the inter-nodal interactions using a $N$-body problem. Diffusion imaging has been used before to study degenerative brain diseases, and group differences have consistently been reported for diffusion indices such as mean diffusivity and fractional anisotropy, as well as more complex network measures of anatomical connectivity. As the AD progresses, some axonal fibers are lost, and prior work has mapped the effects of this loss on brain networks, using concepts such as the $k$-core (a network thresholded by nodal degree) and the rich club (a property whereby the highest degree network nodes are more mutually interconnected than would be expected based on their degree). As connectivity breakdown is typical of AD and other degenerative disorders [16], new connectivity models and metrics are of interest. The $N$-body matrices are effective in detecting AD effects as they combine information on connectivity and volumetric atrophy, as the gravitational force depends on the size of the regions. Information transfer in the brain is impaired by each of these factors, so their use as model properties is likely to lead to metrics that differentiate AD.

A popular model of brain development was advanced by Van Essen [17] who argued that the fissures in the cortex may be formed, in part, due to the physical force of tension along long axonal fibers during embryonic development. In our formulation, the dynamics do not attempt to encode actual forces but instead resemble the flow of information to local hubs and then on to other parts of the network. Currently, the $N$-body problem for brain allows a free-form movement of the particles or nodes of the connectivity matrix. An interesting idea would be to constrain their displacements so that the particles are only restricted to within the brain. In the future, we plan to investigate the particle$^3$-mesh method [18] that will allow us to incorporate morphological constraints along with network topology to simulate the dynamical underpinnings of human brain connectivity.

## References

1. Sporns, O., Tononi, G., Kötter, R.: The human connectome: a structural description of the human brain. PLoS Computational Biology 1(4), 1–42 (2005)
2. Hagmann, P., Cammoun, L., Gigandet, X., Meuli, R., Honey, C., Wedeen, V., Sporns, O.: Mapping the structural core of human cerebral cortex. PLoS Biology 6(7), e159 (2008)
3. Friston, K.: Functional and effective connectivity in neuroimaging: a synthesis. Human Brain Mapping 2(1-2), 56–78 (2004)
4. He, Y., Chen, Z., Evans, A.: Small-world anatomical networks in the human brain revealed by cortical thickness from MRI. Cerebral Cortex 17(10), 2407–2419 (2007)

5. Biswal, B., Zerrin Yetkin, F., Haughton, V., Hyde, J.: Functional connectivity in the motor cortex of resting human brain using echo-planar MRI. Magnetic Resonance in Medicine 34(4), 537–541 (1995)
6. Zhou, C., Zemanová, L., Zamora, G., Hilgetag, C., Kurths, J.: Hierarchical organization unveiled by functional connectivity in complex brain networks. Physical Review Letters 97(23), 238103 (2006)
7. Pollard, H.: Mathematical introduction to celestial mechanics, vol. 1. Prentice-Hall (1966)
8. Dormand, J., Prince, P.: A family of embedded Runge-Kutta formulae. Journal of Computational and Applied Mathematics 6(1), 19–26 (1980)
9. Trojanowski, J., Vandeerstichele, H., Korecka, M., Clark, C., Aisen, P., Petersen, R., Blennow, K., Soares, H., Simon, A., Lewczuk, P.: Update on the biomarker core of the Alzheimer's Disease Neuroimaging Initiative subjects. Alzheimer's & Dementia: The Journal of the Alzheimer's Association 6(3), 230 (2010)
10. Sled, J., Zijdenbos, A., Evans, A.C.: A nonparametric method for automatic correction of intensity nonuniformity in MRI data. IEEE Transactions on Medical Imaging 17(1), 87–97 (1998)
11. Holmes, C., Hoge, R., Collins, L., Woods, R., Toga, A., Evans, A.: Enhancement of MR images using registration for signal averaging. Journal of Computer Assisted Tomography 22(2), 324–333 (1998)
12. Jenkinson, M., Bannister, P., Brady, M., Smith, S.: Improved optimization for the robust and accurate linear registration and motion correction of brain images. NeuroImage 17(2), 825–841 (2002)
13. Fischl, B., Van Der Kouwe, A., Destrieux, C., Halgren, E., Ségonne, F., Salat, D., Busa, E., Seidman, L., Goldstein, J., Kennedy, D.: Automatically parcellating the human cerebral cortex. Cerebral Cortex 14(1), 11–22 (2004)
14. Behrens, T., Berg, H., Jbabdi, S., Rushworth, M., Woolrich, M.: Probabilistic diffusion tractography with multiple fibre orientations: What can we gain? NeuroImage 34(1), 144–155 (2007)
15. Rubinov, M., Sporns, O.: Complex network measures of brain connectivity: uses and interpretations. NeuroImage 52(3), 1059–1069 (2010)
16. Toga, A., Thompson, P.: Connectomics sheds new light on Alzheimer's disease. Biological Psychiatry 73(5), 390–392 (2013)
17. Van Essen, D.: A tension-based theory of morphogenesis and compact wiring in the central nervous system. Nature, 313–318 (1997)
18. Eastwood, J., Hockney, R., Lawrence, D.: P3M3DP-The three-dimensional periodic particle-particle/particle-mesh program. Computer Physics Communications 19, 215–261 (1980)

# Cortical Surface Analysis of Multi-contrast MR Data to Improve Detection of Cortical Pathology in Multiple Sclerosis

Marika Archambault-Wallenburg, Douglas Arnold, Sridar Narayanan, G. Bruce Pike, and D. Louis Collins

Montreal Neurological Institute
McGill University, Montreal

**Abstract.** Cortical multiple sclerosis (MS) lesions are very hard to detect on magnetic resonance images, even though histopathology studies reveal that their extent can be important. Certain pulse sequences are known to help detect the lesions, but this detection is still very incomplete. To aid detection, we propose to use a cortical surface-based analysis of multi-contrast MR data in MS and healthy control subjects. We show that magnetization transfer ratio and T1-weighted scans both show differences at the group level between relapsing-remitting MS patients and healthy controls. This suggests that this approach would be useful to help detect cortical pathology in MS.

**Keywords:** Laminar profile, cortex, multiple sclerosis, intensity standardization.

## 1 Introduction

Multiple sclerosis (MS) is a demyelinating disease of the central nervous system. Focal areas of demyelination in the white matter ("lesions") are readily apparent on conventional magnetic resonance (MR) images as hyperintense spots on T2w scans and on Gadolinium-enhanced T1w scans (in their active phase), and occasionally as hypointense spots on T1w scans (generally in their chronic phase). Subtle changes in normal-appearing white matter can also be detected by more sophisticated MR methods such as magnetization transfer ratio (MTR) [1].

MS pathology in cortical grey matter is much harder to image. Post-mortem histopathology studies have revealed that cortical involvement is present in a large fraction of patients [2] and increases as the disease progresses [3], yet cortical lesions are rarely visible on conventional MR [4,5]. The thinness of the cortex, the presence of partial voluming effects in the voxels adjacent to cerebrospinal fluid (CSF), the low myelin content of the grey matter and absent or low inflammation could all contribute to this effect [5]. Subpial lesions, which extend from the meninges into the cortex, are the most prevalent but also the hardest to see, while juxtacortical lesions, which are mixed with white matter, are the most visible [6,7]. The other types of cortical lesions (intracortical and

L. Shen et al. (Eds.): MBIA 2013, LNCS 8159, pp. 138–149, 2013.

whole-width) represent only 15 and 8 percent of lesions respectively [6]. While difficult to detect, cortical pathology has been linked to cognitive impairment [8], and it is therefore crucial to be able to measure its extent *in vivo*.

Particular MR sequences, including DIR, FLAIR, and high-field MP-RAGE, have been shown to facilitate detection of cortical lesions. However, comparisons with post-mortem scans show that a considerable proportion of lesions are missed by each sequence [5,9,10]. Other methods more adapted to visualizing myelin content in the brain, like myelin water fraction [11] and magnetization transfer ratio [12,13], have been applied to the cortex with some success.

In this paper, we test the hypothesis that cortical surface analysis of MR data can enhance detection of cortical anomalies in multiple sclerosis by comparing multi-contrast data in MS subjects and normal controls. Specifically, our method models the normal distributions of MR intensity features in healthy controls and uses this as a benchmark to compare MR intensity feature values in MS subjects.

## 2 Methods

### 2.1 Subjects

The data used in this paper were taken from the first time point of a longitudinal study of patients with MS conducted at the Montreal Neurological Institute and Hospital (MNI/MNH). Patients were recruited from the MS clinic at the MNH. Recruitment criteria included some degree of cognitive disability as indicated by a score of $\geq 1$ on the cerebral functional system sub scale of Kurtzke's expanded disability status scale (EDSS) [14]. Patients about to start disease-modifying treatment were excluded from the study. Healthy volunteers matched for age and education level (but not gender) were recruited to serve as a healthy control group. The data used for this paper consisted of MR scans of 20 MS subjects (17 relapsing-remitting [RR], 1 primary progressive [PP] and 2 secondary progressive [SP]) and 13 healthy control (HC) subjects.

### 2.2 Data Acquisition

All MR data was acquired on a 3T Siemens TIM Trio scanner at the MNI. For each subject, structural T1-weighted FLASH and dual TSE T2w/PDw scans were performed (see Table 1). MTR was acquired from a PDw MT-OFF/MT-ON image pair (Siemens MT pulse: 1200Hz off-resonance, 9.984 ms duration, 100 Hz bandwidth, 500° effective pulse angle). MTR values were abnormally low in two HC subjects ($\approx 20\%$ lower than in other HC subjects): data from these subjects was ignored for our analysis.

### 2.3 Preprocessing and Lesion in-Painting

In order to compare T1w, T2w and PDw intensities in different scans, it was important to normalize the intensities so they would be in an equivalent range.

**Table 1.** MR acquisition parameters

| Sequence | T1w FLASH | PDw/T2w | MT-ON/OFF |
|---|---|---|---|
| Sequence | 3D FLASH | dual TSE | 3D FLASH |
| Orientation | axial | axial | axial |
| TR (ms) | 20 | 2100 | 33 |
| TE (ms) | 5 | 16/80 | 3.81 |
| Excitation angle | 27 | 12 | 10 |
| Slice thickness (mm) | 1 | 3 | 1 |
| In-plane resolution (mm) | 1 x 1 | 1 x 1 | 1 x 1 |

Note that MTR does not need to be normalized as it is already a semi-quantitative measure. Most intensity standardization techniques in the literature (e.g. Nyul *et al.* [15]) rely on some form of histogram matching that makes the implicit assumption that the underlying composition of tissues in all subjects/brains is the same (so that white matter in all brains should have the same intensity and an equivalent volume, for example). Because in MS the pathology is known to affect properties of the brain tissue even in areas where there are no lesions (so-called normal appearing white/grey matter), such an assumption cannot be made and these methods are inadequate for our purposes. We therefore used non-brain tissue (defined as all tissue visible on the MR scan with the exception of the brain; that is, muscle, bone, fat, skin) to perform intensity scaling, based on the assumption that MS should not significantly affect the composition of these tissues. This standardization was performed after non-uniformity correction using N3 [16]. T1w intensities were linearly rescaled so that the 0.5th percentile and 99.5th percentile of the non-brain tissue intensities were re-mapped to 1 and to 1000 respectively on an arbitrary standard scale. Because both T2w and PDw non-brain tissue intensity histogram had a distinct peak at low intensities, we used this feature for intensity standardization between scans. The intensities were linearly rescaled on both the T2w and PDw scans so that the non-brain low-intensity peak was re-mapped to 500 while the 99.5th non-brain intensity percentile was mapped to 1000.

Because MS lesions in the white matter are often hypointense on T1w images, voxels in white matter lesions adjacent to grey matter structures may be mistaken for grey matter voxels by classification algorithms, which can seriously decrease the quality of a subsequent cortical extraction. To reduce occurrences of this problem, the intensity of voxels in white matter lesions were artificially corrected to match more closely that of the surrounding normal white matter voxels. Lesions masks were defined automatically on the T2w image, and then manually corrected. The T2w lesion masks were resampled to the T1w image space after linear registration of the T1w and T2w images, and the masks were dilated once. An implementation of the in-painting method developed by Criminisi *et al.* [17] was used to in-paint the areas defined by the lesion mask on the T1w volume; this method has the advantage of retaining borders quite well, which is important to maintain the boundary between white and grey matter intact as much as possible.

## 2.4   Cortical Extraction

Pre-processed T1-weighted images were used for cortical extraction. In pre-processing, the images were corrected for non-uniformity using N3 [16], denoised using a non-local means method [18] and lesion in-painted. The FreeSurfer cortical extraction pipeline [19] was run on all subjects. Manual corrections were made at intermediate steps of the cortical extraction as needed (e.g. adjusting the threshold of the initial brain segmentation or manually editing erroneous brain masks). The cortical extraction failed in three subjects (2 RRMS, 1 PPMS): these data were not included in further analysis.

After cortical extraction, each cortical surface was registered to a common template (fsaverage) based on surface curvature pattern as part of the FreeSurfer pipeline [20]. In order to have the same number of vertices in all subjects, we performed an extra registration step in which each point on the spherical template surface was associated with its closest point on the spherical registered subject surface. In this way we obtained for each subject the correspondence between vertices on the native surfaces and on the template surface. This correspondence was used later in our analysis.

## 2.5   Cortical Post-Processing

Cortical profiles were created by extending a straight line from each outer surface vertex to the corresponding inner vertex surface (where correspondence was intrinsically known from the FreeSurfer cortical extraction process). Twenty-one equally spaced points were created along each profile, with point coordinates interpolated from the coordinates of the outer and inner surface vertices. This number was chosen arbitrarily to allow flexibility in the definitions of features, as it allows us to separate the cortical thickness into a two, four, five or ten sections. The cortical thickness at each point was defined as the real-space distance between these vertices.

## 2.6   Features

Nine features were defined at each vertex of the cortical surfaces. These included cortical thickness and two features per contrast (MTR, T1w, T2w, PDw). A value of each contrast was estimated at all profile points (21 per vertex) by linear interpolation on the raw MTR data and after non-uniformity correction and intensity standardization (but not lesion in-painting) for T1w, T2w and PDw data. These values were smoothed along the cortical surface with a smoothing kernel of size 5 (FWHM, in mesh units) using the SurfStatSmooth tool of the SurfStat Toolbox [21] to reduce the noise. Blurring along the cortical surface gives an important advantage over blurring in the 3D volumetric data, as it is possible to blur across the grey matter, white matter and CSF voxels in the latter while blurring is constrained to the cortical grey matter in the former.

The features were defined as the intensity at mid-cortical depth, and the ratio between the intensity in the inner half and outer half of the cortical thickness

**Table 2.** Feature definitions

| Feature | Definition |
|---|---|
| 1 | Cortical thickness (mm) |
| 2 | MTR at mid-cortical surface |
| 3 | ratio of inner to outer MTR |
| 4 | T1w intensity at mid-cortical surface |
| 5 | ratio of inner to outer T1w intensity |
| 6 | T2w intensity at mid-cortical surface |
| 7 | ratio of inner to outer T2w intensity |
| 8 | PDw intensity at mid-cortical surface |
| 9 | ratio of inner to outer PDw intensity |

(see Table 2. These features were selected for their predicted sensitivity to sub-pial, mixed grey-white matter, and whole-cortical width lesions.

## 2.7   Normal Model

Using the set of correspondence between each cortical surface and the template surface (see Section 2.4), features from all subjects were mapped onto a common template surface. The values were smoothed along the template surface using the SurfStatSmooth tool with a kernel size of 8 (FWHM, in mesh units). For each vertex, a model of normal feature value distribution was established by fitting a Gaussian to the distribution of feature values in that vertex across all healthy control subjects. While the distribution of these feature values is not perfectly Gaussian, this representation was deemed adequate for this study. This yielded a very compact description of the model, as it was completely defined by the values of $\mu$ and $\sigma$ at each vertex of the template surface facilitating comparison of the MS patient data to the normal model. After mapping into the common surface space as described above, the MS patient data can be compared in a vertex-to-vertex fashion to obtain a local z-score. In addition, to verify the model, each healthy control subject was compared to a model of normal feature distribution based on all other healthy control subjects in a leave-one-out fashion.

## 2.8   Visualization on MR

The results of the surface-based analysis were finally mapped back to the original MR volumes to allow visualization of the feature (or z-score) values simultaneously with the MR data. The feature values at each vertex of the surfaces were propagated to all voxels that the profile crosses.

## 3   Results

The effects of lesion in-painting are shown in Figure 1. Most lesions are effectively removed, with the exception of very large lesions that sometimes retain a core of low intensity values, but this almost always occurs well away from the cortical surface.

Intensity standardization made the intensities of T1w, PD2w and T2w images much more similar (see Figures 2). The bounds used for re-scaling (percentile values and peak locations) were not significantly different in the HC and MS groups (see Table 3), suggesting that these are good reference intensities since they appear to be independent of disease status.

Figure 3 shows cortical thickness in mm as a z-score for two subjects (one HC and one RR). Figure 4 shows the averaged z-score of all the HC subjects, all the RR subjects and all the SP subjects. Qualitatively, we find that on average,

- cortical thickness is lower in RR, and much lower in SP MS subjects;
- MTR at midsurface is lower in RR and SP MS subjects;
- the ratio of inner to outer cortical MTR is higher in RR and SP MS subjects;
- T1w intensity at midsurface is slightly lower in RR, and much lower in SP MS subjects;
- the ratio of inner to outer cortical T1w intensity is higher in RR, and much higher in SP MS subjects;
- T2w intensity at midsurface is lower in RR, and more extreme (high and low) in SP MS subjects;
- the ratio of inner to outer cortical T2w intensity is higher in SP;
- PDw intensity at midsurface is lower in RR and much lower in SP MS subjects.

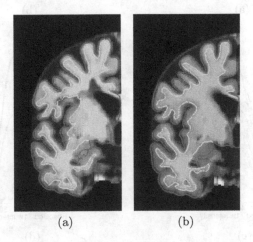

(a)                              (b)

**Fig. 1.** Outer (*red*) and inner (*yellow*) cortical surfaces resulting from cortical extraction on original T1w image (a) and lesion-inpainted T1w image (b)

## 4   Discussion

Our results are in agreement with previously published reports of decreased cortical thickness [22], decreased cortical MTR [12,23]; increased ratio of inner to outer cortical MTR [24]; and decreased cortical T1w intensity [25].

**Table 3.** Reference intensity values used for intensity standardization (mean ± standard deviation)

| Contrast | HC subjects | | MS subjects | |
|---|---|---|---|---|
| | low | high | low | high |
| T1w | 2.3 ± 0.6 | 380 ± 60 | 2.4 ± 0.6 | 390 ± 40 |
| T2w | 240 ± 30 | 1190 ± 80 | 240 ± 40 | 1230 ± 140 |
| PDw | 810 ± 130 | 1800 ± 200 | 810 ± 180 | 1870 ± 80 |

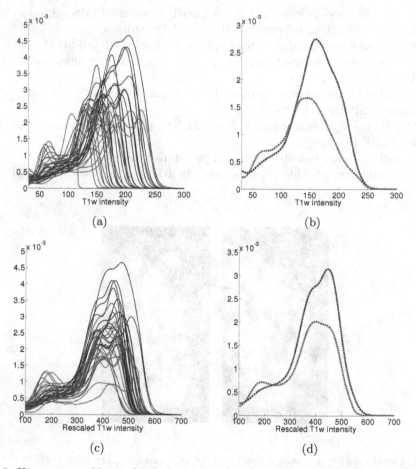

**Fig. 2.** Histograms of brain (excluding lesions) T1w intensity values for MS subjects (*red*) and HC subjects (*blue*) before (a) and after (c) intensity standardization, and corresponding cumulative histograms (b,d) for all MS (*red*) and all HC (*blue*) subjects

A recent post-mortem study by Tardif *et al.* [26] found increased T1 values in subpial lesions compared to normal-appearing cortex, which is consistent with our observation of higher T1w inner-to-outer intensity ratio in MS subjects. Subpial lesions would cause a decrease in T1w intensity along the outer cortical

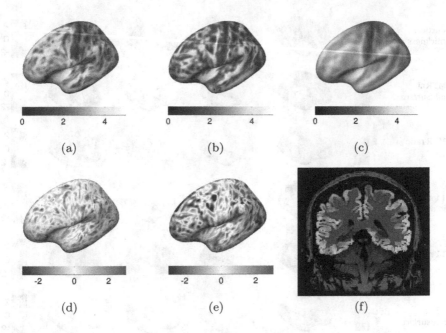

**Fig. 3.** Example results displayed on inflated template surface (left hemisphere only). Cortical thickness in one HC subject (a) and in one RR MS subject (b); model mean cortical thickness (c ); z-score of cortical thickness in same HC subject (d) and RR MS subject (e); overlay of cortical thickness on MR volume (T1w) in same HC subject (f).

surface (as T1 values are known to correlate with myelin content in the cortex [27]).

We find that T2w intensity is lower in RR subjects, while in SP subjects, the T2w intensity was higher in some regions but lower in other (this was a pattern present in both subjects rather than an artefact of averaging) and the ratio of inner to outer cortical T2w intensity was higher. According to Tardif *et al.* [26], the T2 values of cortical lesions are higher than those of normal-appearing cortex, which should result in higher T2w midcortical intensities. The higher ratio of inner to outer cortical T2w intensities could result from T2 increases in mixed grey-white lesions, or might be the result of partial volume effects with CSF in the outer cortical layers. This hypothesis will be tested in future work by evaluating the correlation between cortical thickness and T2w intensity.

Finally, we find that PDw intensity was reduced in MS subjects, in contrast to white matter PDw intensity which is known to be higher in white matter lesions. This could be due to a lack of edema/inflammation in the grey matter combined with neuronal loss, though partial volume effects with CSF could also be at play.

The model presented here is observer independent and therefore provides an unbiased description of changes in the cortical grey matter, as opposed to lesion counts, for example, which might vary across observers. This model also combines

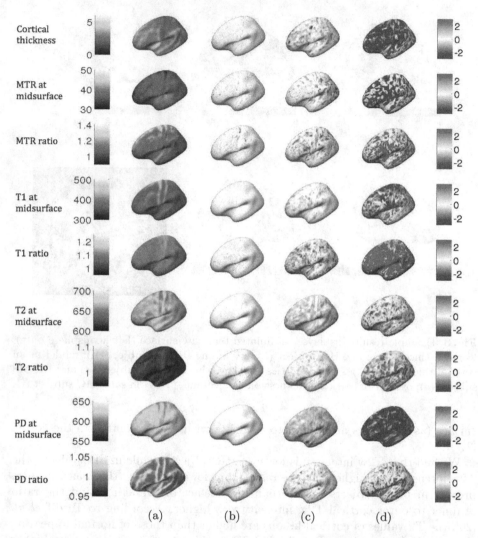

**Fig. 4.** Group averages displayed on inflated template surface (left hemisphere only). Model mean feature value (a), mean z-scores of 11 HC subjects (b), 16 RR subjects (c), and 2 SP subjects (d).

information from multiple contrasts as well as cortical thickness, which should make it more sensitive to cortical pathology than methods that rely on any single measurement/contrast (e.g. cortical thickness, MTR, DIR). Moreover, by considering local feature behaviour along the cortical surface, we eliminate some of the anatomically dependent variation in MR contrast intensities and patterns, though this introduces some dependence on the quality of the surface registration to the template surface.

This method is sensitive to failures of the cortical extraction, as failure to include abnormal cortical tissue (for example, because in subpial lesions, the decreased T1w intensity values at the outer edge of the cortex could shift the detected pial surface inward) would skew our results. A failure of this kind would be difficult to detect by visual inspection of the cortical surface on MRI images, since subpial lesions can be thin and quite extensive and therefore the effect on the cortical extraction would be subtle. Extending all cortical profiles outwards towards the CSF would provide confidence that the entire cortex is included, and could allow detection of subtle differences between low-T1w-intensity cortex and CSF. Similarly, extending cortical profiles towards the white matter would help insure that no mixed white-grey matter lesions are missed.

A specific and sensitive method of detection of cortical disease *in vivo* is essential to study progression and pathology of cortical disease, and this paper presents a novel method to detect cortical lesions and anomalies in multiple sclerosis. We plan to extend this work (1) to consider individual subject classification based on cortical MR features; (2) to evaluate the relationship between cortical features and manually labeled cortical lesions visible on DIR; and (3) to look for correlations of these features with gender and with cognitive impairment. Finally, a better validation will involve applying this technique to post-mortem data for which some histopathology results are available.

**Acknowledgments.** The authors thank Damien Garcia for the inpainting implementation and Mishkin Derakshan for his help with and insights into data processing.

# References

1. Cercignani, M., Bozzali, M., Iannucci, G., Comi, G., Filippi, M.: Magnetisation transfer ratio and mean diffusivity of normal appearing white and grey matter from patients with multiple sclerosis. Journal of Neurology, Neurosurgery & Psychiatry 70(3), 311–317 (2001)
2. Kidd, D., Barkhof, F., McConnell, R., Algra, P., Allen, I., Revesz, T.: Cortical lesions in multiple sclerosis. Brain 122(1), 17–26 (1999)
3. Kutzelnigg, A.: Cortical demyelination and diffuse white matter injury in multiple sclerosis. Brain 128(11), 2705–2712 (2005)
4. Bakshi, R., Thompson, A.J., Rocca, M.A., Pelletier, D., Dousset, V., Barkhof, F., Inglese, M., Guttmann, C.R., Horsfield, M.A., Filippi, M.: MRI in multiple sclerosis: current status and future prospects. The Lancet Neurology 7(7), 615–625 (2008)
5. Geurts, J.J.G., Bo, L., Pouwels, P.J.W., Castelijns, J.A., Polman, C.H., Barkhof, F.: Cortical lesions in multiple sclerosis: combined postmortem MR imaging and histopathology. American Journal of Neuroradiology 26(3), 572–577 (2005)
6. Bo, L., Vedeler, C.A., Nyland, H.I., Trapp, B.D., Mørk, S.J.: Subpial demyelination in the cerebral cortex of multiple sclerosis patients. Journal of Neuropathology & Experimental Neurology 62(7), 723–732 (2003)
7. Peterson, J.W., Bö, L., Mörk, S., Chang, A., Trapp, B.D.: Transected neurites, apoptotic neurons, and reduced inflammation in cortical multiple sclerosis lesions. Ann. Neurol. 50(3), 389–400 (2001)

8. Calabrese, M., Agosta, F., Rinaldi, F., Mattisi, I., Grossi, P., Favaretto, A., Atzori, M., Bernardi, V., Barachino, L., Rinaldi, L.: Cortical lesions and atrophy associated with cognitive impairment in relapsing-remitting multiple sclerosis. Archives of Neurology 66(9), 1144 (2009)
9. Bagnato, F., Yao, B., Cantor, F., Merkle, H., Condon, E., Montequin, M., Moore, S., Quezado, M., Tkaczyk, D., McFarland, H.: Multisequence-imaging protocols to detect cortical lesions of patients with multiple sclerosis: Observations from a post-mortem 3 Tesla imaging study. Journal of the Neurological Sciences 282(1-2), 80–85 (2009)
10. Tallantyre, E.C., Morgan, P.S., Dixon, J.E., Al-Radaideh, A., Brookes, M.J., Morris, P.G., Evangelou, N.: 3 Tesla and 7 Tesla MRI of multiple sclerosis cortical lesions. J. Magn. Reson. Imaging 32(4), 971–977 (2010)
11. Laule, C., Kozlowski, P., Leung, E., Li, D.K.B., MacKay, A.L., Moore, G.R.W.: Myelin water imaging of multiple sclerosis at 7 T: Correlations with histopathology. NeuroImage 40(4), 1575–1580 (2008)
12. Schmierer, K., Scaravilli, F., Altmann, D.R., Barker, G.J., Miller, D.H.: Magnetization transfer ratio and myelin in postmortem multiple sclerosis brain. Ann. Neurol. 56(3), 407–415 (2004)
13. Derakhshan, M., Caramanos, Z., Narayanan, S., Arnold, D.L., Collins, D.L.: Surface-based analysis reveals regions of reduced cortical magnetization transfer ratio in patients with multiple sclerosis. Human Brain Mapping (in press)
14. Kurtzke, J.F.: Rating neurologic impairment in multiple sclerosis: An expanded disability status scale (EDSS). Neurology 33(11), 1444 (1983)
15. Nyul, L.G., Udupa, J.K., Zhang, X.: New variants of a method of MRI scale standardization. IEEE Transactions on Medical Imaging 19(2), 143–150 (2000)
16. Sled, J.G., Zijdenbos, A.P., Evans, A.C.: A nonparametric method for automatic correction of intensity nonuniformity in MRI data. IEEE Transactions on Medical Imaging 17(1), 87–97 (1998)
17. Criminisi, A., Pérez, P., Toyama, K.: Region filling and object removal by exemplar-based image inpainting. IEEE Transactions on Image Processing 13(9), 1200–1212 (2004)
18. Coupé, P., Yger, P., Barillot, C.: Fast non local means denoising for 3D MR images. In: Larsen, R., Nielsen, M., Sporring, J. (eds.) MICCAI 2006. LNCS, vol. 4191, pp. 33–40. Springer, Heidelberg (2006)
19. Fischl, B., Sereno, M.I., Dale, A.M.: Cortical surface-based analysis. NeuroImage (1999)
20. Fischl, B., Sereno, M.I., Dale, A.M.: Cortical Surface-Based Analysis: II: Inflation, Flattening, and a Surface-Based Coordinate System. NeuroImage 9(2), 195–207 (1999)
21. Worsley, K.J.: SurfSt at, http://www.math.mcgill.ca/keith/surfstat/
22. Charil, A., Dagher, A., Lerch, J.P., Zijdenbos, A.P., Worsley, K.J., Evans, A.C.: Focal cortical atrophy in multiple sclerosis: Relation to lesion load and disability. NeuroImage 34(2), 509–517 (2007)
23. Derakhshan, M., Caramanos, Z., Narayanan, S., Collins, D.L., Arnold, D.L.: Regions of reduced cortical magnetization transfer ratio detected in MS patients using surface-based techniques. In: Proceedings of the 17th Annual Meeting of ISMRM, Honolulu, USA, p. 338 (2009)
24. Samson, R., Cardoso, M., Muhlert, N., Sethi, V., Wheeler-Kingshott, C.A.M., Ourselin, S., Ron, M., Miller, D.H., Chard, D.T.: MTR analysis of inner and outer cortical bands in multiple sclerosis. In: ECTRIMS 2012, Lyon, France (2012)

25. Vrenken, H., Geurts, J.J.G., Knol, D.L., van Dijk, L.N., Dattola, V., Jasperse, B., van Schijndel, R.A., Polman, C.H., Castelijns, J.A., Barkhof, F., Pouwels, P.J.W.: Whole-Brain T1 Mapping in Multiple Sclerosis: Global Changes of Normal-appearing Gray and White Matter. Radiology 240(3), 811–820 (2006)
26. Tardif, C.L., Bedell, B.J., Eskildsen, S.F., Collins, D.L., Pike, G.B.: Quantitative Magnetic Resonance Imaging of Cortical Multiple Sclerosis Pathology. Multiple Sclerosis International 2012(7), 1–13 (2012)
27. Eickhoff, S., Walters, N.B., Schleicher, A., Kril, J., Egan, G.F., Zilles, K., Watson, J.D.G., Amunts, K.: High-resolution MRI reflects myeloarchitecture and cytoarchitecture of human cerebral cortex. Human Brain Mapping 24(3), 206–215 (2005)

# *PARP1* Gene Variation and Microglial Activity on [11C]PBR28 PET in Older Adults at Risk for Alzheimer's Disease

Sungeun Kim[1-3,6], Kwangsik Nho[1,2,6], Shannon L. Risacher[1,3],
Mark Inlow[4], Shanker Swaminathan[1], Karmen K. Yoder[1,3,6], Li Shen[1-3,6],
John D. West[1], Brenna C. McDonald[1,3,5,6], Eileen F. Tallman[1,3], Gary D. Hutchins[1,3,6],
James W. Fletcher[1,6], Martin R. Farlow[3,5],
Bernardino Ghetti[3,7], and Andrew J. Saykin[1-3,5,6,8,*]

[1] Center for Neuroimaging, Department of Radiology and Imaging Sciences
[2] Center for Computational Biology and Bioinformatics
[3] Indiana Alzheimer Disease Center, Indiana University School of Medicine,
Indianapolis, IN, USA
[4] Department of Mathematics, Rose-Hulman Institute of Technology, Terre Haute, IN, USA
[5] Department of Neurology
[6] Indiana Institute for Biomedical Imaging Sciences
[7] Department of Pathology and Laboratory Medicine
[8] Department of Medical and Molecular Genetics,
Indiana University School of Medicine, Indianapolis, IN, USA

**Abstract.** Increasing evidence suggests that inflammation is one pathophysiological mechanism in Alzheimer's disease (AD). Recent studies have identified an association between the poly (ADP-ribose) polymerase 1 (*PARP1*) gene and AD. This gene encodes a protein that is involved in many biological functions, including DNA repair and chromatin remodeling, and is a mediator of inflammation. Therefore, we performed a targeted genetic association analysis to investigate the relationship between the *PARP1* polymorphisms and brain microglial activity as indexed by [11C]PBR28 positron emission tomography (PET). Participants were 26 non-Hispanic Caucasians in the Indiana Memory and Aging Study (IMAS). PET data were intensity-normalized by injected dose/total body weight. Average [11C]PBR28 standardized uptake values (SUV) from 6 bilateral regions of interest (thalamus, frontal, parietal, temporal, and cingulate cortices, and whole brain gray matter) were used as endophenotypes. Single nucleotide polymorphisms (SNPs) with 20% minor allele frequency that were within +/- 20 kb of the *PARP1* gene were included in the analyses. Gene-level association analyses were performed using a dominant genetic model with translocator protein (18-kDa) (*TSPO*) genotype, age at PET scan, and gender as covariates. Analyses were performed with and without *APOE* ε4 status as a covariate. Associations with [11C]PBR28 SUVs from thalamus and cingulate were significant at corrected $p<0.014$ and $<0.065$, respectively. Subsequent multi-marker analysis with cingulate [11C]PBR28 SUV showed that

---

\* Corresponding author.

L. Shen et al. (Eds.): MBIA 2013, LNCS 8159, pp. 150–158, 2013.

individuals with the "C" allele at rs6677172 and "A" allele at rs61835377 had higher [¹¹C]PBR28 SUV than individuals without these alleles (corrected $P<0.03$), and individuals with the "G" allele at rs6677172 and "G" allele at rs61835377 displayed the opposite trend (corrected $P<0.065$). A previous study with the same cohort showed an inverse relationship between [¹¹C]PBR28 SUV and brain atrophy at a follow-up visit, suggesting possible protective effect of microglial activity against cortical atrophy. Interestingly, all 6 AD and 2 of 3 LMCI participants in the current analysis had one or more copies of the "GG" allele combination, associated with lower cingulate [¹¹C]PBR28 SUV, suggesting that this gene variant warrants further investigation.

# 1    Introduction

Alzheimer's disease (AD) is the most common form of dementia and a progressive, degenerative disorder resulting in loss of memory at first, and eventually affecting all cognition and behavior. Increasing evidence suggests that failed or dysregulated immune response is one candidate mechanism contributing to the pathogenesis of AD [1-4]. Recent large-scale genome-wide association studies (GWAS) have identified several candidate genetic variants in *CLU, CR1, ABCA7, BIN1, PICALM, CD33, CD2AP, EPHA1* and *MS4A6A/MS4A6E* in addition to the most robust candidate gene, *APOE* [5-8]. Several of these genes are known to be involved in immune system functioning   [2, 3].

The poly (ADP-ribose) polymerase 1 (*PARP1*) gene plays roles in many biological functions including chromatin remodeling, DNA repair, telomere maintenance, and is known to be a mediator of inflammation via regulation of NF-kB and other transcription factors [9]. Several studies have investigated the *PARP1* gene in relation to AD [9-12], reporting risk and protective haplotypes [10], enhanced activity of *PARP1* in AD brain [12], and association with rate of hippocampal atrophy [11].

The peripheral benzodiazepine receptor (PBR; official name – translocator protein (18kDa), *TSPO*) is expressed at low levels in relatively inactive microglia. Microglia play an early critical role in activation of the immune response in the central nervous system [13]. Because activated microglia apparently express higher levels of TSPO than inactive microglia, PBR has been considered a useful marker to detect neuroinflammation. Positron emission tomography (PET) imaging with the radioligand [¹¹C]N-acetyl-N-(2-methoxybenzyl)-2-phenoxy-5-pyridinamine ([¹¹C]PBR28) has shown high selectivity for the TSPO in vivo [14]. The goal of this study was to investigate the relationship between *PARP1* gene variation and microglial activity indexed by [¹¹C]PBR28 PET.

# 2    Materials and Methods

## 2.1    Participants

In order to reduce the potential bias of population stratification, analyses were restricted to 26 non-Hispanic Caucasian participants from the Indiana Memory and Aging Study (IMAS) cohort. IMAS is an ongoing longitudinal study, including euthymic older adults with subjective cognitive decline (SCD), defined by memory concerns (e.g., self-perceived decline) in the context of cognitive test performance that is within the normal range, patients with early and late amnestic mild cognitive impairment (EMCI and LMCI) or mild AD, and age-matched cognitively normal controls (NC) without significant cognitive complaints or concerns. Details regarding participant selection criteria and characterization have been described previously [15, 16]. This study was approved by the Indiana University School of Medicine Institutional Review Board and written informed consent was obtained from all participants. The 26 participants in the study included 7 NC, 6 CC, 4 EMCI, 3 LMCI, and 6 AD. Table 1 shows the sample characteristics. *APOE* ε2/ε3/ε4 genotype, genome-wide genotyping data, and [$^{11}$C]PBR28 PET scans were available for all participants. It has been shown that the rs6971 variant in the *TSPO* gene affects in vivo binding affinity of the [$^{11}$C]PBR28 ligand [17, 18]. Subjects with genotypes corresponding to mixed or high affinity sites at the TSPO were included in the study; one "non-binder" (low-affinity TSPO phenotype) was excluded.

**Table 1.** Sample Characteristics

| Characteristics | All | NC | SCD | EMCI | LMCI | AD |
|---|---|---|---|---|---|---|
| Number of Samples | 26 | 7 | 6 | 4 | 3 | 6 |
| Age at PET scan (years; mean±SD) | 71.3±7.49 | 68.4±2.64 | 70.3±9.81 | 74.5±6.95 | 72.7±5.69 | 72.7±10.48 |
| Education (years; mean±SD) | 16.4±2.78 | 16.3±1.70 | 17.3±1.21 | 15.5±4.12 | 15.3±3.06 | 16.5±4.18 |
| Gender (M/F) | 9/17 | 1/6 | 2/4 | 2/2 | 2/1 | 2/4 |
| *APOE* (ε4-/ε4+) | 15/11 | 3/4 | 4/2 | 3/1 | 2/1 | 3/3 |
| *TSPO* genotype (Mixed/High) | 9/17 | 2/5 | 1/5 | 3/1 | 2/1 | 1/5 |

## 2.2    Data and Quality Control Procedure

**Genetic Data.** Genotyping was performed on genomic DNA from blood using the Illumina HumanOmniExpress BeadChip (Illumina, Inc., San Diego, CA), which contains over 700,000 SNP (single nucleotide polymorphism) markers, according to the manufacturer's protocols (Infinium HD Assay; Super Protocol Guide; Rev. A, May 2008). *APOE* ε2/ε3/ε4 genotyping was separately performed. All genotype data, including two *APOE* SNPs (rs429358 and rs7412), underwent standard quality control (QC) assessment using PLINK v1.07 [19] as described previously [20]. SNPs were imputed using the 1000 Genomes reference panel (http://www.1000genomes.org/) following the Enhancing Neuroimaging Genetics through Meta-Analysis 2 (ENIGMA 2) imputation protocol (http://enigma.loni.ucla.edu/wp-content/uploads/2012/07/ENIGMA2_1KGP_v3.pdf [27 July 2012]). Some imputed SNPs were removed based on the following criteria: $r^2 < 0.5$ between imputed and the nearest genotyped SNPs. After all QC steps, 96 SNPs with 20% minor allele frequency that were within +/- 20 kb of the *PARP1* gene were included in the analyses.

**Imaging Data.** Dynamic PET scans, acquired on a Siemens HR+, were initiated with injection of 512.33±75.83 MBq of [$^{11}$C]PBR28. Data were acquired for 90 min (10x30s, 9x60s, 2x180s, 8x300s, 3x600s). PET data were processed as described previously [18]. In brief, PET data were motion-corrected and normalized to MNI space. Static images were created from data between 40-90 min, and were normalized by injected dose/total body weight to produce standardized uptake value (SUV) images. Regions of interest (ROIs) were generated from each subject's anatomic MRI, which was concurrently acquired on a Siemens Tim Trio using an MPRAGE sequence and post processed using Freesurfer v4.0.1 (http://surfer.nmr.mgh.harvard.edu/). Average [$^{11}$C]PBR28 SUV values were extracted from 6 bilateral ROIs (thalamus, frontal, parietal, temporal, and cingulate cortices, and whole brain gray matter including cingulate and sensory motor areas) and were used as endophenotypes.

## 2.3   Statistical Analyses

In order to investigate the overall influence of *PARP1* variants on microglial activity (as indexed by average [$^{11}$C]PBR28 SUV in 6 bilateral ROIs), a set-based analysis method in PLINK was adopted. In brief, this method evaluates the association of individual SNPs in a given set with a given phenotype and selects a set of independent (based on $r^2$ threshold) and significant (based on p threshold) SNPs to represent the overall effect of the set. Then, the significance of the overall set effect is assessed using permutation to correct for multiple SNPs within a set while taking into account the linkage disequilibrium (LD) structure among SNPs. In this study, the analysis was performed using the following settings: (1) $r^2$ threshold: 0.3, (2) p threshold: 0.05, (3) maximum number of independent and significant SNPs: 99999 in order to use all independent and significant SNPs, and (4) number of permutation: 50,000. Due to the limited number of samples, only a dominant genetic model was assessed. Age at PET scan, gender and TSPO genotype based on the rs6971 SNP were added to the model as covariates. Analysis was performed with and without *APOE* ε4 status as a covariate.

When more than one independent and significant SNP were identified from significant associations, a subsequent multi-marker analysis was performed using a haplotype analysis method in PLINK with the same set of covariates in the model. The association p-value was corrected for multiple testing (the number of SNP combinations) using 50,000 permutations. Although the PLINK set-based approach provides the significance of the *PARP1* gene and the list of independent and significant SNPs in *PARP1*, it does not show the joint influence of multiple SNPs on average

[$^{11}$C]PBR28 SUV values. This multi-marker method allowed us to further study the combinatorial effect of multiple SNPs on average [$^{11}$C]PBR28 SUV values.

## 3    Results

*PARP1* variation was associated with average [$^{11}$C]PBR28 SUV from thalamus at $p<0.014$ after adjusting for *APOE* ε4 status. This association was driven by rs874583, located in the intergenic area downstream of the gene. Samples with one or more minor allele ("C") of rs874583 showed higher SUV in thalamus (Fig.1). Another association with average [$^{11}$C]PBR28 SUV in cingulate showed marginal significance at $p<0.065$ after *APOE* ε4 adjustment and was driven by two SNPs (rs6677172 and rs61835377). Both SNPs are intergenic and downstream of the gene. Minor alleles of these two SNPs (rs6677172: "G", rs61835377: "A") showed an inverse relationship with average [$^{11}$C]PBR28 SUV in cingulate.

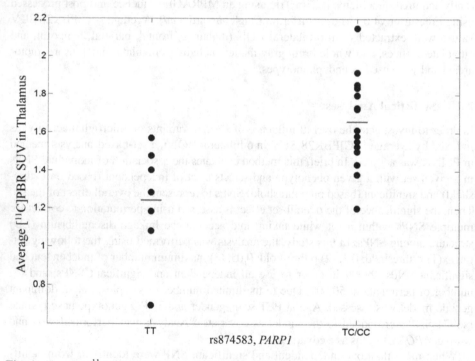

**Fig. 1.** Average [$^{11}$C]PBR28 SUV in thalamus in *PARP1* variant, rs874583 (minor allele: C). SUV was adjusted for age at PET scan, gender, TSPO genotype, and *APOE* ε4 status. The horizontal bars represent the mean PBR SUV for each genotype group.

Two SNPs (rs6677172 and rs61835377) were jointly associated with average [$^{11}$C]PBR28 SUV in cingulate. Therefore, a subsequent multi-marker analysis was performed to investigate influence of the allele combination of the SNPs on the same phenotype. The analysis identified three different combinations of alleles

("CA","CG", and "GG"), of which two were significantly associated with average [¹¹C]PBR28 SUV in cingulate at uncorrected p<0.05. One ("CA") was significant after correction for multiple testing at corrected p<0.05. Table 2 summarizes the multi-marker analysis results. "CA" allele combination was positively correlated with the [¹¹C]PBR28 SUV and "GG" allele combination was negatively correlated with the phenotype. Average [¹¹C]PBR28 SUVs in cingulate are displayed in Fig.2 for samples with and without "CA" allele combination (Fig.2 (a)) and with and without "GG" allele combination (Fig.2 (b)). Interestingly, all 6 AD and 2 out of 3 LMCI participants in the current analysis had one or two copies of the "GG" allele combination, associated with lower average cingulate [¹¹C]PBR28 SUV.

**Table 2.** Multi-marker analysis results. Allele, F, BETA, P, and Corrected P represent allele combination, frequency of allele combination, regression coefficient, uncorrected p, and corrected p for the number of allele combination, respectively.

| PHENOTYPE | Allele | F | BETA | P | Corrected P |
|---|---|---|---|---|---|
| Average [¹¹C]PBR28 SUV Cingulate | CA | 0.212 | 0.204 | 0.0105 | 0.02962 |
| | GG | 0.385 | -0.164 | 0.0241 | 0.06426 |

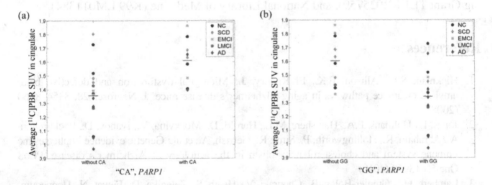

**Fig. 2.** Scatter plots of average [¹¹C]PBR28 SUV in cingulate for (a) "CA" allele group and (b) "GG" allele group. Average PBR SUV was adjusted for age at PET scan, gender, *TSPO* genotype, and *APOE* ε4 status. The horizontal bars represent the mean PBR SUV for each allele group.

## 4  Conclusions

This preliminary study investigated the relationship between variation in *PARP1* and microglial activity indexed by [¹¹C]PBR28 PET and identified significant associations of the gene with average [¹¹C]PBR28 SUVs in thalamus and cingulate. The subsequent multi-marker analysis also identified two allele combinations from the gene-based analysis associated with average [¹¹C]PBR28 SUV in cingulate. These identified associations suggested the role of *PARP1* in immune activation. Microglia can perform different functions [1, 13] and the specific role of microglial activation in the current sample of older adults at risk for AD is not known and may include both adaptive and adverse aspects. However, one interesting observation in the current study is that 8 out of 9 participants with AD or LMCI had one or two copies of the "GG" allele combination, which was associated with lower average $[^{11}C]$PBR28 SUV in cingulate compared to non-"GG" carriers. A previous study with the same cohort showed an inverse relationship between $[^{11}C]$PBR28 SUV and brain atrophy at a follow-up visit, suggesting a possible protective effect of microglial activity against cortical atrophy [21], which warrants further investigation. A major limitation of this preliminary study is the modest sample size which attenuates power, and the findings require replication in larger, independent samples as a future direction. The relationship between *PARP1* and microglial activity also warrants experimental molecular validation. Despite the limited sample size, this preliminary study identified interesting significant in vivo associations in an important pathway related to AD pathobiology. This approach combining neuroimaging and genetics data appears promising and can be applied to many related fields of research.

**Acknowledgment.** This study was supported in part by the National Institutes of Health, National Institute on Aging (R01 AG19771, P30AG10133), National Library of Medicine (R01 LM011360), National Science Foundation (IIS-1117335), NIH Clinical and Translational Sciences Institute Pre-doctoral Training Fellowship (Training Grant TL1 RR025759), and National Library of Medicine (K99 LM011384).

# References

1. Hickman, S.E., Allison, E.K., El Khoury, J.: Microglial dysfunction and defective beta-amyloid clearance pathways in aging Alzheimer's disease mice. J. Neurosci. 28, 8354–8360 (2008)
2. Jones, L., Holmans, P.A., Hamshere, M.L., Harold, D., Moskvina, V., Ivanov, D., Pocklington, A., Abraham, R., Hollingworth, P., Sims, R., Gerrish, A., et al.: Genetic evidence implicates the immune system and cholesterol metabolism in the aetiology of Alzheimer's disease. PLoS One 5, e13950 (2010)
3. Lambert, J.C., Grenier-Boley, B., Chouraki, V., Heath, S., Zelenika, D., Fievet, N., Hannequin, D., Pasquier, F., Hanon, O., Brice, A., Epelbaum, J., Berr, C., Dartigues, J.F., Tzourio, C., Campion, D., Lathrop, M., Amouyel, P.: Implication of the immune system in Alzheimer's disease: evidence from genome-wide pathway analysis. J. Alzheimers Dis. 20, 1107–1118 (2010)
4. Zhang, R., Miller, R.G., Madison, C., Jin, X., Honrada, R., Harris, W., Katz, J., Forshew, D.A., McGrath, M.S.: Systemic immune system alterations in early stages of Alzheimer's disease. J. Neuroimmunol. 256, 38–42 (2013)
5. Harold, D., Abraham, R., Hollingworth, P., Sims, R., Gerrish, A., Hamshere, M.L., Pahwa, J.S., Moskvina, V., Dowzell, K., Williams, A., Jones, N., Thomas, C., et al.: Genome-wide association study identifies variants at CLU and PICALM associated with Alzheimer's disease. Nat. Genet. 41, 1088–1093 (2009)
6. Hollingworth, P., Harold, D., Sims, R., Gerrish, A., Lambert, J.C., Carrasquillo, M.M., Abraham, R., Hamshere, M.L., Pahwa, J.S., Moskvina, V., et al.: Common variants at ABCA7, MS4A6A/MS4A4E, EPHA1, CD33 and CD2AP are associated with Alzheimer's disease. Nat. Genet. 43, 429–435 (2011)

7. Lambert, J.C., Heath, S., Even, G., Campion, D., Sleegers, K., Hiltunen, M., Combarros, O., Zelenika, D., Bullido, M.J., Tavernier, B., Letenneur, L., Bettens, K., et al.: Genome-wide association study identifies variants at CLU and CR1 associated with Alzheimer's disease. Nat. Genet. 41, 1094–1099 (2009)

8. Naj, A.C., Jun, G., Beecham, G.W., Wang, L.S., Vardarajan, B.N., Buros, J., Gallins, P.J., Buxbaum, J.D., Jarvik, G.P., Crane, P.K., Larson, E.B., Bird, T.D., et al.: Common variants at MS4A4/MS4A6E, CD2AP, CD33 and EPHA1 are associated with late-onset Alzheimer's disease. Nat. Genet. 43, 436–441 (2011)

9. Kauppinen, T.M., Suh, S.W., Higashi, Y., Berman, A.E., Escartin, C., Won, S.J., Wang, C., Cho, S.H., Gan, L., Swanson, R.A.: Poly(ADP-ribose)polymerase-1 modulates microglial responses to amyloid beta. J. Neuroinflammation 8, 152 (2011)

10. Liu, H.P., Lin, W.Y., Wu, B.T., Liu, S.H., Wang, W.F., Tsai, C.H., Lee, C.C., Tsai, F.J.: Evaluation of the poly(ADP-ribose) polymerase-1 gene variants in Alzheimer's disease. J. Clin. Lab. Anal. 24, 182–186 (2010)

11. Nho, K., Corneveaux, J.J., Kim, S., Lin, H., Risacher, S.L., Shen, L., Swaminathan, S., Ramanan, V.K., Liu, Y., Foroud, T., Inlow, M.H., Siniard, A.L., et al.: Whole-exome sequencing and imaging genetics identify functional variants for rate of change in hippocampal volume in mild cognitive impairment. Mol. Psychiatry (2013), doi:10.1038/mp.2013.24

12. Strosznajder, J.B., Czapski, G.A., Adamczyk, A., Strosznajder, R.P.: Poly(ADP-ribose) polymerase-1 in amyloid beta toxicity and Alzheimer's disease. Mol. Neurobiol. 46, 78–84 (2012)

13. Gehrmann, J., Matsumoto, Y., Kreutzberg, G.W.: Microglia: intrinsic immuneffector cell of the brain. Brain Res. Brain Res. Rev. 20, 269–287 (1995)

14. Kreisl, W.C., Fujita, M., Fujimura, Y., Kimura, N., Jenko, K.J., Kannan, P., Hong, J., Morse, C.L., Zoghbi, S.S., Gladding, R.L., Jacobson, S., Oh, U., Pike, V.W., Innis, R.B.: Comparison of [(11)C]-(R)-PK 11195 and [(11)C]PBR28, two radioligands for translocator protein (18 kDa) in human and monkey: Implications for positron emission tomographic imaging of this inflammation biomarker. Neuroimage 49, 2924–2932 (2010)

15. Risacher, S.L., Wudunn, D., Pepin, S.M., MaGee, T.R., McDonald, B.C., Flashman, L.A., Wishart, H.A., Pixley, H.S., Rabin, L.A., Pare, N., Englert, J.J., Schwartz, E., Curtain, J.R., West, J.D., O'Neill, D.P., Santulli, R.B., Newman, R.W., Saykin, A.J.: Visual contrast sensitivity in Alzheimer's disease, mild cognitive impairment, and older adults with cognitive complaints. Neurobiol. Aging 34, 1133–1144 (2013)

16. Saykin, A.J., Wishart, H.A., Rabin, L.A., Santulli, R.B., Flashman, L.A., West, J.D., McHugh, T.L., Mamourian, A.C.: Older adults with cognitive complaints show brain atrophy similar to that of amnestic MCI. Neurology 67, 834–842 (2006)

17. Owen, D.R., Yeo, A.J., Gunn, R.N., Song, K., Wadsworth, G., Lewis, A., Rhodes, C., Pulford, D.J., Bennacef, I., Parker, C.A., St Jean, P.L., Cardon, L.R., Mooser, V.E., Matthews, P.M., Rabiner, E.A., Rubio, J.P.: An 18-kDa translocator protein (TSPO) polymorphism explains differences in binding affinity of the PET radioligand PBR28. J. Cereb. Blood Flow. Metab. 32, 1–5 (2012)

18. Yoder, K.K., Nho, K., Risacher, S.L., Kim, S., Shen, L., Saykin, A.J.: Influence of TSPO genotype on [11C]PBR28 standardized uptake values. Journal of Nuclear Medicine (2013), doi:10.2967/jnumed.112.118885

19. Purcell, S., Neale, B., Todd-Brown, K., Thomas, L., Ferreira, M.A., Bender, D., Maller, J., Sklar, P., de Bakker, P.I., Daly, M.J., Sham, P.C.: PLINK: a tool set for whole-genome association and population-based linkage analyses. Am. J. Hum. Genet. 81, 559–575 (2007)

20. Shen, L., Kim, S., Risacher, S.L., Nho, K., Swaminathan, S., West, J.D., Foroud, T., Pankratz, N., Moore, J.H., Sloan, C.D., Huentelman, M.J., Craig, D.W., Dechairo, B.M., Potkin, S.G., Jack Jr., C.R., Weiner, M.W., Saykin, A.J.: Whole genome association study of brain-wide imaging phenotypes for identifying quantitative trait loci in MCI and AD: A study of the ADNI cohort. Neuroimage 53, 1051–1063 (2010)
21. Risacher, S.L., Kim, S., Yoder, K.K., Shen, L., West, J.D., McDonald, B.C., Wang, Y., Nho, K., Tallman, E., Hutchins, G.D., Fletcher, J.W., Ghetti, B., Gao, S., Farlow, M.R., Saykin, A.J.: Relationship of microglial activation measured by [11C]PBR28 PET, atrophy on MRI, and plasma biomarkers in individuals with and at-risk for Alzheimer's disease. In: Alzheimer's Association International Conference 2013 (Abstract number: 39417) (2013)

# A Graph-Based Integration of Multimodal Brain Imaging Data for the Detection of Early Mild Cognitive Impairment (E-MCI)*

Dokyoon Kim[1], Sungeun Kim[2,3], Shannon L. Risacher[2],
Li Shen[2,3], Marylyn D. Ritchie[1], Michael W. Weiner[4,5],
Andrew J. Saykin[2,6,7], and Kwangsik Nho[2,3]

[1] Center for Systems Genomics, Pennsylvania State University
[2] Center for Neuroimaging, Department of Radiology and Imaging Sciences,
Indiana University School of Medicine
{knho,asaykin}@iupui.edu
[3] Center for Computational Biology and Bioinformatics, Indiana University School of Medicine
[4] Department of Radiology, Medicine and Psychiatry, University of California, San Francisco
[5] Department of Veterans Affairs Medical Center, San Francisco
[6] Department of Medical and Molecular Genetics, Indiana University School of Medicine
[7] Department of Neurology, Indiana University School of Medicine

**Abstract.** Alzheimer's disease (AD) is the most common cause of dementia in older adults. By the time an individual has been diagnosed with AD, it may be too late for potential disease modifying therapy to strongly influence outcome. Therefore, it is critical to develop better diagnostic tools that can recognize AD at early symptomatic and especially pre-symptomatic stages. Mild cognitive impairment (MCI), introduced to describe a prodromal stage of AD, is presently classified into early and late stages (E-MCI, L-MCI) based on severity. Using a graph-based semi-supervised learning (SSL) method to integrate multimodal brain imaging data and select valid imaging-based predictors for optimizing prediction accuracy, we developed a model to differentiate E-MCI from healthy controls (HC) for early detection of AD. Multimodal brain imaging scans (MRI and PET) of 174 E-MCI and 98 HC participants from the Alzheimer's Disease Neuroimaging Initiative (ADNI) cohort were used in this analysis. Mean targeted region-of-interest (ROI) values extracted from structural MRI (voxel-based morphometry (VBM) and FreeSurfer V5) and PET (FDG and Florbeta-pir) scans were used as features. Our results show that the graph-based SSL classifiers outperformed support vector machines for this task and the best performance was obtained with 66.8% cross-validated AUC (area under the ROC

* For the Alzheimer's Disease Neuroimaging Initiative (ADNI). Data used in preparation of this article were obtained from the Alzheimer's Disease Neuroimaging Initiative (ADNI) database (adni.loni.ucla.edu). As such, the investigators within the ADNI contributed to the design and implementation of ADNI and/or provided data but did not participate in analysis or writing of this report. A complete listing of ADNI investigators can be found at http://adni.loni.ucla.edu/wpcontent/uploads/how_to_apply/ADNI_Acknowledgement_List.pdf

L. Shen et al. (Eds.): MBIA 2013, LNCS 8159, pp. 159–169, 2013.
© Springer International Publishing Switzerland 2013

curve) when FDG and FreeSurfer datasets were integrated. Valid imaging-based phenotypes selected from our approach included ROI values extracted from temporal lobe, hippocampus, and amygdala. Employing a graph-based SSL approach with multimodal brain imaging data appears to have substantial potential for detecting E-MCI for early detection of prodromal AD warranting further investigation.

**Keywords:** Mild Cognitive Impairment, Multimodal Brain Imaging Data, Data Integration, Graph-based Semi-Supervised Learning, Alzheimer's Disease.

# 1    Introduction

Alzheimer's disease (AD) is a progressive neurodegenerative disease in older adults and at this time, despite incidence rates doubling every 5 years after the age of 65, there is no effective disease modifying treatment for AD to date [1]. AD is predicted to affect 14 million Americans by the year 2050 (www.alz.org) and has become a national priority. The detection and diagnosis of AD at the earliest possible stage is of fundamental importance as early intervention could potentially delay progression to AD and achieve effective disease modification. One of main challenges is to identify and validate biomarkers of AD progression leading to an improved early diagnosis at early symptomatic and especially pre-symptomatic stages. To this end, the concept of mild cognitive impairment (MCI) was introduced [2]. MCI can be classified into early and late stages (E-MCI, L-MCI) based on severity. MCI is thought to be a precursor to the development of early AD, and subjects with late amnestic MCI have a highly elevated probability of developing AD with a conversion rate of approximately 15% per year [3, 4].

New approaches to the search for specific biomarkers to detect MCI/AD compared to healthy controls (HC) have been developed, with neuroimaging (MRI and PET) and cerebrospinal fluid (CSF) biochemical markers showing particular promise [5, 6]. However, in most studies, only patients with L-MCI and AD have been assessed [7]. In order to identify better diagnostic tools that can recognize AD at early symptomatic and especially pre-symptomatic stages, we developed a graph-based semi-supervised learning model to differentiate E-MCI from HC for early detection of AD using multimodal brain imaging scans (MRI and PET) of participants from the ongoing Alzheimer's Disease Neuroimaging Initiative (ADNI).

The semi-supervised learning (SSL) which recently emerged in the machine learning domain, employs a strategy halfway between supervised and unsupervised learning schemes to improve classification performance [8-11]. In particular, the graph-based SSL takes advantage of computational efficiency and representational ease for the biomedical data. Because of the graph structures, it is easy to integrate different types of data for better explaining clinical outcomes [12]. The learning time of graph-based SSL is nearly linear with the number of graph edges while the accuracy remains comparable to the kernel-based methods that suffer from the relative disadvantage of a longer learning time [13, 14]. In addition, the interpretation of bio-logical phenomena can be improved because of the graph structure [15-17], which naturally fits into the graph-based SSL.

## 2    Materials and Methods

### 2.1    Data

**Samples.** The Alzheimer's Disease Neuroimaging Initiative initial phase (ADNI-1) was launched in 2003 to test whether serial magnetic resonance imaging (MRI), posi-tion emission tomography (PET), other biological markers, and clinical and neurop-sychological assessment could be combined to measure the progression of MCI and early AD. This multi-site longitudinal study was intended to aid researchers and clini-cians develop new treatments for MCI and early AD, monitor their effectiveness, and lessen the time and cost of clinical trials. The ADNI-1 has been extended to its subse-quent phases (ADNI-GO and ADNI-2) for follow-up for existing participants and additional new enrollments. Inclusion and exclusion criteria, clinical and neuroimag-ing protocols, and other information about ADNI have been published previously and can be found at www.adni-info.org [18-20]. Demographic information, raw scan data, *APOE* and GWAS genotypes, neuropsychological test scores, and diagnostic informa-tion are available from the ADNI data repository (http://www.loni.ucla.edu/ADNI/). Individuals included in this study were 174 E-MCI (early MCI) and 98 HC (healthy older adults) participants in ADNI-GO or ADNI-2.

**Image Processing.** All available baseline 3T structural brain MRI scans were down-loaded from the ADNI database. As detailed in previous studies [18, 19], two widely employed automated MRI analysis techniques were independently used to process MRI scans: whole-brain voxel-based morphometry (VBM) implemented in the Statis-tical Parametric Mapping 8 (SPM8) software to extract mean grey matter (GM) densi-ty for target regions of interest (ROIs) and FreeSurfer version 5.1 to extract mean cortical thickness and volumetric measure for target ROIs. Pre-processed Florbetapir (also known as AV-45 and Amyloid) PET scans to assess brain amyloid β burden were downloaded from the ADNI database. For each scan, mean regional SUVR (standardized uptake value ratio) values were extracted for target ROIs using Mars-BaR in SPM8, as detailed in previous study [7, 18]. FDG-PET was used to measure the brain's rate of glucose metabolism with the tracer [$^{18}$F] Fluorodeoxyglucose. FDG-PET ROI data was downloaded from the ADNI database. All MRI ROI values were adjusted for the baseline age, gender, education, and intracranial volume (ICV) using a regression model, prior to analyses. All the ROI values of Florbetapir and FDG PET were adjusted for the baseline age, gender, and education.

### 2.2    Classification of Early Mild Cognitive Impairment (E-MCI)

The semi-supervised learning uses both labeled and unlabeled data to improve on the performance of supervised learning. There are several types of SSL algorithms, and the graph-based SSL was used in our study. If two patients' samples were more closely related to others, the algorithm assumed that the diagnosis of E-MCI from those two patients is more likely to be similar. Thus, the classification of E-MCI can be enhanced by considering similarities between patient samples. A natural method of analyzing relationships between entities is a graph, where nodes represent participants and edges show their possible relations. Figure 1 represents an example graph, which was conducted using the brain imaging data. An annotated participant is labeled either by '-1' or '1', indicating the two possible clinical outcomes, either 'healthy older adult' or 'E-MCI'. In order to predict the label of the unannotated patient '?', the edges connected from/to the patient play an important role in influencing propagation of the relation between the patient and its neighbors. This idea can be easily formulated using a graph-based semi-supervised learning [8]. Edges represent relations, more specifically similarities between participants that may be extracted from different brain imaging data. Different brain imaging data produce different graphs. Thus, the classification of E-MCI can be benefit by integrating diverse graphs from multimodal brain imaging data, i.e., incomplete information and noise. Technically, the data-setup of our experiment for the binary classification can be rephrased as $\{x_n, y_n\}_{n=1}^N$ where $x_n \in R^d$ ($d$ is the number of features and $N$ is the number of participants) and $y_n \in \{-1,1\}$.

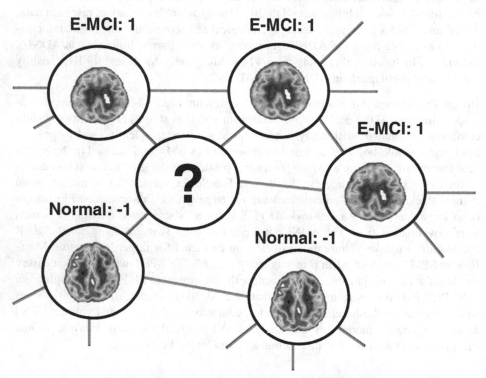

**Fig. 1.** Graph representation of brain imaging data between participants. Nodes represent participants and edges depict relations between samples. An annotated sample is labeled either by −1 or +1. In this example, the negative labels indicate samples from 'healthy older adults'. On the contrary, the positive labels indicate the samples from 'E-MCI'. The diagnosis of the unannotated sample marked as '?' is predicted by employing the graph-based semi-supervised learning.

**Graph-Based Semi-Supervised Learning.** In the graph-based SSL [8], a participant $x_i$ ($i = 1,\ldots,n$) is represented as a node $i$ in a graph, and the relationship between participants is represented by an edge. The edge strength from each node $j$ to other node $i$ is encoded in element $w_{ij}$ of a $n \times n$ symmetric weight matrix $W$. A Gaussian function of Euclidean distance between participants, with length scale hyperparameter $\sigma$, is used to specify connection strength:

$$w_{ij} = \begin{cases} \exp\left( -\dfrac{(x_i - x_j)^T (x_i - x_j)}{\sigma^2} \right) & \text{if } i \sim j, \\ 0 & \text{otherwise.} \end{cases} \tag{1}$$

Nodes $i$ and $j$ are connected by an edge if $i$ is in $j$'s $k$-nearest-neighborhood or vice versa. Thus, nearby participants in Euclidean spaces are assigned large edge weights. The labeled nodes have labels $y_l \in \{-1, 1\}$, while the unlabeled nodes have zeros $y_u = 0$. The graph-based SSL will output an $n$-dimensional real-valued vector $f = [f_l^T f_u^T]^T = (f_1,\ldots,f_l, f_{l+1},\ldots,f_{n=l+u})^T$, which can be thresholded to make label predictions on $f_l = f_1,\ldots,f_n$ after learning. It is assumed that $f_i$ should be close to the given label $y_i$ in labeled nodes (loss condition), and overall, $f_i$ should not be too different from the $f_i$ of adjacent nodes (smoothness condition). One can obtain $f$ by minimizing the following quadratic functional [8, 9, 11]:

$$\min_f (f - y)^T (f - y) + \mu f^T L f \tag{2}$$

where $y = (y_1,\ldots,y_l, 0,\ldots 0)^T$, and the matrix $L$, called the graph Laplacian matrix [21], is defined as $L = D - W$ where $D = \text{diag}(d_i)$, $d_i = \sum_j w_{ij}$. The parameter $\mu$ trades off loss versus smoothness. The solution of this problem is obtained as

$$f = (I + \mu L)^{-1} y \tag{3}$$

where $I$ is the identity matrix.

### 2.3  Integration of Multi-modal Brain Imaging Dataset

In order to combine the graphs from multimodal brain imaging data, four graphs can be integrated from finding optimum combination coefficients. Information from each graph is regarded as partially independent from and partly complementary to others. Reliability may be enhanced by integrating all available data sources using the graph-based SSL, which has been applied to the extended problem of protein function prediction [22] and clinical outcome prediction using multi-levels of genomic data [12]. Based on the method, the integration of multiple graphs is used to find an optimum value of the linear combination coefficient for the individual graphs (Fig. 2). This corresponds to finding the combination coefficients $\alpha$ for the individual Laplacians of the following mathematical formulation:

$$\min_\alpha y^T (I + \sum_{k=1}^{K} \alpha_k L_k)^{-1} y, \sum_k \alpha_k \le \mu \tag{4}$$

, where $K$ is the number of graphs and $L_k$ is the corresponding graph-Laplacian of graph $G_k$. Similar to the output prediction for single graphs, the solution is obtained by

$$f = (I + \sum_{k=1}^{K} \alpha_k L_k)^{-1} y.$$  (5)

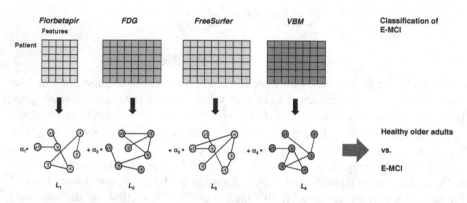

**Fig. 2.** Integration scheme of four different types of brain imaging data. Each brain imaging data can be converted into a graph, and then multiple graphs can be combined through finding the optimal value of the combination coefficient.

## 3   Results

### 3.1   Experiment Setting

The receiver operating characteristic (ROC) curve plots sensitivity (true positive rate) as a function of 1-specificity (false positive rate) for a binary classifier system as its discrimination threshold is varied [23]. An ROC score of 0.5 corresponds to random prediction, and an ROC score of 1.0 implies that the model succeeded in putting all of the positive examples before all of the negatives. For each dataset, we calculated area under the curve (AUC) of ROC as a performance measure. In order to avoid the over-fitting, five-fold cross-validation was conducted. Since some of the brain imaging dataset is high dimensional and noisy, and contains many redundant features, which may incur computational difficulty and low accuracy, a Student $t$-test based feature selection method was used [24]. Even though there are   many feature selection techniques such as filter, wrapper, and embedded method [25], a simple univariate feature selection method was used in order to emphasize not the effect of feature selection but the effect of integration of multimodal brain imaging data. The values of SSL model parameters, $k$ from Equation (1) and $\mu$ from Equation (3), were determined by the results of search over $k \in \{3, 4, 5, 6, 7, 8, 9, 10, 20, 30\}$ and $\mu \in \{0.001, 0.01, 0.05, 0.1, 0.2, 0.3, 0.4, 0.5, 0.6, 0.7, 0.8, 0.9, 1.0, 10, 100, 1000\}$. The optimized combination of model parameters was selected when the greatest AUC was obtained.

## 3.2    Experiment Results

With multimodal brain imaging data, we provide empirical comparison results about which type of brain imaging data is more informative to a given classification problem for diagnosis of E-MCI. Figure 3 shows the AUC performance on the classification of E-MCI. The averages of five-fold AUCs from Florbetapir, FDG, FreeSurfer, and VBM are shown in the figure. Among four types of brain imaging dataset, the performance of FreeSurfer dataset showed the best single modality performance with 0.6576 AUC. In Figure 3, AUC increases in the order of the following dataset, FreeSurfer > VBM > FDG > Florbetapir.

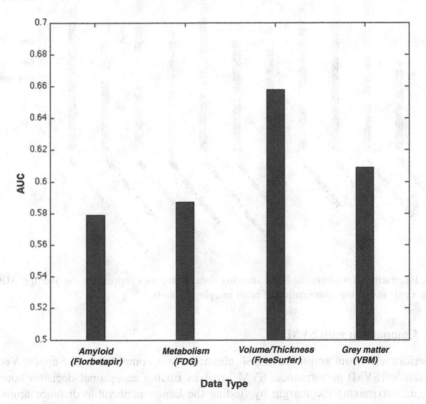

**Fig. 3.** Performance comparison among four types of brain imaging dataset. The y axis represents the average AUC and the x axis shows the date type.

## 3.3    Integration Effects

Since different brain imaging data contain partly independent and partly complementary information content, we integrated across multi-modal brain image datasets for better prediction of E-MCI. We found that multivariate integration across different brain imaging modalities increased the prediction performance for patients with E-MCI. Figure 4 shows the results of the integration with all combination of different types of brain imaging dataset. The model combining Florbetapir and VBM (0.6322 AUC) outperformed the model with VBM only (0.609 AUC). In addition, the integration with FDG and FreeSurfer showed the best performance among all combination of four different types of brain imaging dataset with 0.6681 AUC. However, the integration with all four types of brain image data included did not show the best performance.

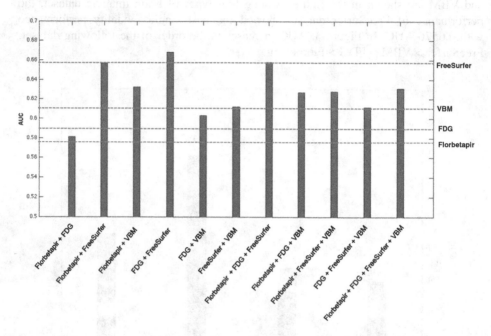

**Fig. 4.** Integration of multimodal brain imaging data. The y axis represents the average AUC and the x axis shows the combination of brain imaging datasets.

### 3.4    Comparison with SVM

The performance from graph-based SSL classifiers was compared with Support Vector Machine (SVM) performance. SVM involves finding an optimal decision boundary, i.e., maximizing the margin by finding the largest achievable distance among the separating hyperplane and the data points on either side. If the data points are separated by a non-linear hyperplane because of some intrinsic property of the problem, it is more appropriate to map the input feature space to a high-dimensional feature space where the data points are separated by a linear hyperplane. This mapping process is conducted by kernel functions. Among kernel functions, the Radial Basis Function (RBF) kernel was used with a wide range of sigma, from $10^{-6}$ to 1, in order to select the best model. In order to fairly compare the performance, we used the same set of features, which was used in the graph-based SSL. The models from the graph-based SSL outperformed the models from SVM except for Florbetapir data (Table 1). The Wilcoxon signed-rank test was used to assess the significance level of difference in performance between the results of the graph-based SSL and SVM [26]. The model with FreeSurfer dataset from the graph-based SSL showed significantly better than the one from SVM.

**Table 1.** Comparison between the graph-based SSL and SVM. *P*-values were calculated using a Wilcoxon signed-rank test between performance (AUC) of the graph-based SSL and SVM.

| Data type | Graph-based SSL | SVM | *P*-value |
|---|---|---|---|
| Florbetapir | 0.5789 (± 0.0732) | **0.5825** (± 0.0372) | 1.0000 |
| FDG | **0.5873** (± 0.0587) | 0.5664 (± 0.0643) | 0.8413 |
| FreeSurfer | **0.6576** (± 0.0905) | 0.5163 (± 0.0552) | 0.0159 |
| VBM | **0.609** (± 0.1059) | 0.5709 (± 0.0916) | 0.5476 |

## 4     Discussions and Conclusions

Using automatic whole-brain ROI analysis techniques and a graph-based semi-supervised learning (SSL) method, we developed a classification model to differentiate E-MCI from HC for early detection of AD. In this study, we used MRI (FreeSurfer and VBM) and PET (Florbetapir and FDG) scans from 174 E-MCI and 98 HC in the ADNI cohort. The graph-based SSL technique was used to integrate multimodal brain imaging data and select imaging-based phenotypes for optimizing E-MCI prediction accuracy. The data integration framework for multimodal brain imaging data has scalability to easily extend to additional types of brain imaging data. In addition, it preserves type-specific properties from the brain imaging data since the matrices from different types of brain imaging data were not simply merged but combined after conversion into a graph for the integration (Fig. 2).

Our results showed that 1) the graph-based SSL classifiers outperformed support vector machines (SVM) for this task; 2), we obtained the best results when using ROI values extracted by FreeSurfer from structural MRI scans; (3) the overall best performance was obtained with 66.8% cross-validated AUC when FDG PET and FreeSurfer data were combined; (4) the integration with all four types of brain image data included did not show the best performance; and (5) selected imaging-based phenotypes included ROI values extracted from temporal lobe, hippocampus, and amygdala. It has been showed that regional brain atrophy occurs initially and most severely in the entorhinal cortex and hippocampus before spreading throughout the neocortex [27]. These findings suggest that the predictive model may be combined with various data sources from different types of brain imaging data. Integration of independent or complementary information content may improve the chances of successful early diagnosis of AD. The graph-based SSL approach with multimodal brain imaging data has substantial potential for enhanced early detection of AD.

**Acknowledgements.** Data collection and sharing for this project was funded by the Alzheimer's Disease Neuroimaging Initiative (ADNI) (National Institutes of Health Grant U01 AG024904). ADNI is funded by the National Institute on Aging, the National Institute of Biomedical Imaging and Bioengineering, and through generous contributions from the following: Abbott; Alzheimer's Association; Alzheimer's Drug Discovery Foundation; Amorfix Life Sciences Ltd.; AstraZeneca; Bayer HealthCare; BioClinica, Inc.; Biogen Idec Inc.; Bristol-Myers Squibb Company; Eisai Inc.; Elan Pharmaceuticals Inc.; Eli Lilly and Company; F. Hoffmann-La Roche Ltd and its affiliated company Genentech, Inc.; GE Healthcare; Innogenetics, N.V.; Janssen Alzheimer Immunotherapy Research & Development, LLC.; Johnson & Johnson Pharmaceutical Research & Development LLC.; Medpace, Inc.; Merck & Co., Inc.; Meso Scale Diagnostics, LLC.; Novartis Pharmaceuticals Corporation; Pfizer Inc.; Servier; Synarc Inc.; and Takeda Pharmaceutical Company. The Canadian Institutes of Health Research is providing funds to support ADNI clinical sites in Canada. Private sector contributions are facilitated by the Foundation for the National Institutes of Health (www.fnih.org). The grantee organization is the Northern California Institute for Research and Education, and the study is coordinated by the Alzheimer's Disease Cooperative Study at the University of California, San Diego. ADNI data are disseminated by the Laboratory for Neuro Imaging at the University of California, Los Angeles. This research was also supported by NIH grants P30 AG010129, K01 AG030514, and the Dana Foundation.

Samples from the National Cell Repository for AD (NCRAD), which receives government support under a cooperative agreement grant (U24 AG21886) awarded by the National Institute on Aging (NIA), were used in this study. Additional support for data analysis was provided by NLM K99 LM011384, NIA R01 AG19771, P30 AG10133, NCI R01 CA101318, NLM R01 LM011360, NSF IIS-1117335, and RC2 AG036535, and U01 AG032984 from the NIH, Foundation for the NIH, and NINDS (R01NS059873).

# References

1. Alzheimer's, Association, Thies, W., Bleiler, L.: Alzheimer's disease facts and figures. Alzheimer's & Dementia: The Journal of the Alzheimer's Association 7, 208–244 (2011)
2. Petersen, R.C., Smith, G.E., Waring, S.C., et al.: Mild cognitive impairment: clinical characterization and outcome. Archives of Neurology 56, 303–308 (1999)
3. Stephan, B.C., Hunter, S., Harris, D., et al.: The neuropathological profile of mild cognitive impairment (MCI): a systematic review. Mol. Psychiatry 17, 1056–1076 (2012)
4. Petersen, R.C., Roberts, R.O., Knopman, D.S., et al.: Mild cognitive impairment: ten years later. Archives of Neurology 66, 1447–1455 (2009)
5. Wang, H., Nie, F., Huang, H., Kim, S., Nho, K., et al.: Identifying quantitative trait loci via group-sparse multitask regression and feature selection: an imaging genetics study of the ADNI cohort. Bioinformatics 28, 229–237 (2012)
6. Meda, S.A., Narayanan, B., Liu, J., Perrone-Bizzozero, N.I., et al.: A large scale multivariate parallel ICA method reveals novel imaging-genetic relationships for Alzheimer's disease in the ADNI cohort. NeuroImage 60, 1608–1621 (2012)
7. Risacher, S.L., Kim, S., et al.: The role of apolipoprotein E (APOE) genotype in early mild cognitive impairment (E-MCI). Frontiers in Aging Neuroscience 5, 11 (2013)
8. Zhou, D., Bousquet, O., Weston, J., Scholkopf, B.: Learning with local and global consistency. In: Advances in Neural Information Processing Systems (NIPS), vol. 16, pp. 321–328 (2004)

9. Belkin, M., Matveeva, I., Niyogi, P.: Regularization and Semi-supervised Learning on Large Graphs. In: Shawe-Taylor, J., Singer, Y. (eds.) COLT 2004. LNCS (LNAI), vol. 3120, pp. 624–638. Springer, Heidelberg (2004)

10. Zhu, X., Ghahramani, Z., Lafferty, J.: Semi-supervised learning using Gaussian fields and harmonic functions. In: Proceedings of the Twenty-first International Conference on Machine Learning (ICML), pp. 912–919. AAAI Press, Washington, DC (2003)

11. Chapelle, O., Weston, J., Scholkopf, B.: Cluster kernels for semi-supervised learning. In: Advances in Neural Information Processing Systems (NIPS), vol. 15, pp. 585–592 (2003)

12. Kim, D., Shin, H., Song, Y.S., Kim, J.H.: Synergistic effect of different levels of genomic data for cancer clinical outcome prediction. J. Biomed Inform. 45, 1191–1198 (2012)

13. Tsuda, K., Shin, H., Scholkopf, B.: Fast protein classification with multiple networks. Bioinformatics 21(suppl. 2), ii59–ii65 (2005)

14. Shin, H., Tsuda, K.: Prediction of Protein Function from Networks. In: Chapelle, O., Schölkopf, B., Zien, A. (eds.) Semi-Supervised Learning, ch. 20, pp. 339–352. MIT Press (2006)

15. Spellman, P.T., Sherlock, G., et al.: Comprehensive identification of cell cycle-regulated genes of the yeast Saccharomyces cerevisiae by microarray hybridization. Mol. Biol. Cell 9, 3273–3297 (1998)

16. Segal, E., Shapira, M., et al.: Module networks: identifying regulatory modules and their condition-specific regulators from gene expression data. Nat. Genet. 34, 166–176 (2003)

17. Ohn, J.H., Kim, J., Kim, J.H.: Genomic characterization of perturbation sensitivity. Bioinformatics 23, i354–i358 (2007)

18. Risacher, S.L., Shen, L., West, J.D., et al.: Longitudinal MRI atrophy biomarkers: relationship to conversion in the ADNI cohort. Neurobiology of Aging 31, 1401–1418 (2010)

19. Risacher, S.L., Saykin, A.J., West, J.D., et al.: Baseline MRI predictors of conversion from MCI to probable AD in the ADNI cohort. Current Alzheimer Research 6, 347–361 (2009)

20. Weiner, M.W., Veitch, D.P., et al.: The Alzheimer's Disease Neuroimaging Initiative: a review of papers published since its inception. Alzheimer's & Dementia: The Journal of the Alzheimer's Association 8, S1–S68 (2012)

21. Chung, F.R.K.: Spectral Graph Theory. Regional Conference Series in Mathematics, vol. 92 (1997)

22. Shin, H., Lisewski, A.M., Lichtarge, O.: Graph sharpening plus graph integration: a synergy that improves protein functional classification. Bioinformatics 23, 3217–3224 (2007)

23. Gribskov, M., Robinson, N.L.: Use of receiver operating characteristic (ROC) analysis to evaluate sequence matching. Comput. Chem. 20, 25–33 (1996)

24. Jafari, P., et al.: An assessment of recently published gene expression data analyses: reporting experimental design and statistical factors. BMC Med. Inform. Decis. Mak. 6, 27 (2006)

25. Saeys, Y., Inza, I., Larranaga, P.: A review of feature selection techniques in bioinformatics. Bioinformatics 23, 2507–2517 (2007)

26. Demsar, J.: Statistical comparisons of classifiers over multiple data sets. Journal of Machine Learning Research 7, 1–30 (2006)

27. Scahill, R.I., Schott, J.M., et al.: Mapping the evolution of regional atrophy in Alzheimer's disease: unbiased analysis of fluid-registered serial MRI. Proc Natl. Acad. Sci. U. S. A. 99, 4703–4707 (2002)

# Whole Brain Functional Connectivity Using Multi-scale Spatio-Spectral Random Effects Model

Hakmook Kang[1,*], Xue Yang[2], Frederick W. Bryan[2], Christina M. Tripp[1], and Bennett A. Landman[2]

[1] Biostatistics, Vanderbilt University, Nashville TN, 37232 USA
[2] Electrical Engineering, Vanderbilt University, Nashville TN, 37235 USA
{Hakmook.Kang,Xue.Yang,Frederick.W.Bryan,Christina.M.Tripp,
Bennett.Landman}@vanderbilt.edu

**Abstract.** Functional brain networks produce connected low frequency patterns of activity when the brain is at rest which can be analyzed with resting state functional MRI (rs-fMRI) by fitting general linear models for signals acquired at a pre-defined seed region and other regions of interest (ROIs). However, typical rs-fMRI analysis tends to ignore spatial correlations in rs-fMRI data, hence biases the standard errors of estimated parameters and leads to incorrect inference. Spatio-temporal or spatio-spectral models can incorporate the spatial correlations in fMRI data. To date, these models have not targeted rs-fMRI connectivity analysis. Herein, we expand a spatio-spectral model from fMRI analysis based on several ROIs to whole brain rs-fMRI connectivity analysis. Our model captures distance-dependent local correlation (within an ROI), distance-independent global correlation (between ROIs), and temporal correlations for whole brain rs-fMRI connectivity analysis with or without confounders. Simulated and empirical experiments demonstrate that this spatio-spectral model yields valid inference for whole brain rs-fMRI connectivity analysis.

**Keywords:** fMRI connectivity analysis, seed analysis, spatial correlations, spectral analysis.

## 1  Introduction

Neuroscience and patient care have been transformed by quantitative inference of spatial-temporal brain correlations in normal and patient populations with millimeter resolution and second precision using functional MRI (fMRI) [1]. Classical statistical approaches allow mapping of brain regions associated with planning/execution, response, and default mode behaviors through task, event, and resting state paradigms, respectively [2]. When the brain is at rest (i.e., not task driven), functional networks produce correlated low frequency patterns of activity that can be observed with resting state fMRI (rs-fMRI). These correlations define one measure of functional connectivity which may be estimated by regression of activity in a region of interest (ROI) against that of the remainder of the brain [3].

Absolute voxel-wise MRI intensities (arbitrary values) are rarely used in isolation for inference – rather, the temporal and spatial patterns/correlations of changes over time are of primary interest. Statistical analyses enable *inference* of the probability

L. Shen et al. (Eds.): MBIA 2013, LNCS 8159, pp. 170–179, 2013.
© Springer International Publishing Switzerland 2013

that observed signals are not observed by chance (i.e., that there exist *significant* associations between the observed signals and model of brain activity). The techniques in wide-spread use (e.g., Gaussian noise models, auto-regressive temporal correlation) ignore spatial correlations in estimating model parameters [4]. Ignoring intrinsic spatial correlation will distort the variance of estimated parameters, leading to Type I errors in the presence of positive spatial correlation or Type II errors in the presence of negative spatial correlation [5]. Traditionally, pre-processing and post-processing steps in the statistical parametric mapping pipeline partially account for the spatial correlations. For example, data are spatially smoothed with a Gaussian kernel before estimation [6] and the correlation is taken account in the inference procedures through random field theory [7].

Recently, Kang et al. [8] proposed a spatio-spectral mixed-effects model to overcome the main barrier of incorporating spatial correlations in fMRI data analysis. This model consists of fixed and random effects that capture within-ROI and between-ROI correlations. The authors demonstrated capturing the spatial and temporal correlation through simulation and empirical experiments, but the framework was limited to consideration of up to five ROIs.

Herein, we proposed a new functional connectivity analysis method incorporating the voxel-wise general linear model and ROI connectivity results (Fig. 1). By alleviating a key estimation limitation, we can expand the Kang et al spatio-spectral mixed-effects model for an arbitrary number of ROIs to a generalized model for the whole brain rs-fMRI connectivity analysis. Briefly, (1) the whole brain is shattered into small ROIs, (2) estimation is performed on each voxel accounting for within-ROI and between-ROI correlations, and (3) statistical significance is inferred on the ROI level. We evaluate our model through simulation and empirical experiments on the whole gray matter.

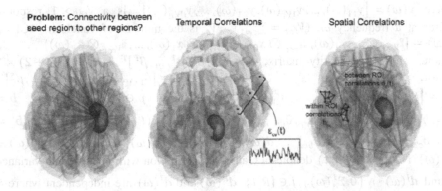

**Fig. 1.** The spatial and temporal model. Our goal is to discover the connectivity between a seed region and every other region in the brain. Spatial correlations model within-ROI correlations and inter-ROI correlations – these are not typically addressed in rs-fMRI. Temporal correlations are voxel-wise correlations across time – these are typically addressed in rs-fMRI analysis.

## 2    Theory

### 2.1    Model

We consider the following general spatio-temporal mixed-effects model for rs-fMRI:

$$y_{cv}(t) = \beta_{cv}^0 + (\beta_c^s + b_{cv})x_{seed}(t) + \sum_{p=1}^{P} \beta_{cv}^p x_p(t) + d_c(t) + \epsilon_{cv}(t), \qquad (1)$$

where $y_{cv}(t)$ is the rs-fMRI intensity at voxel $v$ in ROI $c$ at time $t$, $x_p$ can be any confounders, e.g., motion parameters, $t = 1, ..., T$, $c = 1, ..., C$, and $v = 1, ...,V_c$ in ROI $c$. Additionally, $x_{seed}$ is the mean time course within the seed region, $\beta_{cv}^0$ is the constant value at voxel $v$ in ROI $c$ across time, $\beta_c^s$ is the connectivity between the seed ROI and ROI $c$, $\beta_{cv}^p$ ($p = 1, ..., P$) is the coefficient associated with the $p$-$th$ confounder at voxel $v$ in ROI $c$, $b_{cv}$ is a zero-mean voxel-specific random deviation of the seed connectivity within an ROI $c$ and this random deviation is assumed to be independent across ROIs, $d_c(t)$ is a zero-mean ROI-specific random effect which models the remaining connectivity of all other ROIs after regression of the seed ROI connectivity, and $\epsilon_{cv}(t)$ is noise that takes into account intra-voxel temporal correlation.

Under the assumption of the stationary error series $\{\epsilon_{cv}(t)\}$, the spectrum, analogous to temporal covariance matrix in the time domain, is a diagonal matrix in the Fourier domain. Therefore, we transform the model in the time domain to the frequency domain. Let the Fourier coefficients of the series $\{x_{seed}(t)\},\{x_p(t)\},\{d_c(t)\}$, and $\{\epsilon_{cv}(t)\}$ be $x_{seed}(\omega), x_p(\omega), d_c(\omega)$ and $\epsilon_{cv}(\omega), (\omega = \omega_1, \omega_2, ..., \omega_T)$, respectively. Then, using matrix notation in the frequency domain,

$$y(\omega) = X(\omega)(\beta + b) + Kd(\omega) + \epsilon(\omega), \qquad (2)$$

where $y(\omega) = [y_{11}(\omega), ..., y_{1V_1}(\omega), y_{21}(\omega), ..., y_{CV_C}(\omega)]^T$ is a $V_{tot} \times 1$ response vector at a frequency $\omega$, ($V_{tot} = \sum_{c=1}^{C} V_c$, $V_c$ is the number of voxels in ROI $c$), $X(\omega) = [\mathbb{I}_{V_{tot}} \otimes x_{seed}(\omega), \mathbb{I}_{V_{tot}} \otimes x_0(\omega), \mathbb{I}_{V_{tot}} \otimes x_1(\omega), ..., \mathbb{I}_{V_{tot}} \otimes x_P(\omega)]$, $\mathbb{I}_n$ denotes an $n \times n$ identity matrix, $\beta = [\beta^s, \beta^0, \beta^1, ..., \beta^P]^T$ is a $V_{tot}(P + 2) \times 1$ vector, $\beta^s = [\beta_1^s, ..., \beta_1^s, \beta_2^s, ..., \beta_2^s, ..., \beta_C^s]^T$, $\beta^p = [\beta_{11}^p, \beta_{12}^p, ..., \beta_{1V_1}^p, \beta_{21}^p, ..., \beta_{2V_2}^p, ..., \beta_{CV_C}^p]^T$ for $p \in \{0,1,...,P\}$, $b = [b_{11}, b_{12}, ..., b_{1V_1}, b_{21}, ..., b_{CV_C}, 0, ..., ..., ...,0]^T$ is a $V_{tot}(P + 2) \times 1$ vector, $b_c^* = [b_{c1}, b_{c2}, ..., b_{cV_c}]^T \sim N(0, \Sigma_{bc})$, $d(\omega) = [d_1(\omega), ..., d_C(\omega)]^T$, $d_j(\omega) = d_j^R(\omega) + id_j^I(\omega)$. Note that $N(\mu, \tau)$ denotes a Gaussian distribution with mean $\mu$ and variance $\tau$, and $d^j(\omega) \sim N\left(0, \Sigma_d^j(\omega)\right), j \in \{R, I\}$, $d^R(\omega)$ and $d^I(\omega)$ are independent where $R$ and $I$ denote the real and imaginary part of a complex number, respectively. $K = K_1 \oplus K_2 \oplus ... \oplus K_C$, where $\oplus$ denotes direct sum and $K_j = [1, ..., 1]^T$ is a vector of length $V_j$ whose elements are all one, $j = 1,...,C$. $\epsilon(\omega) = [\epsilon_{11}(\omega), ..., \epsilon_{1V_1}(\omega), \epsilon_{21}(\omega), ..., \epsilon_{CV_C}(\omega)]$ and $\epsilon(\omega) = \epsilon^R(\omega) + i\epsilon^I(\omega)$. N.b. $[\epsilon^R(\omega), \epsilon^I(\omega)]^T \sim N\left(0, \frac{1}{2}f(\omega)\mathbb{I}_{2V_{tot}}\right)$, where $f(\omega)$ is the spectrum at frequency $\omega$.

## 2.2    Estimation

We define $\boldsymbol{\gamma}_{cv} = [\gamma_{cv}^s, \beta_{cv}^0, \beta_{cv}^1, \ldots, \beta_{cv}^P]^T, \gamma_{cv}^s = \beta_c^s + b_{cv}^s$. The ordinary least square (OLS) estimator of $\boldsymbol{\gamma}$ is

$$\hat{\boldsymbol{\gamma}} = \left[ \sum_{k=1}^T X^T(\omega_k) X(\omega_k) \right]^{-1} \left[ \sum_{k=1}^T X^T(\omega_k) \boldsymbol{y}(\omega_k) \right]. \tag{3}$$

Now we need to estimate $\boldsymbol{\beta}^s$ and $\boldsymbol{b}$. To simplify, rewrite $\boldsymbol{\beta}^{s*} = [\beta_1^s, \beta_2^s, \ldots, \beta_C^s]^T, \boldsymbol{b}^* = [b_{11}, b_{12}, \ldots, b_{1V_1}, b_{21}, \ldots, b_{CV_C}]^T$, $\Sigma_b = \Sigma_{b1} \oplus \Sigma_{b2} \oplus \ldots \oplus \Sigma_{bC}$, and $\hat{\boldsymbol{\gamma}}^s = K\boldsymbol{\beta}^{s*} + \boldsymbol{b}^*$.

To estimate $\boldsymbol{\beta}$, we do not need to estimate the exact value of $\boldsymbol{b}$ but the covariance. The covariance of $\boldsymbol{b}$ can be estimated using spatial variogram [9]. If we use empirical variogram estimation, the estimation of $\Sigma_b$ will only depend on the variance of $\hat{\boldsymbol{\gamma}}^s$ across voxels within each ROI, which can be noisy. We model the spatial dependence using an exponential variogram and estimate the parameters using restricted maximum likelihood [10].

$$\hat{\boldsymbol{\beta}}^{s*} = \left[ K^T \widehat{\Sigma}_b^{-1} K \right]^{-1} \left[ K^T \widehat{\Sigma}_b^{-1} \hat{\boldsymbol{\gamma}}^s \right]. \tag{4}$$

### Estimation of $Cov(d(\omega))$ and $f(\omega)$

Define $z_{cv}(\omega) = y_{cv}(\omega) - X(\omega)\boldsymbol{\gamma}_{cv}$. $z_{cv}(\omega)$ can be expressed as $d_c(\omega) + \epsilon_{cv}(\omega)$.

$$\widehat{Var}(d_c(\omega)) = \widehat{Var}(z_{c1}(\omega), \cdots, z_{cV_c}(\omega)), \tag{5}$$

where given locally stationary spatial process within an ROI, we compute the variance of $\boldsymbol{z}_c(\omega)$ at each frequency, which guarantees that the estimated variance is always greater than or equals to zero.
When $c \neq c'$,

$$\widehat{Cov}(d_c(\omega), d_{c'}(\omega)) = \widehat{Cov}(\bar{y}_c(N(\omega)), \bar{y}_{c'}(N(\omega))), \tag{6}$$

where $\bar{y}_c(\cdot)$ denotes the average of $y$ across all the voxels in ROI $c$ and $N(\omega)$ denotes the frequencies around a frequency $\omega$. The size of neighbors of a frequency $\omega$, i.e., $N(\omega)$, can be arbitrarily chosen between 1 and $T/2$ and we choose $T/8$.
The resulting covariance matrix of $\boldsymbol{d}(\omega)$ is guaranteed to be semi-positive definite. The spectrum for the real part or imaginary part is

$$\hat{f}^j(\omega) = [1/V_{tot}] \sum_{c=1}^C \sum_{v=1}^{V_c} \{\widehat{Var}(z_{cv}(\omega)) - \hat{\sigma}_{d_c}^2\}, \tag{7}$$

where $\hat{f}^j(\omega) = \frac{1}{2} f(\omega)$, $j \in \{R, I\}$, using either the real parts or the imaginary parts of $z_{cv}(\omega)$ and $\widehat{Var}(d_c(\omega)) \equiv \hat{\sigma}_{d_c}^2$, respectively. Then, a more robust estimator of the spectrum will be $\hat{f}(\omega) = [1/2]\left(\hat{f}^R(\omega) + \hat{f}^I(\omega)\right)$.

## Estimation of $\mathrm{Cov}(\widehat{\beta})$

One of the limitations of the spatio-spectral mixed-effects model in [8] is the procedure for estimating $\mathrm{Cov}(\widehat{\beta})$ scales quadratically with the number of ROIs. Since we are interested in the coefficients for the seed time course $\beta^{s*}$, we can simplify the covariance equations to perform the analysis on the whole brain. From OLS estimation, $\mathrm{Cov}(\widehat{\gamma})$ is:

$$
\begin{aligned}
&\mathrm{Cov}(\widehat{\gamma}) \\
&= \left[\sum_{k=1}^{T} X^T(\omega_k)X(\omega_k)\right]^{-1} \left[\sum_{k=1}^{T} X^T(\omega_k)\mathrm{Cov}(y(\omega_k))X(\omega_k)\right] \left[\sum_{k=1}^{T} X^T(\omega_k)X(\omega_k)\right]^{-1}.
\end{aligned}
\tag{8}
$$

The $\mathrm{Cov}(\widehat{\gamma})$ can be arranged so that each regressor is separated: $\mathrm{Cov}(\widehat{\gamma}) = \begin{bmatrix} \mathrm{Cov}(\widehat{\gamma}^s) & \mathrm{Cov}(\widehat{\gamma}^s, \widehat{\gamma}^{0\sim P}) \\ \mathrm{Cov}(\widehat{\gamma}^s, \widehat{\gamma}^{0\sim P}) & \mathrm{Cov}(\widehat{\gamma}^{0\sim P}) \end{bmatrix}$, from which we can write the covariance of the estimated seed coefficients as

$$
\mathrm{Cov}(\widehat{\beta}^{s*}) = \left[K^T \widehat{\Sigma}_b^{-1} K\right]^{-1} K^T \widehat{\Sigma}_b^{-1} \mathrm{Cov}(\widehat{\gamma}^s) \widehat{\Sigma}_b^{-1} K \left[K^T \widehat{\Sigma}_b^{-1} K\right]^{-1}.
\tag{9}
$$

Let's define terms to further simplify (9) to achieve computational efficiency:

(1.) $x(\omega) = [x_{seed}(\omega), x_0(\omega), x_1(\omega), \ldots, x_P(\omega)]$,

(2.) $X^* = [x(\omega_1) \quad x(\omega_2) \quad \cdots \quad x(\omega_T)]^T$,

(3.) $(X^{*T}X^*)^{-1} \left(\sum_{k=1}^{T} \left(x_{seed}(\omega)^2 (x(\omega_k)^T x(\omega_k))\right)\right)(X^{*T}X^*)^{-1} \equiv A$,

(4.) $\left((X^{*T}X^*)^{-1} x(\omega_k)^T x(\omega_k)(X^{*T}X^*)^{-1}\right) \equiv H(\omega_k)$,

(5.) $(X^{*T}X^*)^{-1} \sum_{k=1}^{T} \left(f(\omega_k)x(\omega_k)^T x(\omega_k)\right)(X^{*T}X^*)^{-1} \equiv Q$,

(6.) $A = \{a_{i,j}\}$, $H(\omega_k) = \{h(\omega_k)_{i,j}\}$, $Q = \{q_{i,j}\}$.

Define an operator $sum(\mathbf{M})$ that adds up all the elements in a matrix $\mathbf{M}$. Then after simplification and using the notations (1.) – (6.) above, we arrive at

$$
\begin{aligned}
\mathrm{Cov}(\widehat{\beta}^{s*}) = \; &a_{11} \begin{bmatrix} sum\left(\widehat{\Sigma}_{b1}^{-1}\right) & 0 & 0 \\ 0 & \ddots & 0 \\ 0 & 0 & sum\left(\widehat{\Sigma}_{bC}^{-1}\right) \end{bmatrix}^{-1} + \sum_{k=1}^{T} \left(h(\omega_k)_{11}\widehat{\Sigma}_d(\omega_k)\right) \\
&+ \widehat{q}_{11} \begin{bmatrix} sum\left(\widehat{\Sigma}_{b1}^{-2}\right) & 0 & 0 \\ 0 & \ddots & 0 \\ 0 & 0 & sum\left(\widehat{\Sigma}_{bC}^{-2}\right) \end{bmatrix}.
\end{aligned}
\tag{10}
$$

## 2.3 Inference

The t-test can be performed based on the estimated coefficient parameters and the covariance. Since we considered both the multi-scale spatial correlations, i.e., distance-independent between-ROI and distance-dependent within-ROI correlations, and the temporal correlations, the standard errors of parameter estimates are less likely biased. Since there are more than one ROI, it is necessary to do correction for multiple comparisons. Two widely used multiple correction methods are random field theory (RFT) and false discovery rate (FDR). RFT requires spatial smoothing of the data and is not appropriate here because we do not employ spatial smoothing but do model the underlying spatial dependence. Therefore, we employed the FDR method for the inference on the whole brain ROIs.

# 3  Methods

## 3.1  Simulation

We simulated rs-fMRI images from Gray Matter (GM) labels with one seed ROI and 95 other ROIs. The mean connectivity coefficient for each ROI was randomly chosen from {-0.8, 0, 0.8} and no confounder was included. The connectivity coefficient for each voxel was simulated as the mean coefficient plus a zero-mean voxel-specific random effect with standard deviation 0.1. The number of voxels and the coordinates varied from ROI to ROI but the within-ROI Euclidian distance-dependent correlation structures were the same (i.e., the variogram function was the same). The between-ROI covariance was defined by a positive definite matrix in which the mean correlation was 0.2859, and minimum and maximum were -0.3652 and 0.8821, respectively. The temporal correlation was modeled by an autoregressive model (AR(1)) with the model coefficient of 0.3. The temporal signal to noise ratio (SNR) was simulated from 10 to 100 with the step size 10. The temporal SNR was defined as the ratio between mean intensity of the images to the standard deviation of the noise across time. It is noteworthy that the SNR mentioned in this paper is the temporal SNR that is typically high in rs-fMRI experiments. For each SNR level, 100 Monte Carlo simulations were performed. We calculated the false positive rate (FPR) and false negative rate (FNR) while controlling FDR at 0.05. The accuracies of estimated ROI connectivity coefficient $\widehat{\beta^s}$, within-ROI covariance $\widehat{\Sigma_b}$, and between-ROI correlations are evaluated with root mean squared error (RMSE). See Fig. 2.

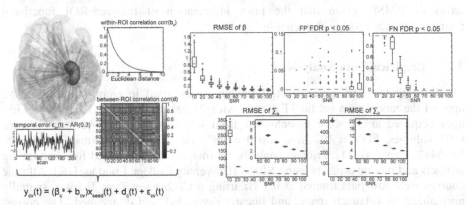

**Fig. 2.** Simulation setting and results. The left part displays the setting of the simulation experiment. The red region is selected as the seed region, and our interest is the connectivity between the seed region and every other 95 regions. The within-ROI correlation is plotted as a function of Euclidean distance, the between-ROI correlation is a 95 by 95 matrix, and the temporal error follows an AR(1) model with the model coefficient of 0.3. The RMSE of $\widehat{\beta^s}$, $\widehat{\Sigma_b}$ and $\widehat{\Sigma_d}$, the FP and FN with FDR correction are plotted in the right part as a function of SNR. The RMSE plots of $\widehat{\Sigma_b}$ and $\widehat{\Sigma_d}$ are enlarged for SNR from 50 to 100.

The RMSE of $\widehat{\beta^s}$ decreases exponentially as the SNR increases. The FPR of connectivity coefficients is under control for all SNR settings at FDR = 0.05. However, the FNR is 1 when SNR is very low (SNR = 10), then it decreases exponentially toward lower level as SNR increases. The RMSEs of $\widehat{\Sigma_b}$ and $\widehat{\Sigma_d}$ decrease exponentially as SNR increases.

The widely accepted seed-based method in which the time series in each ROI are averaged across voxels and functional connectivity is defined as correlation between a seed time series and the average time series in an ROI, was also applied to the simulated data at SNR = 80. Because of high SNR, the conventional method results in FNR = 0 as our method does. However, in terms of FPR, the spatio-spectral random effects model outperforms the conventional approach, i.e., FPR of 0.0327 from the conventional approach and 0.0287 from our method. This 12 percent gain in FPR confirms that ignoring the underlying positive correlation in an ROI tends to inflate false positive findings.

To further improve estimation accuracy, we considered incorporating a connectivity prior for the ROIs. In the above simulations the between-ROI correlations $\Sigma_d$ could be decomposed in three components as shown in Fig. 3. We used these three components (but not their magnitudes) as a basis for $\widehat{\Sigma_d}$ in the estimation for 100 Monte Carlo simulations when SNR is 80 and compared the results with the previous results. In Fig. 3, the box plots labeled as 'no components' are our previous results and the box plots labeled as 'components' using the prior information to estimate the between ROI-correlations. As expected, the estimation of $\widehat{\Sigma_d}$ becomes more accurate while the estimation of $\widehat{\beta^s}$ and $\widehat{\Sigma_b}$ stay the same. Employing the component priors reduces FPR but increases FNR compared to 'no component'. However, the gain and loss in terms of FPR and FNR seem to be negligible. This simulation results demonstrate that utilizing additional information enhances estimation accuracy in terms of RMSE, given that the prior information of between-ROI functional connectivity is accessible and reliable.

## 3.2    Empirical Data Analysis

To illustrate that our spatio-spectral model can be used in empirical studies, we applied the model on a public 3T dataset with 25 healthy subjects. The rs-fMRI images acquired at 3T were downloaded from http://www.nitrc.org/projects/nyu_trt/ (197 volumes, FOV = 192 mm, flip $\theta$ = 90°, TR/TE = 2000/25 ms, 3x3x3 mm, 64x64x39 voxels) [11]. Prior to analysis, all images were corrected for slice timing artifacts and motion artifacts using SPM8 (University College London, UK). All time courses were low pass filtered at 0.1 Hz using a Chebychev Type II filter, spatially normalized to Talairach space, and linearly detrended, and de-meaned. The corresponding high resolution T1-weighted anatomical images (FOV = 256mm, flip $\theta$ = 8°, TR/TE = 2500/4.3 ms, TI = 900 ms, 176 slices) were used to acquire label images following the method described in [12,13]. The right hippocampus was selected as the seed region for each subject. The six estimated motion parameters were used as confounders. The mean estimated seed connectivity coefficient $\widehat{\beta^s}$ and the mean between-ROI correlations $\widehat{\Sigma_d}$ across 25 subjects are shown in Fig. 4. Although neither

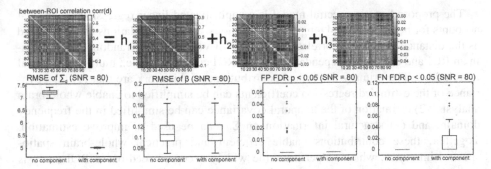

**Fig. 3.** Estimation with component priors. The first line shows the predefined between-ROI correlations can be decomposed by three components. The second line displays the results comparing the previous estimation without priors and the estimation with priors.

our multi-scale spatio-spectral random effects model nor the conventional approach (not presented here) can claim statistically significant functional connection to the seed region at FDR = 0.05, we demonstrate the capacity for performing the whole-brain analysis while properly considering both spatial and temporal correlations in rs-fMRI data.

## 4    Discussion

The proposed ROI-level analysis enables inference of brain activity associations taking into account voxel- and ROI-level dependence structure in rs-fMRI data, while typical ROI analyses narrow the problem to focus on the average time series, which ignores within- and between-ROI correlations. ROI analyses are easier to interpret since the significant regions can be mapped to and explained by the known neuroanatomy but averaging the voxel intensities reduces some voxel-wise specificity and results in incorrect inference. The proposed multi-scale spatio-spectral random effects model overlaps voxel-based and ROI-based analyses so that inference is tested on the ROI-level while the voxel-wise effects are incorporated through the random effects.

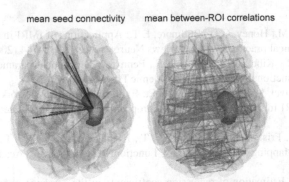

**Fig. 4.** Empirical Results. The red region is the seed region. The left brain shows the mean connectivity coefficient across 25 subjects. The right brain shows the mean between ROI correlations across 25 subjects.

The proposed spatio-spectral model is a sophisticated linear regression model that accounts for both spatial and temporal correlations. Spatial correlations are considered as the distance-dependent correlation structure of voxel-specific random effects within an ROI and distance-independent between-ROI correlations, i.e., multi-scale spatial correlations. The primary theoretical contributions of this work are that (1) the covariance of the estimated regression coefficients can be simplified to enable whole-brain analysis, (2) estimation of the temporal covariance can be simplified in the frequency domain, and (3) structural information on $\Sigma_d$ can be used to improve estimation. Together, these contributions enable efficient and practical whole-brain spatio-spectral inference, which outperforms the widely accepted seed-based ROI analysis with averaged time series across voxels. Although the proposed framework is based on different theoretical underpinnings, the random effects general linear models of scientific interest may be used interchangeably with traditional massively univariate statistical parametric mapping (SPM).

Our model to incorporate component prior information regarding between-ROI functional dependence deserves further research in order to utilize structural information in multi-modal MRI, e.g., Diffusion Tensor Images and rs-fMRI. However, it requires caveat to use this component-based approach because non-reliable or incorrect prior information can severely distort the results, even though this can be considered as one of a few non-Bayesian approaches to directly combine functional and structural connectivity information.

**Acknowledgements.** This work was supported in part by NIH N01-AG-4-0012, NIH 1T32EB014841,and the National Center for Research Resources, Grant UL1 RR024975-01 (now at the National Center for Advancing Translational Sciences, Grant 2 UL1 TR000445-06). The content is solely the responsibility of the authors and does not necessarily represent the official views of the NIH. This work was conducted in part using the resources of the Advanced Computing Center for Research and Education at Vanderbilt University, Nashville, TN.

# References

1. Matthews, P.M., Honey, G.D., Bullmore, E.T.: Applications of fMRI in translational medicine and clinical practice. Nature Reviews Neuroscience 7, 732–744 (2006)
2. Asburner, J.T., Kibel, S.J., Nichols, T.E., Penny, W.D.: Statical parametric mapping: the analysis of functional brain images. Academic Press (2007)
3. Van Den Heuvel, M.P., Hulshoff Pol, H.E.: Exploring the brain network: a review on resting-state fMRI functional connectivity. European Neuropsychopharmacology 20, 519–534 (2010)
4. Penny, W.D., Friston, K.J., Ashburner, J.T., Kiebel, S.J., Nichols, T.E. (eds.): Statistical Parametric Mapping: The Analysis of Functional Brain Images. Academic Press, New York (2006)
5. Dubin, R.A.: Estimation of regression coefficients in the presence of spatially autocorrelated error terms. The Review of Economics and Statistics 70, 466–474 (1988)

6. Worsley, K.J., Marrett, S., Neelin, P., Vandal, A.C., Friston, K.J., Evans, A.C.: A unified statistical approach for determining significant signals in images of cerebral activation. Human Brain Mapping 4, 58–73 (1996)
7. Worsley, K.J., Evans, A.C., Marrett, S., Neelin, P.: A three-dimensional statistical analysis for CBF activation studies in human brain. Journal of Cerebral Blood Flow and Metabolism 12, 900 (1992)
8. Kang, H., Ombao, H., Linkletter, C., Long, N., Badre, D.: Spatio-spectral mixed-effects model for functional magnetic resonance imaging data. Journal of the American Statistical Association 107, 568–577 (2012)
9. Cressie, N.: Statistics for Spatial Data. Wiley (1993)
10. Lark, R., Cullis, B.: Model-based analysis using REML for inference from systematically sampled data on soil. European Journal of Soil Science 55, 799–813 (2004)
11. Shehzad, Z., Kelly, A.M.C., Reiss, P.T., Gee, D.G., Gotimer, K., Uddin, L.Q., Lee, S.H., Margulies, D.S., Roy, A.K., Biswal, B.B.: The resting brain: unconstrained yet reliable. Cerebral Cortex 19, 2209–2229 (2009)
12. Asman, A.J., Landman, B.A.: Non-local statistical label fusion for multi-atlas segmentation. Medical Image Analysis 17, 194–208 (2013)
13. Asman, A.J., Landman, B.A.: Formulating spatially varying performance in the statistical fusion framework. IEEE Transactions on Medical Imaging 31, 1326–1336 (2012)

# Modeling Cognitive Processes via Multi-stage Consistent Functional Response Detection

Jinglei Lv[1,2], Dajiang Zhu[2], Xi Jiang[2], Kaiming Li[3], Xintao Hu[1], Junwei Han[1], Lei Guo[1], and Tianming Liu[2]

[1] School of Automation, Northwestern Polytechnical University, Xi'an, China
[2] Department of Computer Science and Bioimaging Research Center,
The University of Georgia, Athens, GA, USA
[3] Biomedical Imaging Technology Center, Emory University, Atlanta, GA, USA

**Abstract.** Recent neuroscience research suggested that cognitive processes can be viewed as functional information flows on a complex neural network. However, computational modeling of cognitive processes based on fMRI data has been rarely explored so far due to two key challenges. First, there has been a lack of universal and individualized brain reference system, on which computational modeling of cognitive processes can be performed, integrated, and compared. Second, there has been a lack of ground-truth of cognitive processes. This paper presents a novel framework for computational modeling of working memory processes via a multi-stage consistent functional response detection. We deal with the above two challenges by using a publicly released large-scale cortical landmark system as a universal and individualized brain reference system and as a statistical data integration platform. Specifically, in the first-stage analysis, for each corresponding landmark we measure the consistency of its fMRI BOLD signals from a group of subjects, and the landmarks with high group-wise consistency are found to be highly task-related. In the second stage, the consistency of dynamic functional connection (DFC) time series of each landmark pair from the same group of subjects are measured, and those connections with high consistent patterns are declared as the active interactions during the cognitive task. Here, the group-wise consistent responses inferred from statistical pooling of data from multiple subjects via the universal brain reference system are considered as the benchmark to evaluate the multi-stage framework. Experimental results on working memory task fMRI data revealed that our methods can detect meaningful cognitive processes.

**Keywords:** cognitive processes, task fMRI, functional response detection.

## 1 Introduction

Recent neuroscience research has suggested that cognitive processes can be considered as functional information flows on complex neural networks [1-3]. A critical characteristic of cognitive processes is that they are dynamic and hierarchical [7]. With modern advancements of fMRI techniques, researchers are now able to map brain regions involved in the brain's cognitive processes such as working memory with decent spatial and temporal resolutions [4, 5]. However, computational modeling of cognitive processes based on fMRI data has been rarely explored in the literature so far due to at least two key challenges. First, there has been a critical lack of

L. Shen et al. (Eds.): MBIA 2013, LNCS 8159, pp. 180–188, 2013.

universal and individualized brain reference system on which computational modeling of cognitive processes can be performed, integrated, pooled and compared across individuals. The Brodmann brain map and associated atlases have been used for over 100 years in neuroscience, however, the brain regions in Brodmann map at the gyral or sulcal scale are relatively coarse to map and represent fMRI BOLD signals. Second, there is no ground-truth for both cognitive processes and fMRI data. Actually, it has been a longstanding challenge to evaluate results in fMRI-based mapping of brain function and computational modeling of cognitive processes.

In this paper, we present a novel framework for computational modeling of cognitive processes (using working memory as a test-bed) via multi-stage consistent functional response detection. Specifically, we deal with the abovementioned two challenges by using a publicly released large-scale cortical landmark system [6] with 358 common and individualized cortical landmarks, named DICCCOL (Dense Individualized and Common Connectivity-based Cortical Landmarks), as a universal and individualized brain reference system. Experimental results have shown that this DICCCOL brain reference system offers much finer granularity, much better functional homogeneity, and intrinsically-established correspondences across individuals and populations, in comparison with the Brodmann map and atlases [6]. Therefore, the DICCCOL system not only can be used for the computational modeling of dynamic and hierarchical cognitive processes, but also can be used as a statistical data integration platform. As a result, the group-wise consistent functional responses inferred from statistical pooling of data from multiple subjects can be considered as the benchmark to evaluate the multi-stage framework. Given the lack of ground-truth of cognitive processes, group-wise consistency and reproducibility across individuals are probably the desired choice at the current stage.

Specifically, in the first-stage modeling, for each corresponding DICCCOL landmark from a group of subjects, we measure the consistency of its fMRI BOLD signals, and the landmarks with high group-wise consistency are determined as highly task-related ones. These landmarks are thus considered as the first-stage information processing centers. In the second-stage modeling, the consistency of dynamic functional connectivity (DFC) time series of each landmark pair from the same group of subjects are quantitatively measured, and those connections with highly consistent patterns are regarded as the active functional interactions during the cognitive task. The proposed multi-stage consistent response detection framework has been applied on a working memory task-based fMRI dataset [8] to computationally model the dynamic and hierarchical working memory process, and experimental results revealed that our methods can detect meaningful cognitive processes.

## 2    Materials and Methods

### 2.1    Overview

The computational framework of our multi-stage fMRI data analysis and modeling based on large-scale cortical landmarks are summarized in Fig.1. First, the structurally and functionally corresponding 358 DICCCOL landmarks are localized and optimized via the methods in [6] for each subject in a group based on DTI data. The DTI images are co-registered with the working memory task-based fMRI data [8] for each subject in order to extract fMRI signals for the cortical landmarks [6]. Second, we calculate the dynamic functional connections (DFC) between each pair of cortical landmarks, which are used to represent the time-varying functional interaction responses to external block-based stimulus. In general, the consistent response detection framework consists of two stages. In the first stage, we conduct group-wise consistency analysis directly on fMRI BOLD signals of each corresponding DICCCOL landmark from a group of subjects, based on which we determine the first-stage information centers for the working memory cognitive task. In the second stage, we perform group-wise consistent response detection on the DFC time series of corresponding cortical landmark connections across subjects. Based on the results in this stage, we detect active interactions and determine second-stage information processing centers. Then, the landmarks and connections that exhibit either consistent BOLD response or consistent functional connectivity responses are integrated to represent hierarchical working memory cognitive processes, in comparison with traditional activation detection results by group-wise GLM method [5, 12].

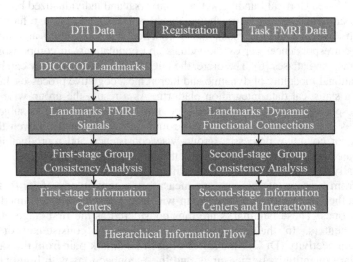

**Fig. 1.** The pipeline of task-based fMRI data processing, analysis and modeling

## 2.2    Data Acquisition and Pre-Processing

In a working memory task-based fMRI experiment under IRB approval [8], fMRI images of 19 healthy young adult subjects are scanned on a 3T GE Signa scanner. The acquisition parameters are as follow: fMRI: 64×64 matrix, 4mm slice thickness, 220mm FOV, 30 slices, TR=1.5s, TE=25ms, ASSET=2. Each participant performed the modified version of the OSPAN task (3 block types: OSPAN (30 TRs) with a response (10 TRs), Arithmetic (20 TRs), and Baseline (20 TRs)), while fMRI data was acquired. DTI data was acquired with dimensionality 128×128×60, spatial resolution 2mm×2mm×2mm; parameters are TR 15.5s and TE 89.5ms, with 30 DWI gradient directions and 3 B0 volumes acquired. The DTI data was co-registered to the fMRI space via FSL FLIRT. For fMRI images, the pre-processing pipeline includes motion correction, slice time correction, temporal pre-whitening, spatial smoothing, and global drift removal. For DTI data, pre-processing includes skull removal, motion correction and eddy current correction. The brain tissue segmentations were performed on the DTI-derived images via the similar approaches in [9]. The fiber tracking was performed using the MEDINRIA package. For each subject, the 358 DICCCOL landmarks with structural correspondences are localized and optimized on white matter cortical surface via the computational framework in [6].

## 2.3 FMRI Signal Extraction for Each Landmark

DTI images of each subject were first registered into the fMRI space via FSL FLIRT [10]. As DICCCOL landmarks were localized and optimized on the DTI white surfaces, which were reconstructed from DTI-derived tissue maps, we first translate the landmark locations into voxels of DTI tissue maps. With the registration of DTI and fMRI data, we then locate the landmarks on fMRI images and extract corresponding fMRI signal for each landmark. As our work majorly focuses on the relative fluctuation of fMRI signals and their inter-relationship, we normalize each

extracted signal $S = [s_1, s_2, \ldots \ldots, s_n]$ before all the analyses as: $S_{norm} = \dfrac{S - \frac{\sum_{i=1}^{n} s_i}{n}}{\sigma_S}$ (1)

## 2.4 Cortical Landmarks' Dynamic Functional Connections

A sliding window method was applied to measure the temporally dynamic functional interaction of two cortical landmarks based on their fMRI signals, and the generated time series is defined as the dynamic functional connection (DFC) of these two landmarks, as illustrated in Fig.2. Specifically, given an fMRI signal with the total length of $T$ (units in fMRI image volume), and the sliding window with the width of $t_w$, at each time point $t_n$, we extracted a signal window with length $t_w$ centered at $t_n$ (Fig.2(b)). With two signal windows obtained from different fMRI signals of two cortical landmarks, we calculated the Pearson's correlation between them and defined it as the dynamic functional connection at $t_n$ (Fig.2(b)). Note that for the first and last few time points in the fMRI BOLD signal, the window length is shortened to calculate the correlation. After sliding over all the time points, the resulted DFC time series have the same length of $T$ as the original fMRI signals. Thus, we can measure the functional interactions among cortical landmarks through DFC time series signals, as illustrated at the bottom of Fig.2(b).

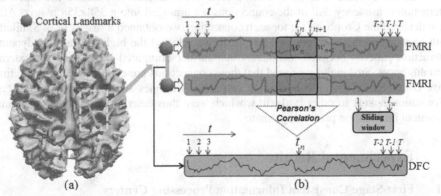

**Fig. 2.** DFC calculation for an example landmark pair. (a) Green spheres are 358 DICCCOL landmarks. An exemplar connection of landmark pair is illustrated as a yellow line in the yellow dashed frame. (b) A sliding window approach is applied on two fMRI signals of a landmark pair and the DFC is then calculated.

## 2.5     Multi-stage Consistent Functional Response Detection

To measure a set of time series signals' consistency, e.g., a group of fMRI BOLD signals for the same cortical landmark in 19 subjects' brains, we calculated the Cronbach's $\alpha$ [11] of them. Specifically, for a set of signals $X$, which consists of $K$ signals, $S_i$ represents each signal column with $n$ time points in Eq.(2).

$$X = [S_1, S_2, \ldots \ldots S_K], \quad S_i = [s_{i1}, s_{i2}, \ldots \ldots s_{in}]^T \tag{2}$$

The Cronbach's $\alpha$ is calculated as below, where $\sigma_{S_i}^2$ is the variance of each signal, and $\sigma_X^2$ is the variance of the signal set of $X$ in Eq.(3).

$$\alpha = \frac{K}{K-1}\left(1 - \frac{\sum_{i=1}^K \sigma_{S_i}^2}{\sigma_X^2}\right) \tag{3}$$

In the following paragraphs, the Cronbach's $\alpha$ will be calculated as a measurement of the consistency of fMRI signals for each corresponding landmark, and it is also used as the measurement of the consistency of DFCs for each landmark-pair.

Specifically, in the first-stage, we extracted 358 cortical landmarks' fMRI signals for each subject in a group of $n$ subjects. As each landmark possesses structural and functional correspondence across different subjects, for $n$ fMRI signals of the same cortical landmark, we calculated their Cronbach's $\alpha$ to measure their consistency across subjects. With an experimentally determined threshold, we selected those landmarks with high fMRI signal consistency, and compared the averaged multi-subjects' signals of each selected landmark with the external stimuli curve. From this stage of analysis, we can determine the first-stage information processing centers.

In the second stage, we calculated the DFC time series with the sliding window length of 15 TRs (which is shorter than the length of any block type) via the methods in Section 2.4 for each landmark pair, in order to obtain their dynamic functional interaction patterns. Since the correspondences of cortical landmarks also apply to their corresponding connections, the group-wise consistent functional response analysis to corresponding connections is meaningful. Then for each landmark-pair connection $i$-$j$, we calculated the Cronbach's $\alpha$ of DFC time series from a group of $n$ subjects to measure the functional interaction consistency. All of the connections are arranged into a 358×358 matrix. After we calculated the Cronbach's $\alpha$ for each connection, we obtained a matrix of $\alpha$. Similarly, with an experimentally determined threshold, we selected the highly consistent dynamic interaction patterns between landmarks, and further compared them with the external stimulus curve. Strikingly, we found that these connections are either linked with the first-stage consistent information processing centers, or the ones starting from the first-stage information centers to other landmarks, which were thus determined as the second-stage consistent information processing centers.

# 3     Experimental Results

## 3.1     First-Stage Consistent Information Processing Centers

As described in Section 2.5, we calculated the Cronbach's $\alpha$ of fMRI signals for each corresponding landmark, and plotted them in Fig.3(a). Then, we used an empirical threshold of $\alpha$ to select landmarks with high consistency of fMRI signals across subjects. In this way, we derived 35 consistently corresponding landmarks and further plotted their Cronbach's $\alpha$ values with blue stars in Fig.3(b). For each of the selected 35 landmarks, we averaged its fMRI signals from a group of 19 subjects and calculated the Pearson's correlation with external stimulus curve convolved with the hemodynamic response function (Fig.3(d)), which are represented by the red stars in Fig.3(b). From Fig.3(b), we can infer that most of the selected 35 landmarks with high Cronbach's $\alpha$ also exhibited high correlation (>0.5) with the stimulus curve. There are also 3 landmarks (illustrated by the black arrow in Fig.3(b)) that showed high anti-correlation (< -0.7) with the block-based stimulus. For visualization, we presented the locations of the 35 landmarks in Fig.3(g). Also, exemplar fMRI signal curves of the 35 landmarks are shown in Figs.3(e)-3(f), in which the green and yellow blocks correspond to the landmarks in green and yellow circles in Fig.3(g), respectively. These results demonstrate that the landmarks with high consistencies of fMRI signals across subjects either fit well with the stimuli curve as shown in Fig.3(e), or exhibit high anti-correlation with the stimuli curve as shown in Fig.3(f). Most of these selected landmarks either locate on the visual cortex or the frontal lobe, which are determined as the first-stage information processing centers. From a neuroscience perspective, it is reasonable that the 35 landmarks are selected as the first-stage information center since visual and frontal regions are likely to be the origins of bottom-up and top-down information sources in working memory processes [1-3].

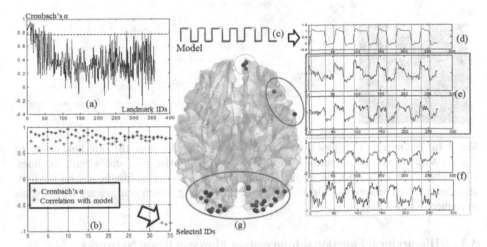

**Fig. 3.** (a) The curve of Cronbach's $\alpha$ for 358 cortical landmarks. (b) Selected 35 landmarks with high $\alpha$ values above the red dashed line in (a) and their Pearson's correlations with the stimulus curve. (c) Stimulus curve model. (d) Model convolved with HRF (hemodynamics response function). (e) Exemplar average fMRI signals of landmarks in green circles of (g). (f) Exemplar average fMRI signals of the landmarks in yellow circles of (g).

## 3.2    Second-Stage Consistent Functional Responses

In this stage, the consistency of DFC signals of each connection *i-j* was calculated via the method in Section 2.5 and the matrix of $\alpha$ is presented in Fig.4(a). We thresholded the matrix of α and selected connections with high consistency of DFCs across subjects, as highlighted by the white elements in Fig.4(b). For neuroscience interpretation, they are further visualized in Fig.4(c), in which, the red spheres are the first-stage information centers obtained in Section 3.1 and the red lines are the connections with high consistency of DFCs. Figs.4(e)-4(g) show exemplar DFC signals of the selected connections and comparisons with the stimulus model. We found that these connections exhibit either high positive strength (Figs.4(e)-4(f)) or negative strength (Fig.4(g)) around the task change points, as illustrated by blue, green and red dashed lines. These results showed evidence that there are group-wise consistent interaction patterns among cortical landmarks, and these interactions exhibit high strength around task change points. From Fig.4(c), we can also infer that many of these interactions are among the first-stage information centers, and there are also some interactions spread to other cortical landmarks, which are determined as the second-stage information centers and will be discussed in details in the next section.

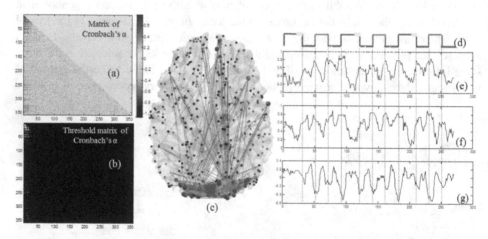

**Fig. 4.** (a) The matrix of Cronbach's α of DFCs among 358 landmarks. (b) Threshold matrix of (a). (c) Visualization of connections exhibiting high group-wise consistency with red lines. Blue spheres are 358 DICCCOL landmarks and larger red spheres are highlighted for the first-stage information centers. (d) Stimulus model. (e), (f), and (g): Exemplar average DFC signals of connections (red lines) in (c).

### 3.3     Hierarchical Functional Information Flows on Brain Networks

With the two-stage analyses discussed above, we detected the first-stage information centers with high consistency of fMRI BOLD responses (red spheres in Fig.5(a)) and second-stage connections with consistent functional interaction responses (red lines in Fig.5(a)). Furthermore, there are many other cortical landmarks (yellow spheres in Fig.5(a)) that are involved in the responding functional interactions, but not detected in the first-stage analysis. Here, we consider those yellow landmarks in Fig.5(a) as the second-stage information processing centers with more complex functional behaviors such as reverberation processes [1-3]. Essentially, they receive and process information through the functional interactions with the first-stage information centers, and perform higher-level cognitive processes. Therefore, the visualizations of the two-stage information processing centers in Fig.5(a) reveal dynamic and hierarchical information flows during working memory task on large-scale landmarks.

In addition, for comparison, we performed group-wise activation detection using the FSL FEAT based on the GLM model and mixed-effect model [12] on fMRI volumes of the same dataset. We mapped the detected activations (p-value=0.05, z-value>3.5) to the cortical surface as red regions in Figs.5(b-d). We also overlaid our first-stage (red spheres) and second-stage (yellow spheres) information centers onto the same cortical surface. The comparison shows that the detected activations from FSL FEAT [12] coincide with most of our first-stage information centers. This means our first-stage information centers are mostly in agreement with traditional activation detection method. However, many second-stage information centers are outside of the activation areas by the traditional FSL FEAT. Quantitative results are provided in Fig.5(e). Here, 27 out of 35 first-stage information centers are overlaid with traditional activations, but only 9 out of 37 second-stage information centers are covered by traditional activations. These results demonstrate the advantages of our two-stage consistent response detection methods: it not only detects the responding brain regions that well follow the stimulus curve, but also other responding regions (*whose fMRI signals do not necessarily follow the external task stimulus curve*) that are in the down-streams of the dynamic and hierarchical cognitive processes.[1-3]

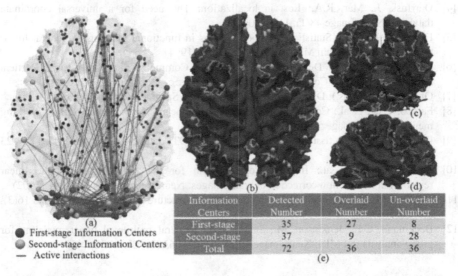

| Information Centers | Detected Number | Overlaid Number | Un-overlaid Number |
|---|---|---|---|
| First-stage | 35 | 27 | 8 |
| Second-stage | 37 | 9 | 28 |
| Total | 72 | 36 | 36 |

(a)
● First-stage Information Centers
◐ Second-stage Information Centers
— Active interactions

(e)

**Fig. 5.** (a) Illustration of dynamic and hierarchical information flows during working memory processes on cortical landmarks. (b) Comparison with traditional voxel-wise activation detection result by the FSL FEAT. Red areas of the cortical surface are activations and blue areas are not. (c)-(d) are two additional views of (b). (e) Numbers of information centers detected from two stages of analyses, and the number of overlaid landmarks with detected activations (red regions) in (b).

# 4    Conclusion

We presented a novel multi-stage consistent functional response detection framework to computationally model the dynamic and hierarchical cognitive processes. We used the publicly available DICCCOL brain localization and reference system to characterize the dynamic information flows on brain networks and determine the consistent functional responses. The working memory task-based fMRI data was used as an example, and experimental results demonstrated meaningful information flows during working memory task. In particular, qualitative and quantitative comparisons with traditional voxel-based activation detection via GLM demonstrated the superiority of computational modeling of dynamic and hierarchical cognitive processes, which is the major novelty and contribution of this work.

# References

[1]  Ward, L.M.: Synchronous neural oscillations and cognitive processes. Trends in Cognitive Sciences 7(12), 553–559 (2003)
[2]  Lamme, V.A.F., Roelfsema, P.R.: The distinct modes of vision offered by feedforward and recurrent processing. Trends Neurosci. 23, 571–579 (2000)
[3]  Varela, F., et al.: The brainweb: phase synchronization and large scale integration. Nat. Rev. Neurosci. 2, 229–239 (2001)
[4]  Derrfuss, J., Mar, R.A.: Lost in localization: The need for a universal coordinate database. NeuroImage 48(1), 1–7 (2009)
[5]  Friston, K.J., et al.: Statistical parametric maps in functional imaging: A general linear approach. Human Brain Mapping 2(4), 189–210 (1994)
[6]  Zhu, D.: DICCCOL: Dense Individualized and Common Connectivity-based Cortical Landmarks. Cerebral Cortex (2012), http://dicccol.cs.uga.edu/
[7]  Ohta, N., et al. (eds.): Dynamic cognitive processes. Springer (2005)
[8]  Faraco, C.C., et al.: Complex span tasks and hippocampal recruitment during working memory. NeuroImage 55(2), 773–787 (2011)
[9]  Liu, T., et al.: Brain tissue segmentation based on DTI data. NeuroImage 38(1), 114–123 (2007)
[10]  Jenkinson, M., et al.: Improved optimization for the robust and accurate linear registration and motion correction of brain images. Neuroimage 17(2), 825–841 (2002)
[11]  Cronbach, L.J.: Coefficient alpha and the internal structure of tests. Psychometrika 16(3), 297–334 (1951)
[12]  Beckmann, C.F., Jenkinson, M., Smith, S.M.: General multilevel linear modeling for group analysis in FMRI. Neuroimage 20(2), 1052–1063 (2003)

# Bivariate Genome-Wide Association Study of Genetically Correlated Neuroimaging Phenotypes from DTI and MRI through a Seemingly Unrelated Regression Model

Neda Jahanshad[1,**], Priya Bhatt[1,**], Derrek P. Hibar[1], Julio E. Villalon[1], Talia M. Nir[1], Arthur W. Toga[1], Clifford R. Jack, Jr.[2], Matt A. Bernstein[2], Michael W. Weiner[3,4], Katie L. McMahon[5], Greig I. de Zubicaray[6], Nicholas G. Martin[7], Margaret J. Wright[7], and Paul M. Thompson[1,*]

[1] Imaging Genetics Center, Laboratory of Neuro Imaging,
Department of Neurology, UCLA School of Medicine, Los Angeles, CA
[2] Department of Radiology, Mayo Clinic, Rochester, Minnesota, USA
[3] Department of Radiology, Medicine, and Psychiatry, UC San Francisco, CA, USA
[4] Department of Veterans Affairs Medical Center, San Francisco, CA, USA
[5] University of Queensland, Centre for Advanced Imaging, Brisbane, Australia
[6] University of Queensland, School of Psychology, Brisbane, Australia
[7] Queensland Institute of Medical Research, Brisbane, Australia

**Abstract.** Large multisite efforts (e.g., the ENIGMA Consortium), have shown that neuroimaging traits including tract integrity (from DTI fractional anisotropy, FA) and subcortical volumes (from T1-weighted scans) are highly heritable and promising phenotypes for discovering genetic variants associated with brain structure. However, genetic correlations ($r_g$) among measures from these different modalities for mapping the human genome to the brain remain unknown. Discovering these correlations can help map genetic and neuroanatomical pathways implicated in development and inherited risk for disease. We use structural equation models and a twin design to find $r_g$ between pairs of phenotypes extracted from DTI and MRI scans. When controlling for intracranial volume, the caudate as well as related measures from the limbic system - hippocampal volume - showed high $r_g$ with the cingulum FA. Using an unrelated sample and a Seemingly Unrelated Regression model for bivariate analysis of this connection, we show that a multivariate GWAS approach may be more promising for genetic discovery than a univariate approach applied to each trait separately.

**Keywords:** Neuroimaging genetics, brain connectivity, bivariate analysis, GWAS, genetic correlation.

---

* The Alzheimer's Disease Neuroimaging Initiative (ADNI).
** Equally contributing authors.

L. Shen et al. (Eds.): MBIA 2013, LNCS 8159, pp. 189–201, 2013.
© Springer International Publishing Switzerland 2013

# 1    Introduction

In many case-control genome-wide association studies (GWAS) of neurological diseases and disorders, such as Alzheimer's disease and schizophrenia, single genetic variations in the genome have been found to associate with the presence of the disease. While extremely popular, genetic association studies do not reveal what causes the disease or the neurological systems affected by the risk genes. On the other hand, if quantitative traits derived from brain imaging measures are used as a target for such genetic studies (e.g., GWAS), specific genetic loci can be mapped to specific features of the brain that may modulate disease risk.

Even so, single-nucleotide variations generally have small effects on any phenotype – carriers of different genetic variants may differ in the mean value of a brain measure by as little as 1-2%, or even less. Because of this, large populations are needed for genome-wide association analyses – making it very difficult to collect enough data at a single site to detect the effects on the brain of single-letter changes in the genome. Efforts to boost power in imaging genetics studies are therefore highly beneficial. Consortia that bring together information from multiple sites, such as the ENIGMA (Enhancing Neuro Imaging Genetics through Meta Analysis) Project (http://enigma.loni.ucla.edu/), draw on information from tens of thousands of subjects [1] to boost the power to discover genetic influences on brain structure. These consortia require that the phenotype of interest be easily measurable, stable, robust to imaging acquisition parameters, and heritable across multiple cohorts. These studies often focus on bilaterally averaged measures of regional brain volumes with high signal-to-noise ratios, limiting the scope of possible phenotypes to those obtainable rapidly and routinely in many image analysis labs [2]. Despite these constraints on the kinds of brain measures that can be assessed in vast samples, several phenotypes from T1-weighted structural scans, and fractional anisotropy maps from diffusion tensor imaging scans, have been found to be feasible targets for large-scale genetic analysis. Large scale GWAS analyses have been applied to individual measures from brain MRI and DTI, analyzed one at a time, such as average bilateral subcortical volumes, and averaged bilateral mean FA values in tract-based regions of interest (ROIs).

Genetic epidemiological studies show that bivariate rather than univariate methods can improve power to identify and localize chromosomal regions associated with genetically correlated traits (in the case of linkage analysis, for example) [3]. Intuitively, if the same genetic variants influence two or more different imaging measures – even measures from different imaging modalities – it should be possible to measure the overlap and use it to boost the power to find which specific genetic variants are associated with each measure. This "genetic correlation" principle has been used recently to boost power in a variety of genetic analyses. It is especially valuable in imaging genetics because of the extreme difficulty of amassing samples large enough to pick up the effects of single genetic variants on the brain.

Even within an imaging modality such as DTI, Chiang et al. [4] recently used cross-twin cross-trait analysis to find sets of voxels in the brain that had common genetic influences. By clustering these voxels according to their genetic correlation, it was possible to screen the genome for variants that affected different regions of the image, yielding higher power than simply considering each voxel on its own. The use of genetic correlation to discover coherent patterns of genetic influence in an image can also be extended to pick up common genetic influences on data from different imaging modalities. Recently, classical methods from quantitative genetics have been used to reveal bivariate genetic correlations among brain measures from T1-weighted MRI and DTI [5] - the two modalities used in this paper. The prior study by Kochunov et al., proved successful in using a large pedigree sample to find genetic correlations between brain measures from two imaging modalities, and localizing loci on the genome that had suggestive associations to phenotypes from both modalities, including average global FA and cortical thickness. Additionally, these prior works used genetic correlations to boost power to find specific genetic variants of interest. We set out to expand this type of analysis to multiple regions and phenotypes extractable in large cohorts and consortia such as ENIGMA. The overarching goal of our work is to discover genetic variants that affect brain measures that can be extracted efficiently from large neuroimaging databases worldwide. One tactic to do so, as shown in this paper, is to probe multiple imaging modalities for common genetic influences, and use these patterns as a coherent target to hunt for influential genes.

The Seemingly Unrelated Regression (SUR; [6]) bivariate model has proven to be a successful model to evaluate simultaneous GWASs of correlated traits. Unlike other multivariate methods, the SUR model is a system of linear equations that enables an unrestricted bivariate association test of genetic effects on each trait. In addition, the SUR model provides a great deal of flexibility as it includes a set of simultaneous regression equations that can have different sets of dependent variables and predictors. SUR can be thought of as a generalization of multiple regression, in which several multiple regression equations are all satisfied at once. The idea behind SUR is to fit a number of regression equations at once – not necessarily with the same outcome measure – and use the information on the covariance in the errors from each equation to update the others. Here we aimed to study genes affecting brain measures computed from T1-weighted MRI and DTI scans. It is logical that the size and white matter integrity of different parts of the brain might share some degree of genetic correlation, and we set out to find these patterns. We studied a cohort of healthy young twins to determine the genetic correlations between the different MRI and DTI measures. We then followed through with a bivariate SUR genome-wide association analysis of some of the most correlated regions in an unrelated elderly cohort (ADNI) with various degrees of cognitive impairment, including the FA of the cingulum and the volume of the caudate and the hippocampus.

## 2 Methods

### 2.1 Image Acquisition and Subject Information

We analyzed MRI and DTI data from two separate cohorts of human subjects: QTIM and ADNI; the details of these cohorts and the methods used to scan them are summarized below. QTIM, a large dataset of twins imaged with both MRI and high angular resolution diffusion imaging, was used to assess the genetic correlations between phenotypes from the different modalities using a bivariate twin modeling design. ADNI, a publicly available dataset that includes subject genotypes, neuroimaging scans (MRI, DTI, rsfMRI, etc.), and a whole host of biological and clinical assessments, was used for the genome-wide association study.

*QTIM (Queensland Twin IMaging study)* -- Whole-brain 3D anatomical MRI and HARDI scans were acquired from over 600 healthy genotyped twins and siblings (age: 23.1±2.0) with a high magnetic field (4T) Bruker Medspec MRI scanner. T1-weighted images were acquired with an inversion recovery rapid gradient echo sequence. Acquisition parameters were: TI/TR/TE=700/1500/3.35 ms; flip angle=8 degrees; slice thickness = 0.9mm, with a 256x256 acquisition matrix. Diffusion-weighted images (DWI) were acquired using single-shot echo planar imaging with a twice-refocused spin echo sequence to reduce eddy-current induced distortions. Imaging parameters were: 23 cm FOV, TR/TE 6090/91.7 ms, with a 128x128 acquisition matrix. Each 3D volume consisted of 55 2-mm thick axial slices with no gap and 1.79x1.79 mm$^2$ in-plane resolution. 105 images were acquired per subject: 11 with no diffusion sensitization (i.e., $b_0$ images) and 94 DWI ($b$=1159 s/mm$^2$) with gradient directions evenly distributed on the hemisphere. Scan time was 14.2 minutes. In total, images from 224 of the entire group of right-handed young adults (mean age: 23.4 years, s.d. 2.0) were analyzed in this study, including 51 pairs of monozygotic twins and 56 pairs of dizygotic twins. Remaining subjects included non-twin siblings, singletons, and those subjects whose image processing and volume extraction did not pass rigorous quality control. This set of data comprised the Queensland Twin Imaging dataset, QTIM.

*ADNI* -- The Alzheimer's Disease Neuroimaging Initiative (ADNI), is a multisite longitudinal study comprised of clinical, genetic and neuroimaging data of AD, MCI and normal elderly patients with varying degrees of cognitive impairment. ADNI recently launched a second phase (ADNI-2) of longitudinal data collection to include diffusion-weighted scans, among other newly added imaging modalities, with the goal of studying microstructural integrity and anatomical connectivity (among other measures) in elderly individuals. Whole-brain MRI scans were collected using 3-Tesla GE Medical Systems scanners, at 14 sites across North America. T1-weighted SPGR (spoiled gradient echo) anatomical scans were collected in addition to DWIs. For each diffusion MRI scan, there were 41 DWIs ($b$=1000 s/mm$^2$) and 5 T2-weighted images acquired with no diffusion gradient ($b_0$ images). This protocol was selected to optimize the signal-to-noise ratio given a fixed scan time [7]. At the time of writing (June 2013), approximately 200 subjects have been scanned with DTI. Of those scanned so far with DTI, 65 of them possessed sufficient genetic data and imaging data, including data from both DTI and MRI scans. A blood draw for genomic DNA extraction of each subject was obtained at the screening or baseline visit and was genotyped using the Illumina HumanOmniExpress BeadChip (Illumina, Inc, San Diego, CA, USA) for each subject (620,901 SNPs). Any SNP with a minor allele frequency less than 0.1 was excluded from the study. Table 1 shows a summary of relevant demographic information for this study.

**Table 1.** The highest degree of genetic correlation was shared between the FA of the cingulum and the volume of the caudate nucleus of the brain. Additionally the cingulum mean FA was also the tract measure most highly genetically correlated with the volume of the hippocampus, both of which make up the circuitry of the limbic system – a key target of pathology in the development of Alzheimer's disease. Average volume, FA, and standard deviation of structures are shown.

| | Caudate Volume Mean (SD) | Hippocampal Volume Mean (SD) | Cingulum FA Mean (SD) | Age (yrs) Mean (SD) | ICV |
|---|---|---|---|---|---|
| Total n = 65 | 3288.5 mm³ (481.8) | 3367.9 mm³ (497.7) | 0.362 (0.04) | 74.42 (7.4) | 0.765 (0.09) |
| Males n = 36 | 3455.5 mm³ (500.6) | 3460.8 mm³ (550.2) | 0.370 (0.04) | 73.57 (7.1) | 0.817 (0.06) |
| Females n = 29 | 3081.1 mm³ (369.9) | 3252.5 mm³ (403.8) | 0.351 (0.03) | 75.48 (7.8) | 0.701 (0.06) |

## 2.2 DTI and MRI Processing and Phenotype Extraction

Non-brain regions were automatically removed from each T1-weighted MRI scan, and from a T2-weighted image from the DWI set using the FSL tool "BET" (http://fsl.fmrib.ox.ac.uk/fsl/). A trained neuroanatomical expert manually edited the T1-weighted scans to further refine the brain extraction. All T1-weighted images were linearly aligned using FSL (with 9 DOF) to a common space with 1mm isotropic voxels and a 220×220×220 voxel matrix. DWI data were corrected for eddy current distortions using the FSL tools (http://fsl.fmrib.ox.ac.uk/fsl/). For each subject, the images with no diffusion sensitization were averaged, and elastically registered to the T1 scan to compensate for susceptibility artifacts.

For both datasets, single tensor-based FA maps were computed from the DW images and registered to the ENIGMA-DTI mean template [2, 8] as outlined at http://enigma.loni.ucla.edu/ongoing/dti-working-group/. Skeletonized maps were created using tract-based spatial statistics (TBSS [9]) and regions along the skeleton were parcellated according to the Johns Hopkins University DTI Atlas [10]. The FA of partial tracts and bilateral regions were averaged. The regions analyzed (ROIs) included the full skeleton, GCC – the *genu* of the corpus callosum, BCC – the body of the corpus callosum, SCC – the *splenium* of the corpus callosum, FX – the fornix, CGC – the bilateral cingulate, CR – *corona radiata*, EC – bilateral external capsule, IFO – bilateral inferior fronto-occipital fasciculus, PTR – posterior thalamic radiation, SFO – bilateral superior fronto-occipital fasciculus, SLF – bilateral superior longitudinal fasciculus, SS – bilateral sagittal stratum, and CST – the bilateral corticospinal tract.

Subcortical regions were segmented using FSL's FIRST according to protocols found at http://enigma.loni.ucla.edu/protocols/imaging-protocols/ [11]. These regions included average bilateral volumes for the amygdala, nucleus accumbens, hippocampus, caudate, thalamus, pallidum, and putamen.

## 2.3     Calculating the Genetic Correlation

Using the QTIM sample, we used a "cross-twin cross-trait" analysis to detect common genetic or environmental factors influencing all pairs of subcortical structure volumes and the mean FA for all regions of interest examined. Covariance matrices for these phenotypes were computed for the monozygotic twins (MZ) who share all the same genes, and the dizygotic twins (DZ) who share on average half of their genetic polymorphisms. These covariance matrices were then entered into a multivariate structural equation model (SEM) using OpenMx [12] (http://openmx.psyc.virginia.edu) to fit the relative contributions of additive genetic (A), shared environmental (C), and unshared or unique environmental and error (E) components to the population variances and covariances of the observed variables.

If the correlation between the volume in one twin and the FA in the other twin is greater in MZ pairs (sharing 100% of their genome) than in DZ pairs (sharing approximately 50% of their genome), then, in the classical twin design, we assume that the greater correlation may be attributable to common genetic factors that influence the two traits. Using a multivariate SEM, we can compute the additive genetic and shared environmental influences on the correlations between the two phenotypes, denoted as $r_A$ and $r_C$, respectively. Significant associations were determined if removal of the additive genetic correlation component of the model ($r_A$ in the path diagram seen in Figure 1) resulted in a significantly poorer fit to the data. Using this model, we were able to narrow down regions where a strong bivariate genetic association was detectable. This would imply that both the FA and the volumes of the respective brain regions are influenced by a common subset of additive genetic factors, or that these two imaging traits exhibit "pleiotropy". Pleiotropic effects of genes in this case would imply that a trait in twin #1 of a pair is able to predict the other trait in the twin #2 of the pair, and that the predictions tend to be better in identical than fraternal twins; if common genes are responsible for driving some of the correlation, the cross-twin prediction would be more accurate in the case of MZ twins than DZ twins as they share more of their genome. With a large enough sample size, recent methods show that it may be possible to estimate the shared genetic correlation of different traits using the full genome even in unrelated individuals [13].

## 2.4     Seemingly Unrelated Regression Model for GWAS

A standard univariate genome-wide association test uses the general linear regression model to test the additive effect of all genotyped variants on the phenotype of interest.

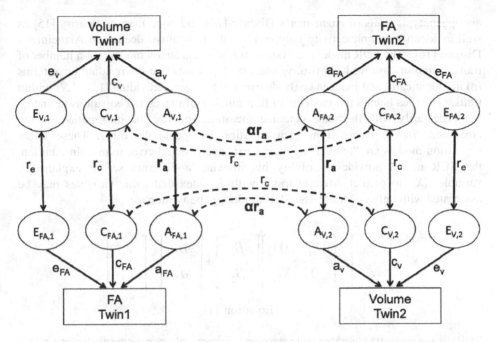

**Fig. 1.** Cross-twin cross-trait diagram for computing genetic correlations. In this method from classical quantitative genetics, a trait in one twin (such as the volume of part of the brain) is used to predict a different trait in the other twin (such as the integrity of a fiber tract on DTI). If these "cross-twin cross-trait" predictions can be made more accurately in identical twins, who share all their genes, than in fraternal twins, who do not, there is a basis to begin to model the additive genetic influences on both traits, as well as many other components that account for the correlations between the imaging modalities.

Using ADNI, a neuroimaging dataset independent of the one we used to calculate genetic correlations, we ran a univariate genome-wide association study (GWAS) on subcortical volume measures (the caudate and the hippocampus), which were found to have highest genetic correlations with the FA of the cingulum (see Results). As we searched the full genome, i.e., we tested approximately 500,000 SNPs (with a minor allele frequency (MAF) greater than 0.1) for any statistical association with each volume of interest; a stringent threshold is set for determining significance (as is standard practice in a GWAS study). We selected all variants that showed any sign of suggestive associations ($p < 10^{-4}$) to test in our SUR model. We hypothesized that some of these variants are also associated with the FA of the cingulum; we expected that joint bivariate analysis would allow an improvement in the significance of the tested associations.

The seemingly unrelated regression (SUR) model was originally developed for applications in econometrics [6]. Recently, the SUR model has been applied in a biomedical framework, i.e., identifying genetic variants associated with endophenotypic traits of Alzheimer's Disease [14] and bone marrow density [15] as well as identifying connectivity failures related to cognitive decline in Alzheimer's Disease [16]. The SUR model is a system of linear regression models for a number of traits, $n$ (in our case we have two, $y_1$ and $y_2$). It assumes that the residual error terms ($\varepsilon$) are identically and independently distributed for each individual (1, ..., $N$) within traits. The idea behind the model is to fit a number of regression equations at once – not necessarily with the same outcome measure, and use the information on the covariance in the errors from each equation to update the other. These linear regression models are "related" by their correlated residual error terms. In addition, the SUR model provides flexibility by allowing a different set of explanatory variables ($X_i$) to predict different traits, with the idea that some variables may be associated with only one trait. The SUR model can be written as:

$$
\begin{bmatrix} y_1 \\ y_2 \end{bmatrix} = \begin{bmatrix} X_1 & 0 \\ 0 & X_2 \end{bmatrix} \begin{bmatrix} \beta_1 \\ \beta_2 \end{bmatrix} + \begin{bmatrix} a_1 \\ a_2 \end{bmatrix} + \begin{bmatrix} \varepsilon_1 \\ \varepsilon_2 \end{bmatrix}
$$

(Equation 1)

SUR allows us to fit a number of regression equations at once, using the solution of a set of simultaneous equations to improve the accuracy of all the fitted models. For the purposes of this study, we used a bivariate SUR model of correlated brain measures to help boost the power to detect those genetic associations often too difficult to discover due to their small effect sizes. The two traits examined are a given subcortical volume (e.g., the volume of the hippocampus, averaged across the left and right hemispheres) and an average tract FA (e.g., the mean FA of the cingulum). Specifically for the purposes of this study, we examined two bivariate models: (1) the average volume of the hippocampus and the average tract FA and (2) the average volume of the caudate and the average FA tract. In our regression models that are assumed to hold simultaneously, the regional brain volumes are predicted by sex, age and intracranial volume and FA is predicted by sex and age, where coefficients for all variables remained unrestricted. Additionally (not shown in the equation) we control for the first four components derived from the multi-dimensional scaling (MDS) plots to control for differences in population structure, an important factor in genetic association studies. This correction makes sure that differences in ethnicity among participants do not lead to spurious genetic associations with brain measures of interest that would not hold up within any one ethnic group.

$$
\begin{aligned}
y_{hvol} &= Age * \beta_{age} + Sex * \beta_{sex} + IVC * \beta_{IVC} + a_{hvol} + \varepsilon_{hvol} \\
y_{CGC} &= Age * \beta_{age} + Sex * \beta_{sex} + a_{CGC} + \varepsilon_{CGC}
\end{aligned} \quad + \varepsilon
$$

(Equation 2)

SUR regressions were carried out using the 'systemfit' package in R (version 2.15.1).

# 3    Results

The cross-twin cross-trait model was fitted between all pairs of bilateral volume measures and FA measures. When controlling for the intracranial volume, this model revealed a high genetic correlation between the average caudate volume and the mean FA in the bilateral cingulum (Figure 2). This relationship is of interest, as it is not obvious *a priori* that measures from DTI will correlate with morphometry on standard anatomical MRI, and it is even less obvious that the correlations will be due to common variants in the genome. The presence of genetic correlations across imaging modalities shows that both of these situations are indeed true of our datasets.

Additionally, the FA of the cingulum is the connection most genetically correlated with the hippocampus - a region previously used as the phenotype of interest to discover novel genetic associations in the largest meta-analytical brain imaging studies to date (N>20,000 subjects) [1, 17]. Although the genetic correlation is much lower, it is still significant.

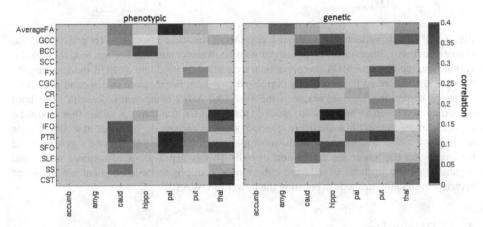

**Fig. 2. Left:** phenotypic correlations between different brain measures, and **Right:** genetic correlations between bilateral subcortical structure volumes (from anatomical MRI) and mean tract FAs (from DTI scans of the same subjects) while controlling for the intracranial volume, where *red colors* indicate high genetic correlation and *blue* indicates low detectable correlations. Note that the phenotypic correlation is the standard correlation between any of the two brain measures, here taking into account the non-independence of siblings by using a random-effects model. The genetic correlation will be zero if the correlation is zero, or if it is non-zero but there are no genetic variants with detectable effects on both measures.

A univariate GWAS was performed for each of the caudate and the hippocampal volumes. We controlled for age, sex, intracranial volume, and the first four components of the multidimensional scaling (MDS) plots. All SNPs that showed a suggestive association ($p<10^{-4}$) were carried forward into an SUR model. This included 39 SNPs for the caudate and 30 SNPs for hippocampal volume. The bivariate SUR model involved the volume of interest and also the FA of the cingulum, which was the DTI measure found to have the highest genetic correlation with both volumes. In Figure 3, results from both univariate and bivariate analyses are plotted relative to the (uniform) *p*-values that would be expected under the null hypothesis. In general, while it appears the bivariate assessment does not improve association *p*-values for the most associated variants, there is a general trend for improving the power for association overall.

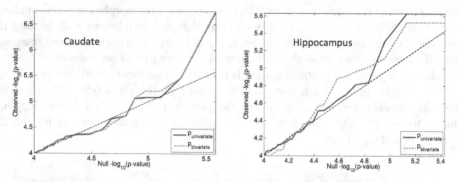

**Fig. 3.** All genetic variants that showed a suggestive statistical association ($p < 10^{-4}$) with (a) caudate nucleus volume, or (b) hippocampal volume, when controlling for age, sex, intracranial volume and the first four MDS components, were carried forward into an SUR model using the effect of the variant on the genetically correlated cingulum FA measure as a second predictive equation, controlling for age, sex, and the first four MDS components. Results from both univariate and bivariate analyses are plotted relative to the (uniform) *p*-values that would be expected under the null hypothesis. In general, while it appears the bivariate assessment does not improve association *p*-values for the most associated variants, there may be a general trend for improving the power for association overall. This is just a proof of concept study, and expansion of the methods to a larger cohort may corroborate the theoretical advantage of bivariate correlation methods in boosting the power of GWAS.

# 4    Discussion

Here we developed a new method to find genetic factors that affect two different brain imaging modalities, after showing that measures from each are genetically correlated. This leads to the remarkable conclusion that common variants in the human genome are partly responsible for driving the correlation between measures in two very different imaging modalities. To show this correlation, we first determined the genetic correlation between various neuroimaging measures obtained from DTI and MRI, using a structural equation model and a twin design. Next, we show that these genetically correlated measures can be used in a bivariate genome-wide association test. This may, at least in principle, provide boosted power in identifying additional genetic loci involved in determining and influencing brain structure.

Using genetic correlations to cluster imaging phenotypes has previously been helpful in discovering brain regions influenced by the same underlying genetic variants. One study clustered regions of the cortex with common underlying genetic determination [18,19]. It is logical that after clustering, this new regions of interest can be useful for boosting the power of univariate genome-wide association studies to discover genetic variants that may modulate brain structure using measures obtained from a single modality including DTI [4] or details of subcortical structures segmented from standard MRI [20]. Here, the joint use of the DTI and MRI measures offers additional advantages, as they are already measures known to be reliable and heritable [2, 21]. They are also the target biomarkers and phenotypes of several multisite projects and consortia, particularly of the ENIGMA group [22]. In such consortia, meta-analysis of genetic effects can discover and validate the effect of specific genetic variants on specific brain structures. These discovered variants may hold the key to identifying new genetic markers that put the brain at risk for developmental and degenerative disorders, while also allowing us to identify the neuroanatomical and molecular pathways involved.

A bivariate analysis such as the one proposed here – if conducted on a multi-site, meta-analytic scale – could boost power to discover genetic associations, and could help to identify molecular pathways in which these genes exert their effects. The same approach of clustering genetically correlated features in images could allow us to map the trajectory of effects on connected brain regions or even hubs and subnetworks in brain connectivity maps. Our SUR model even allows us to use different predictive covariates for different phenotypes of interest (i.e., using ICV as a covariate for volume measures, but not for FA measures from DTI scans).

ADNI, in particular, focuses on discovering genetic markers associated with brain degeneration in Alzheimer's disease. As such, the genetic correlations between measures from the cingulum in the limbic system and the hippocampus is of interest. The cingulum is the main white matter pathway connecting limbic structures (i.e., hippocampus, amygdala) with the cingulate cortex and the striatum. Our test set was comprised of only 65 unrelated subjects, so power is obviously extremely limited. While no genome-wide significant results are expected, our methods could be used to pick up trends for better identifying loci of interest. As the ADNI-2 DTI database grows, a future analysis involving more subjects is feasible.

A related idea to that in this paper is the use of very large sets of phenotypes to fit models, without requiring any of the subjects to have all the measures collected. Using imaging data from multiple sources, [23] were able to classify ADNI subjects into diagnostic groups, even when very large amounts of data are missing. The use of sparse regression models that allow "block-wise" missing data is a considerable advantage in epidemiology, as there are many cohorts with "deep phenotyping" – many measures assessed – without being able to rely on having all measures in all subjects. When the available sample sizes become truly vast (such as the 10,000+ subjects analyzed in the ENIGMA efforts [22,24-26]), it should be possible to fit bivariate correlation matrices between all pairs of points in a pair of imaging modalities, followed by clustering of the resulting genetic correlation matrix. Such an approach has already been found to boost power for GWAS studies within a modality [17], but the current paper suggests that it is possible to draw upon a very large body of multi-modal biomarker data and apply genetic screening to pick out coherent inherited patterns that run through all imaging modalities. Among all the ways to boost power in imaging genetics, it seems that the joint and simultaneous use of many modalities of data may help pick up genetic signals. In this way, imaging genetics offers some advantages over clinical genetic association studies, as the target signal is a vast and high-dimensional signal with latent structure. The better we exploit the underlying statistical coherence in the target signals, the more rapidly and efficiently we will detect the genetic variants that influence them.

# References

1. Stein, J.L., et al.: Identification of common variants associated with human hippocampal and intracranial volumes. Nat. Genet. 44(5), 552–561 (2012)
2. Jahanshad, N., et al.: Multi-site genetic analysis of diffusion images and voxelwise heritability analysis: A pilot project of the ENIGMA-DTI working group. Neuroimage (2013)
3. Almasy, L., Dyer, T.D., Blangero, J.: Bivariate quantitative trait linkage analysis: pleiotropy versus co-incident linkages. Genetic Epidemiology 14(6), 953–958 (1997)
4. Chiang, M.C., et al.: Gene network effects on brain microstructure and intellectual performance identified in 472 twins. J. Neurosci. 32(25), 8732–8745 (2012)
5. Kochunov, P., et al.: Genetic analysis of cortical thickness and fractional anisotropy of water diffusion in the brain. Frontiers in Neuroscience 5, 120 (2011)
6. Zellner, A.: An Efficient Method of Estimating Seemingly Unrelated Regressions and Tests for Aggregation Bias. Journal of the American Statistical Association 57(298), 348–368 (1962)
7. Zhan, L., et al.: Angular versus spatial resolution trade-offs for diffusion imaging under time constraints. Hum. Brain Mapp. (2012)
8. Kochunov, P., et al.: Genome-wide association of full brain white matter integrity – from the ENIGMA DTI working group. In: Organization of Human Brain Mapping, Beijing, China (2012)
9. Smith, S.M., et al.: Tract-based spatial statistics: voxelwise analysis of multi-subject diffusion data. NeuroImage 31(4), 1487–1505 (2006)
10. Mori, S., et al.: Stereotaxic white matter atlas based on diffusion tensor imaging in an ICBM template. Neuroimage 40(2), 570–582 (2008)
11. Hibar, D.P., +200-co-authors, ENIGMA-Consortium: ENIGMA2: Genome-wide scans of subcortical brain volumes in 16,125 subjects from 28 cohorts worldwide. In: Organization of Human Brain Mapping, Seattle, WA (2013)
12. Boker, S., et al.: OpenMx: An Open Source Extended Structural Equation Modeling Framework. Psychometrika 76(2), 306–317 (2011)
13. Lee, S.H., Yang, J., Goddard, M.E., Visscher, P.M., Wray, N.R.: Estimation of pleiotropy between complex diseases using single-nucleotide polymorphism-derived genomic relationships and restricted maximum likelihood. Bioinformatics 28, 2540–2542 (2012)
14. Bhatt, P., et al.: Multivariate analysis of GWAS for identification for genetic variants in Endophenotypes related to Alzheimer's Disease, Master's thesis. Oregon Health and Science University (2012)

15. Saint-Pierre, A., et al.: Bivariate association analysis in selected samples: application to a GWAS of two bone mineral density phenotypes in males with high or low BMD. Eur. J. Hum. Genet. 19(6), 710–716 (2011)
16. Jahanshad, N., et al.: Boosting power to associate brain connectivity measures and dementia severity using Seemingly Unrelated Regressions (SUR). In: Wang, L., Yushkevich, P., Ourselin, S. (eds.) MICCAI Workshop on Novel Imaging Biomarkers in Alzheimer's Disease, Nice, France. LNCS, pp. 103–112 (2012)
17. Bis, J.C., et al.: Common variants at 12q14 and 12q24 are associated with hippocampal volume. Nat. Genet. 44(5), 545–551 (2012)
18. Chen, C.H., et al.: Hierarchical genetic organization of human cortical surface area. Science 335, 1634–1636 (2012)
19. Chen, C.H., et al.: Genetic influences on cortical regionalization in the human brain. Neuron 72, 537–544 (2011)
20. Hibar, D.P., et al.: Genetic clustering on the hippocampal surface for genome-wide association studies. In: Mori, K., et al. (eds.) MICCAI 2013, Part II. LNCS, vol. 8150, pp. 674–681. Springer, Heidelberg (2013)
21. den Braber, A., Bohlken, M.M., Brouwer, R.M., van 't Ent, D., Kanai, R., Kahn, R.S., de Geus, E.J., Hulshoff Pol, H.E., Boomsma, D.I.: Heritability of subcortical brain measures: A perspective for future genome-wide association studies. Neuroimage (2013)
22. Thompson, P.M., et al.: The ENIGMA Consortium: Large-scale Collaborative Analyses of Neuroimaging and Genetic Data. Special Issue of Brain Imaging and Behavior, Invited Review (in submission, 2013)
23. Yuan, L., Wang, Y., Thompson, P.M., Narayan, V.A., Ye, J.: Multi-source feature learning for joint analysis of incomplete multiple heterogeneous neuroimaging data. Neuroimage 61, 622–632 (2012)
24. Hibar, D.P., et al., ENIGMA-Consortium: ENIGMA2: Genome-wide scans of subcortical brain volumes in 16,125 subjects from 28 cohorts worldwide. In: Organization of Human Brain Mapping, Seattle, WA (2013)
25. Turner, J.A., et al., ENIGMA-Schizophrenia: A Prospective Meta-Analysis of Subcortical Brain Volumes in Schizophrenia via the ENIGMA Consortium. In: Organization of Human Brain Mapping, Seattle, WA (2013)
26. Hibar, D.P., et al., ENIGMA-BipolarDisorder: Meta-analysis of structural brain differences in bipolar disorder: the ENIGMA-Bipolar Disorder. In: Organization of Human Brain Mapping, Seattle, WA (2013)

# Network-Guided Sparse Learning for Predicting Cognitive Outcomes from MRI Measures[*]

Jingwen Yan[1,2], Heng Huang[3], Shannon L. Risacher[1], Sungeun Kim[1],
Mark Inlow[4], Jason H. Moore[5], Andrew J. Saykin[1], and Li Shen[1,2,**]

[1] Radiology and Imaging Sciences, Indiana University School of Medicine, IN, USA
[2] School of Informatics, Indiana University Indianapolis, IN, USA
shenli@iu.edu
[3] Computer Science and Engineering, University of Texas at Arlington, TX, USA
[4] Department of Mathematics, Rose-Hulman Inst. of Tech., IN, USA
[5] The Geisel School of Medicine at Dartmouth College, NH, USA

**Abstract.** Alzheimer's disease (AD) is characterized by gradual neurodegeneration and loss of brain function, especially for memory during early stages. Regression analysis has been widely applied to AD research to relate clinical and biomarker data such as predicting cognitive
outcomes from MRI measures. In particular, sparse models have been
proposed to identify the optimal imaging markers with high prediction
power. However, the complex relationship among imaging markers are
often overlooked or simplified in the existing methods. To address this
issue, we present a new sparse learning method by introducing a novel
network term to more flexibly model the relationship among imaging
markers. The proposed algorithm is applied to the ADNI study for predicting cognitive outcomes using MRI scans. The effectiveness of our
method is demonstrated by its improved prediction performance over
several state-of-the-art competing methods and accurate identification
of cognition-relevant imaging markers that are biologically meaningful.

## 1 Introduction

Characterized by gradual loss of brain function, especially the memory and cognitive capabilities, Alzheimer's disease (AD) is a neurodegenerative disorder that
has attracted tremendous research attention due to its significant public health
impact and unknown disease mechanisms. Neuroimaging data, which characterize brain structure and function and its longitudinal changes, have been studied

---

[*] For the Alzheimer's Disease Neuroimaging Initiative. Data used in preparation of this article were obtained from the Alzheimer's Disease Neuroimaging Initiative (ADNI) database adni.loni.ucla.edu. As such, the investigators within the ADNI contributed to the design and implementation of ADNI and/or provided data but did not participate in analysis
or writing of this report. A complete listing of ADNI investigators can
be found at: http://adni.loni.ucla.edu/wp-content/uploads/how_to_apply/
ADNI_Acknowledgement_List.pdf
[**] Corresponding author.

L. Shen et al. (Eds.): MBIA 2013, LNCS 8159, pp. 202–210, 2013.
© Springer International Publishing Switzerland 2013

as potential biomarkers for early detection of AD. Regression models have been studied to relate imaging markers to AD phenotypes such as cognitive outcomes.

Early applications focused on traditional regression models such as stepwise regression [6], which predicted cognitive outcomes one at a time. To address the relationships among multiple outcomes, multi-task learning strategies were recently proposed for achieving improved prediction performance. For example, $\ell_{2,1}$-norm [8, 11] was employed to extract features that have impact on all or most clinical scores; and a sparse Bayesian method [7] was proposed to explicitly estimate the covariance structure among multiple outcome measures.

Despite of the above achievements, few regression models take into account the covariance structure among predictors. Since brain structures tend to work together to achieve a certain function, brain imaging measures are often correlated with each other. A recent study proposed a prior knowledge guided regression model, using the group information to enforce the intra-group similarity [10]. However, the relationships among brain structures are much more complicated than a simple partitioning of all the structures into non-overlapping groups. To overcome this limitation, we present a new sparse learning method by introducing a novel network term to more flexibly model the relationship among brain imaging measures. This new model not only preserves the strength of $\ell_{2,1}$-norm to enforce similarity across multiple scores from a cognitive test, but also takes into account the complex network relationship among imaging predictors. We empirically demonstrate its effectiveness by applying it to the ADNI data.

## 2   Network-Guided Sparse Regression

Throughout this section, we write matrices as boldface uppercase letters and vectors as boldface lowercase letters. Given a matrix $\mathbf{M} = (m_{ij})$, its $i$-th row and $j$-th column are denoted as $\mathbf{m}^i$ and $\mathbf{m}_j$ respectively. The Frobenius norm and $\ell_{2,1}$-norm (also called as $\ell_{1,2}$-norm) of a matrix are defined as $||\mathbf{M}||_F = \sqrt{\sum_i ||\mathbf{m}^i||_2^2}$ and $||\mathbf{M}||_{2,1} = \sum_i \sqrt{\sum_j m_{ij}^2} = \sum_i ||\mathbf{m}^i||_2$, respectively.

We focus on multi-task learning paradigm, where imaging measures are used to predict one or more cognitive outcomes. Let $\{\mathbf{x}_1, \cdots, \mathbf{x}_n\} \subseteq \Re^d$ be imaging measures and $\{\mathbf{y}_1, \cdots, \mathbf{y}_n\} \subseteq \Re^c$ cognitive outcomes, where $n$ is the number of samples, $d$ is the number of predictors (feature dimensionality) and $c$ is the number of response variables (tasks). Let $\mathbf{X} = [\mathbf{x}_1, \ldots, \mathbf{x}_n]$ and $\mathbf{Y} = [\mathbf{y}_1, \ldots, \mathbf{y}_n]$.

Motivated by using the $\ell_1$ norm (Lasso, [5]) to impose sparsity on relevant features, the $\ell_{2,1}$ norm [3] was first proposed to taking into account the relationship among responses while still preserving the sparsity advantage of Lasso. The object function is:

$$\min_{\mathbf{W}} ||\mathbf{W}^T\mathbf{X} - \mathbf{Y}||_F^2 + \gamma||\mathbf{W}||_{2,1} . \tag{1}$$

This approach couples multiple tasks together, with $\ell_2$ norm within tasks and $\ell_1$ norm within features. While the $\ell_2$ norm enforces the selection of similar features across tasks, the $\ell_1$ norm helps achieve the final sparsity. It has been widely applied to capture biomarkers having affects across most or all responses. Yet in

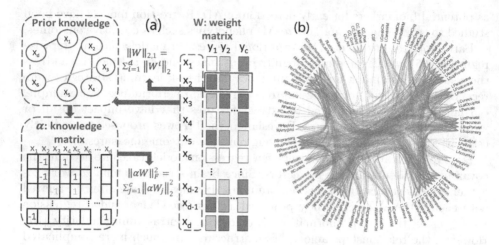

**Fig. 1.** (a) Illustration of the proposed NG-L21 model: This model enforces $\ell_{2,1}$-norm regularization ($\|\mathbf{W}\|_{2,1}$) to jointly select prominent predictors for all response variables, and introduces a new regularization term ($\|\alpha\mathbf{W}\|_F^2$) to flexibly model the relationship among predictors based on prior knowledge. (b) Correlation network among 99 FreeSurfer measures in an example cross-validation trial: Two measures are connected if their Pearson correlation coefficient, calculated from the training data, is $\geq 0.5$.

this model the rows of $\mathbf{W}$ are equally treated, which implies that the underlying structures among predictors are ignored. To address this issue, Group-Sparse Multi-task Regression and Feature Selection (G-SMuRFS) method [9] was proposed to exploit the interrelated structures within and between the predictor and response variables. It assumes 1) possible partition exists among predictors, and 2) predictors within one partition should have similar weights.

However, in practice the relationship among predictors may not be as simple as a straightforward partition. For example, imaging markers can be grouped by different brain circuitries, which may overlap with each other. In addition, instead of partitioning predictors into groups, the relationship among predictors can be represented more generally by a network (e.g., Figure 1(a)). To model these more complicated but more flexible structures among predictors, we propose a new *Network-Guided $\ell_{2,1}$ Sparse Learning (NG-L21)* model as follows.

The key idea here is to introduce a new regularization term ($\|\alpha\mathbf{W}\|_F^2$) to the $\ell_{2,1}$ model (Eq (1)) and formulate the objective function as:

$$\min_{\mathbf{W}} \|\mathbf{W}^T\mathbf{X} - \mathbf{Y}\|_F^2 + \gamma_1\|\alpha\mathbf{W}\|_F^2 + \gamma_2\|\mathbf{W}\|_{2,1} , \qquad (2)$$

where $\alpha$ is a sparse matrix in which each row indicates a neighborhood relationship within a network of connected predictors.

Fig. 1(a) shows a schematic example of $\alpha$ as well as the entire NG-L21 model. A network is given as prior knowledge, where nodes are predictors. In this study, the network is constructed as follows: An edge $(i, j)$ is inserted to the network if and only if $r(i, j)$ exceeds a given threshold (e.g., 0.5 used in our experiments), where $r(i,j)$ is the Pearson correlation coefficient between predictors $i$ and $j$ calculated based on the training data. Fig. 1(b) shows an example correlation network. Based on the network, we can define the knowledge matrix $\alpha$ as follows: for each edge $i, j$ in the network, we create a row in $\alpha$ with $i$-th entry as $-1$, $j$-th entry as $1$ and all the other entries as zeros. The intuition is that the weight difference between two correlated predictors should be minimized, which is reflected by the new regularization term of $\|\alpha \mathbf{W}\|_F^2$. We call this model *NG-L21*. Instead of using $-1$ and $1$ in $\alpha$, we can fill in the actual $-r(i,j)$ and $r(i,j)$ values for each edge $(i,j)$. Thus, the more correlated a feature pair is, the more constraint the pair is imposed by. We call this *weighted* model *NG-L21$_w$*.

Eq. (2) can be solved by taking the derivative w.r.t $\mathbf{W}$ and setting it to 0:

$$\mathbf{X}\mathbf{X}^T\mathbf{W} - \mathbf{X}\mathbf{Y}^T + \gamma_1\mathbf{D_1}\mathbf{W} + \gamma_2\mathbf{D_2}\mathbf{W} = 0, \tag{3}$$

where $\mathbf{D_1} = \alpha^T\alpha$, a matrix in which each row integrates all the neighboring relationships. For $i$-th row, it is the sum of all the rows in $\alpha$ whose $i$-th element is not zero. $\mathbf{D_2}$ is a diagonal matrix with the $i$-th diagonal element as $\frac{1}{2\|\mathbf{w}^i\|_2}$. Thus, we have

$$\mathbf{W} = (\mathbf{X}\mathbf{X}^T + \gamma_1\mathbf{D_1} + \gamma_2\mathbf{D_2})^{-1}\mathbf{X}\mathbf{Y}^T, \tag{4}$$

where $\mathbf{W}$ can be efficiently obtained by solving the linear equation $(\mathbf{X}\mathbf{X}^T + \gamma_1\mathbf{D_1} + \gamma_2\mathbf{D_2})\mathbf{W} = \mathbf{X}\mathbf{Y}^T$. Following [9], an efficient iterative algorithm based on Eq. (4) can be easily developed as follows.

**Input: X, Y**
Initialize $\mathbf{W}^1 \in \mathbb{R}^{d\times c}$, $t = 1$ ;
**while** *not converge* **do**
  1. Calculate the diagonal matrices $\mathbf{D}_2^{(t)}$, where the $i$-th diagonal element of $\mathbf{D}_2^{(t)}$ is $\frac{1}{2\|\mathbf{w}_t^i\|_2}$ ;
  2. $\mathbf{W}^{(t+1)} = (\mathbf{X}\mathbf{X}^T + \gamma_1\mathbf{D_1} + \gamma_2\mathbf{D}_2^{(t)})^{-1}\mathbf{X}\mathbf{Y}^T$ ;
  3. $t = t + 1$ ;
**end**
**Output:** $\mathbf{W}^{(t)} \in \mathbb{R}^{d\times c}$.

Next, we prove that the above algorithm converges to the global optimum. According to Step 2 in the algorithm, we have

$$W_{t+1} = \min_W Tr(X^TW - Y)^T(X^TW - Y) + \gamma_1 Tr(W^TD_1W) + \gamma_2 Tr(W^TD_{2(t)}W)$$

$$Tr(X^TW_{t+1} - Y)^T(X^TW_{t+1} - Y) + \gamma_1 Tr(\alpha W_{t+1})^T\alpha W_{t+1} + \gamma_2\sum_{i=1}^d\|w_{t+1}^i\|_2$$

$$\leq Tr(X^TW^{(t)} - Y)^T(X^TW^{(t)} - Y) + \gamma_1 Tr(\alpha W_t)^T\alpha W_t + \gamma_2\sum_{i=1}^d\|w_t^i\|_2$$

Finally we have:

$$\left\|X^T W_{t+1} - Y\right\|_F^2 + \gamma_1 \left\|\alpha W_{t+1}\right\|_F^2 + \gamma_2 \left\|W_{t+1}\right\|_{2,1}$$
$$\leq \left\|X^T W_t - Y)\right\|_F^2 + \gamma_1 \left\|\alpha W_t\right\|_F^2 + \gamma_2 \left\|W_t\right\|_{2,1}$$

The last but one step holds, because [8] for any vector $w$ and $w_0$, we have $\|w\|_2 - \frac{\|w\|_2^2}{2\|w_0\|_2} \leq \|w_0\|_2 - \frac{\|w_0\|_2^2}{2\|w_0\|_2}$. Thus, the algorithm decreases the objective value in each iteration. Since the problem is convex, satisfying the Eq. (2) indicates that $W$ is the global optimum solution. Therefore, this algorithm will converge to the global optimum of the problem.

# 3    Experimental Results

## 3.1    Data and Experimental Setting

The magnetic resonance imaging (MRI) and cognitive data were downloaded from the Alzheimer's Disease Neuroimaging Initiative (ADNI) database. One goal of ADNI has been to test whether serial MRI, positron emission tomography (PET), other biological markers, and clinical and neuropsychological assessment can be combined to measure the progression of mild cognitive impairment (MCI) and early AD. For up-to-date information, see www.adni-info.org.

This study included 179 AD and 205 healthy control (HC) participants (Table 1). For each baseline MRI scan, FreeSurfer V4 was employed for brain segmentation and cortical parcellation, and extracted 73 thickness measures and 26 volume measures. These 99 imaging measures were used to predict three sets of cognitive scores [1] separately: Mini-Mental State Exam (MMSE), Rey Auditory Verbal Learning Test (RAVLT, including 5 scores shown in Table 2 as joint response variables), and Wechsler Memory Scale III logical memory (LogMem). Using the regression weights derived from the HC participants, all the imaging measures were pre-adjusted for the baseline age, gender, education, handedness, and intracranial volume, and all the cognitive measures were pre-adjusted for the baseline age, gender, education and handedness.

Regression was performed separately on each cognitive task (MMSE, RAVLT, or LogMem) using the MRI measures as predictors, where the proposed NG-L21 and NG-L21$_w$ methods and three competing regression methods (Linear, Ridge and L21) were evaluated. Pearson correlation coefficients $r$ between the actual

**Table 1.** Participant characteristics

| Category | HC | AD |
|---|---|---|
| Number | 205 | 179 |
| Gender(M/F) | 112/93 | 98/81 |
| Handness(R/L) | 191/14 | 167/12 |
| Age(mean±std) | 76.07±4.98 | 75.58±7.51 |
| Education | 16.17±2.74 | 14.85±2.10 |

**Table 2.** RAVLT scores

| Score ID | Description |
|---|---|
| TOTAL | Total score of the first 5 learning trials |
| TOT6 | Trial 6 total number of words recalled |
| TOTB | List B total number of words recalled |
| T30 | 30 minute delay number of words recalled |
| RECOG | 30 minute delay recognition score |

**Table 3.** Mean prediction performance over five cross-validation trials is reported for each experiment, where the performance is measured by correlation coefficients between the actual and predicted cognitive scores in each trial. The p values, calculated from the paired sample t test between two sets of cross-validation correlation coefficients, are shown for comparing two proposed methods with L21.

| | | TOTAL | T30 | RECOG | TOT6 | TOTB | MMSE | LogMem |
|---|---|---|---|---|---|---|---|---|
| Correlation Coefficients | NG-L21$_w$ | 0.6511 | 0.5926 | 0.5636 | 0.6137 | 0.4630 | 0.7574 | 0.7076 |
| | NG-L21 | 0.6505 | 0.5925 | 0.5634 | 0.6130 | 0.4606 | 0.7575 | 0.7068 |
| | L21 | 0.6306 | 0.5792 | 0.5469 | 0.5967 | 0.4441 | 0.7488 | 0.6977 |
| | Ridge | 0.6215 | 0.5415 | 0.5368 | 0.5814 | 0.4406 | 0.7478 | 0.6870 |
| | Linear | 0.5396 | 0.4299 | 0.4533 | 0.4741 | 0.3525 | 0.6708 | 0.6071 |
| p values | L21 vs NG-L21$_w$ | 0.0029 | 0.0488 | 0.0476 | 0.0105 | 0.0021 | 0.0104 | 0.0119 |
| | L21 vs NG-L21 | 0.0037 | 0.0469 | 0.0577 | 0.0129 | 0.0024 | 0.0088 | 0.0098 |

and predicted cognitive scores were computed to measure the prediction performance. Five-fold cross validation was employed to obtain an unbiased estimate of regression performance. Paired t-test was applied to the cross-validation results to evaluate whether performance significantly differ between two methods.

## 3.2 Network Construction

Each MRI measure was treated as a network node, and the connectivity network among 99 MRI measures was constructed based on their pairwise Pearson correlation coefficients. Rather than including all pairwise links, threshold 0.5 was applied to connect only highly correlated nodes. For nodes that were not very correlated, constraints should not be imposed to make their regression weights similar to each other. A network was created using only the training data. Thus, our 5 cross-validation trials yielded 5 networks that were almost identical. One example was shown in Fig. 1(b), where totally 85 structures out of 99 had qualified links with correlation coefficient higher than 0.5. To incorporate this connectivity information into the proposed models, we examined the weighted network in NG-L21$_w$ and non-weighted one in NG-L21. While in the weighted network each link between structures was assigned the value of their correlation coefficient, non-weighted network treated all the links equally.

## 3.3 Prediction Performance and Biomarker Identification

Shown in Table. 3 is the performance comparison among all five methods. NG-L21 and NG-L21$_w$ both demonstrated an improved performance over the other three methods, while L21 performed the best among the three competing methods. The difference between NG-L21 and NG-L21$_w$ was minor, and the weighted method only led to slight improvements than non-weighted one for TOTAL, TOT6 and LogMem. This could be partially due to the small range of the edge

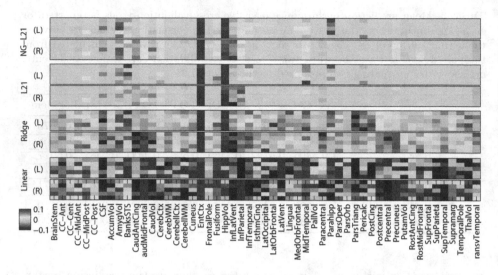

**Fig. 2.** Heat maps of regression weights for predicting MMSE scores using MRI measures. Five-fold cross-validation regression weights are plotted for NG-L21, L21, Ridge and Linear regression models respectively. Each panel corresponds to the measures from the left (L) or right (R) hemisphere. The measures shown in the first seven column (highlighted in blue) are unilateral, and the remaining ones are bilateral.

weights (0.5-1.0). To further make sure the improvements of the proposed methods were not by chance, we calculated p-values from the paired sample t test between two sets of cross-validation correlation coefficients from two different methods. According to the last two rows in Table 3, both NG-L21 and NG-L21$_w$ outperformed L21 significantly for predicting all the tested cognitive outcomes.

Finally, we examined the biomarkers identified by different methods. Shown in Fig. 2 was an example comparison of resulting regression coefficients among four methods (NG-L21$_w$ was extremely similar to NG-L21 and thus not shown), where 99 MRI measures were used to predict MMSE score. Each methods occupied two panels, representing the left and right hemispheres respectively. Apparently NG-L21 and L21 both showed sparse patterns while Linear and Ridge methods yielded non-sparse patterns that were hard to interpret. In addition, NG-L21 tended to select slightly more features than L21 as correlated measures were forced to be selected together in NG-L21, which yielded not only more stable patterns across cross-validation trials but also more biologically meaningful and more interpretable results. The MRI markers identified by NG-L21 yielded promising patterns that matched prior knowledge on neuroimaging and cognition. MMSE measured overall cognitive impairment; and thus its result (Fig. 2) included important AD-relevant imaging markers such as hippocampus, amygdala, inferior lateral ventricle, entorhinal cortex, and middle temporal gyri. Both LogMem and RAVLT were memory tests; and thus their results (Fig. 2) included regions relevant to memory, such as hippocampus, amygdala, entorhinal cortex, middle temporal gyri and parahippocampal gyri.

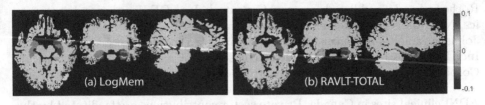

**Fig. 3.** NG-L21 weight maps on brain for (a) RAVLT-TOTAL and (b) LogMem scores

## 4    Conclusions

We presented a new network-guided sparse learning model NG-L21 and demonstrated its effectiveness by applying it to the ADNI data for predicting cognitive outcomes from MRI scans. While spatial correlation had been considered in several voxel-based feature selection and learning models [2, 4], the existing studies on predicting cognitive outcomes from ROI-based MRI measures often ignored [7, 8] or simplified [10] the relationships among these ROI predictors. The proposed NG-L21 model aimed to bridge this gap and introduced a novel network term to flexibly model the relationship among imaging markers. An efficient algorithm was developed to implement this model and was shown to be able to achieve global optimum. Its application to the ADNI data exhibited the following strengths of the NG-L21 model: (1) It could flexibly take into account the complex relationship among imaging markers in a network format rather than a simple grouping scheme used in [10]. (2) As a multi-task sparse learning framework, it could identify a compact set of imaging markers related to multiple cognitive outcomes. (3) By considering the correlation among predictors, it yielded not only improved prediction performance but also more stable cross-validation feature selection patterns. Different from traditional Lasso and L21 methods that tended to select only one relevant feature from a group of highly correlated ones, the NG-L21 model could jointly identify these correlated features, making the results more stable and easier to interpret.

**Acknowledgement.** This research was supported by NIH R01 LM011360, U01 AG024904, RC2 AG036535, R01 AG19771, P30 AG10133, and NSF IIS-1117335 at IU, by NSF CCF-0830780, CCF-0917274, DMS-0915228, and IIS-1117965 at UTA, and by NIH R01 LM011360, R01 LM009012, and R01 LM010098 at Dartmouth.

Data collection and sharing for this project was funded by the Alzheimer's Disease Neuroimaging Initiative (ADNI) (National Institutes of Health Grant U01 AG024904). ADNI is funded by the National Institute on Aging, the National Institute of Biomedical Imaging and Bioengineering, and through generous contributions from the following: Abbott; Alzheimer's Association; Alzheimer's Drug Discovery Foundation; Amorfix Life Sciences Ltd.; AstraZeneca; Bayer HealthCare; BioClinica, Inc.; Biogen Idec Inc.; Bristol-Myers Squibb Company; Eisai Inc.; Elan Pharmaceuticals Inc.; Eli Lilly and Company; F. Hoffmann-La

Roche Ltd and its affiliated company Genentech, Inc.; GE Healthcare; Innogenetics, N.V.; Janssen Alzheimer Immunotherapy Research & Development, LLC.; Johnson & Johnson Pharmaceutical Research & Development LLC.; Medpace, Inc.; Merck & Co., Inc.; Meso Scale Diagnostics, LLC.; Novartis Pharmaceuticals Corporation; Pfizer Inc.; Servier; Synarc Inc.; and Takeda Pharmaceutical Company. The Canadian Institutes of Health Research is providing funds to support ADNI clinical sites in Canada. Private sector contributions are facilitated by the Foundation for the National Institutes of Health (www.fnih.org). The grantee organization is the Northern California Institute for Research and Education, and the study is coordinated by the Alzheimer's Disease Cooperative Study at the University of California, San Diego. ADNI data are disseminated by the Laboratory for Neuro Imaging at the University of California, Los Angeles. This research was also supported by NIH grants P30 AG010129, K01 AG030514, and the Dana Foundation.

# References

1. Aisen, P.S., Petersen, R.C., et al.: Clinical core of the Alzheimer's Disease Neuroimaging Initiative: progress and plans. Alzheimers Dement 6(3), 239–246 (2010)
2. Liu, M., Zhang, D., Yap, P.-T., Shen, D.: Tree-guided sparse coding for brain disease classification. In: Ayache, N., Delingette, H., Golland, P., Mori, K. (eds.) MICCAI 2012, Part III. LNCS, vol. 7512, pp. 239–247. Springer, Heidelberg (2012)
3. Obozinski, G., Taskar, B., Jordan, M.: Multi-task feature selection. Technical Report, Statistics Department, UC Berkeley (2006)
4. Sabuncu, M.R., Van Leemput, K.: The relevance voxel machine (RVoxM): A bayesian method for image-based prediction. In: Fichtinger, G., Martel, A., Peters, T. (eds.) MICCAI 2011, Part III. LNCS, vol. 6893, pp. 99–106. Springer, Heidelberg (2011)
5. Tibshirani, R.: Regression shrinkage and selection via the lasso. J. R. Stat. Soc. Ser. B 58, 267–288 (1996)
6. Walhovd, K., Fjell, A., et al.: Multi-modal imaging predicts memory performance in normal aging and cognitive decline. Neurobiol Aging 31(7), 1107–1121 (2010)
7. Wan, J., et al.: Sparse Bayesian multi-task learning for predicting cognitive outcomes from neuroimaging measures in Alzheimer's disease. In: CVPR 2012, pp. 940–947 (2012)
8. Wang, H., Nie, F., et al.: Sparse multi-task regression and feature selection to identify brain imaging predictors for memory performance. In: ICCV 2011, pp. 557–562 (2011)
9. Wang, H., Nie, F., et al.: Identifying quantitative trait loci via group-sparse multitask regression and feature selection: an imaging genetics study of the ADNI cohort. Bioinformatics 28(2), 229–237 (2012)
10. Yan, J., et al.: Multimodal neuroimaging predictors for cognitive performance using structured sparse learning. In: Yap, P.-T., Liu, T., Shen, D., Westin, C.-F., Shen, L. (eds.) MBIA 2012. LNCS, vol. 7509, pp. 1–17. Springer, Heidelberg (2012)
11. Zhang, D., Shen, D.: Multi-modal multi-task learning for joint prediction of multiple regression and classification variables in Alzheimer's disease. Neuroimage 59(2), 895–907 (2012)

# A Framework to Compare Tractography Algorithms Based on Their Performance in Predicting Functional Networks

Fani Deligianni, Chris A. Clark, and Jonathan D. Clayden

Imaging and Biophysics Unit, Institute of Child Health, University College London,
London, United Kingdom
{f.deligianni,j.clayden,christopher.clark}@ucl.ac.uk
http://www.ucl.ac.uk/ich/research-ich/imaging-and-biophysics

**Abstract.** Understanding the link between brain function and structure is of paramount importance in neuroimaging and psychology. In practice, inaccuracies in recovering brain networks may confound neurophysiological factors and reduce the sensitivity in detecting statistically robust links. Hence, reproducibility and inter-subject variability of tractography approaches is currently under extensive investigation. However, a reproducible network is not necessarily more accurate. Here, we build a statistical framework to compare the performance of local and global tractograpy in predicting functional brain networks. We use a model selection framework based on sparse canonical correlation analysis and an appropriate metric to evaluate the similarity between the predicted and the observed functional networks. We demonstrate compelling evidence that global tractography outperforms local tractography in a cohort of healthy adults.

**Keywords:** structural connectivity, global tractography, prediction.

## 1 Introduction

Investigating the relationship between functional and structural brain connectivity is vital in understanding and interpreting neurophysiological findings. It is well established that during rest the brain shows spontaneous activity that is highly correlated between multiple brain regions. This activity can be captured with resting-state functional magnetic resonance imaging (rs-fMRI) and it results in reproducible functional networks across subjects. On the other hand, diffusion weighted images (DWI) measure the anisotropic diffusion of water molecules in the brain and carry valuable information regarding interregional brain connections. However, reconstructing the neuronal pathways relies on tractography algorithms that generate networks with poor reproducibility across subjects and studies. Although compelling evidence has emerged that there are strong structural connections between regions that are functionally linked [1], it is challenging to quantify the influence of fiber reconstruction errors.

L. Shen et al. (Eds.): MBIA 2013, LNCS 8159, pp. 211–221, 2013.

Tractography algorithms are tested for their reproducibility within and across subjects. However, reproducibility does not necessarily correlate with accuracy. For example, deterministic tractrography algorithms provide reproducible results but they are inaccurate when fibers cross and diverge. Phantom evaluation is a principled way of examining the performance of tractography algorithms [2]. Phantoms are made based on simplified assumptions that aim to test the performance of tractography under certain scenarios. Nevertheless, the increased fiber complexity of real tissues cannot be captured with the fiber cup phantom, which is an over-simplified scenario of a few crossing fibers.

In this work, we aim to compare the performance of two well known tractography algorithms [3, 4], which are categorised as local and global, respectively. Tractography techniques are categorised as global or local according to whether they account for information along the whole tract or not, respectively. The main advantages of local tracking are the low time complexity and that each tract is independent of the others. However, a major drawback that limits their robustness is that errors in propagating can accumulate along the local steps [3]. This can significantly affect the results and also contributes to distance-related biases. On the other hand, global tracking represents a new approach for identifying brain networks, which involves the simultaneous reconstruction of all the neuronal fibers by finding a solution that best fits the measured diffusion data. This approach has a better ability to resolve ambiguous fiber orientations, since it considers information along the whole neuronal pathway.

A phantom evaluation demonstrated that global tracking is superior to local tractography approaches [4, 5]. However, further experiments based on tracing results in macaques and a cohort of healthy subjects showed only a small improvement in the results [5]. Here, we suggest a systematic way to examine how different tractography approaches affect the observed relationship between structure and function. To our knowledge, this is the first systematic approach to examine whether a predictive framework based on resting-state fMRI is sensitive to differences in tractography.

To this end, we have developed a predictive framework based on sparse canonical correlation analysis (SCCA) [6]. SCCA is a special case of sparse reduced rank regression [7]. Firstly, we characterise functional connectivity as the inverse covariance matrix based on a shrinkage approach that guarantees well-defined, symmetric positive definite (SPD) matrices [8]. Subsequently, we introduce a model selection framework based on cross-validation to quantify the out-of-sample error related to each tractography approach. Finally, the distance between the predicted functional networks and the 'ground truth' rs-fMRI brain networks is estimated based on an intrinsic metric suitable to quantify differences in covariance matrices, independently of their parameterisation, ie. covariance versus the inverse of covariance [9–11].

This work builds upon previous inference approaches to investigate influences between structural connections and functional links [11, 12]. Deligianni et al. presented a framework based on principal component analysis (PCA) and canonical correlation analysis (CCA). Whereas this approach achieves dimensionality reduction, SCCA is based on a lasso penalty that aims to select the most relevant connections resulting in simultaneous dimensionality reduction and model selection. Model selection based on an $l1$ penalty is also presented in [11]. However, [11] relies on structural networks to regularise the estimation of functional connectivity based on the assumption that a functional connection between two regions only exists when there is a direct structural connection. An advantage of our approach is that it combines a multivariate technique, CCA, with model selection. Therefore, the predicted functional connectivity is well conditioned and it does not necessarily requires further regularisation to be constrained into symmetric positive definite space of matrices.

We apply the proposed approach in a cohort of healthy subjects with multiple structural and functional scans. We demonstrate that a prediction framework based on resting-state fMRI data can capture systematic differences between global and local tractogaphy. We present detailed quantitative results suggesting that global connectivity outperforms local connectivity in predicting functional networks from structural brain networks. Our results suggest that a prediction framework based on functional data could potentially be applied to compare the performance of tractography algorithms in *in-vivo* human imaging data and highlight specific connections that influence prediction.

## 2   Methods

### 2.1   Brain Network Construction

**Defining Regions of Interest (ROIs).** To define corresponding nodes in both functional and structural networks we used atlas-based regions of interest (ROIs) derived from Freesurfer cortical parcellation of the T1-weighted images [13]. BOLD fluctuations are profound in gray matter (GM), whereas tractography is more reliable in delineating white matter (WM) fibers. Hence, we focus on brain networks defined by cortical GM ROIs that are connected via WM fibers. We propagate the anatomical labels from T1 space to native space for both fMRI and DWI using non-rigid registration [14].

**Preprocessing.** The first five volumes of rs-fMRI data are removed to avoid T1 effects and preprocessing of the functional data involves motion correction, low pass filtering and spatial smoothing with FSL [15]. To construct corresponding functional networks the fMRI signal is averaged across voxels within each GM ROI. The signal in WM and cerebrospinal fluid (CSF) is also averaged and along with the six motion parameters provided from FSL is linearly regressed out.

We used TractoR for preprocessing of the diffusion weighted images (DWI) [16]. This involves converting DICOM files into a 4D NIfTI, identifying the volume with no diffusion weighting to use as an anatomical reference, creating a mask to identify voxels which are within the brain and correcting the data set for eddy current induced distortions. The last two stages are performed using FSL. Furthermore, the gradient vectors are corrected retrospectively to account for the eddy current correction.

**Functional Brain Networks.** Assuming that the brain activity patterns are described by a Gaussian multidimensional stationary process, the covariance matrix characterizes fully the statistical dependencies among the underlying signals [17]. Hence, we use the inverse covariance, normalised to unit diagonal to characterise functional connectivity. The inverse covariance is directly related to partial correlation, which provides a measure of connectivity strength between two regions once the influence of the others has been regressed out. This is particularly suited to relate functional connectivity with structural brain connectivity, since the latter describes direct pathways between cortical regions. To produce a well-conditioned, symmetric positive definite, $(\mathcal{Sym}_p^+)$, sample covariance matrix we use the shrinkage estimator [8]:

$$\hat{\Sigma}_\lambda = \lambda\hat{\mathbf{T}} + (1-\lambda)\hat{\Sigma} \tag{1}$$

where the sample covariance matrix $\hat{\Sigma}_\lambda$ is estimated as a convex linear combination of the unrestricted sample covariance matrix $\hat{\Sigma}$ and the estimator $\hat{\mathbf{T}}$, which is the identity matrix $\mathbf{I}$. In this case, the optimal regularization parameter $\lambda \in [0,1]$ is determined analytically based on the Ledoit-Wolf theorem [18]. This approach provides a systematic way to regularise the sample covariance matrix and it has been shown to greatly enhance inference of gene association networks [19], where the number of variables $n$ is much greater than the number of observations $p$. Therefore, it is suited to examine brain networks where the number of connections grow quadratically with the number of ROIs.

**Structural Brain Networks.** Two sets of structural networks are derived based on local and global tractography, respectively. The local tractography is implemented in TractoR based on the classic ball and stick model [3].

Global tractography is used to produce a second set of brain networks from the same DWI. Global tractography approaches try to reconstruct neuronal fibers simultaneously by finding line configurations that describe best the measured data. This makes them robust to noise, crossing fibers and imaging artefacts. However, their practical application was hindered by the computational complexity and time requirements. Reisert et al. proposed a time efficient approach that minimises a sum of two energies with respect to the fiber model, $M$, and the observed data, $D$. These energies control for the length of fibers (internal energy, $E_{int}$) and the difference between the model and the observed data (external energy, $E_{ext}$), respectively [4].

$$E(M) = E_{int}(M) + E_{ext}(M,D) \tag{2}$$

The model consists of small line segments. Each segment is described as a spatial location and orientation. From the arrangement of all segments a predicted MR-signal is computed based on the ball and stick model. The internal energy is based on attraction forces between connected segments that encourages them to stay together and have similar orientation. The external energy is the square difference between the actual signal and the predicted signal after the local mean is subtracted from both model and measured data. The optimisation is done based on the Metropolis-Hasting sampler.

To produce the corresponding structural connectivity matrices we consider only fibers that connect cortical regions via white matter and disregard the rest. We estimate the 'strength' of connection between two cortical regions as the number of fibers that connect the regions divided by the average number of white matter voxels that surround them.

## 2.2   A Predictive Framework Based on Sparse Canonical Correlation

**Sparse Canonical Correlation.** Canonical correlation analysis (CCA) is generally applied when one set of predictor variables $\mathbf{X}$ is to be related to another set of predicted variables $\mathbf{Y}$ and observations are available for both groups. Note that CCA is designed to deal with situations where the underlying variables are not statistically independent and, hence, they are inherently inter-correlated. The ultimate goal of CCA is to find two basis vectors (canonical vectors) $u$, $v$, one for each variable, so that the projections of $\mathbf{X}$, $\mathbf{Y}$ onto these vectors, respectively are maximally linearly correlated.

In CCA all variables from both sets are included in the fitted canonical vectors. However, for the purpose of studying brain connectivity, we are interested in sparse sets of associated variables, that would allow interpretable links between function and structure to emerge. Hence, we adapt sparse canonical correlation analysis (SCCA) to optimise the CCA criterion, subject to certain constrains [6]:

$$\text{maximise}_{u,v} u^T \mathbf{X}^T \mathbf{Y} v$$
$$\text{subject to}: \|u\|^2 \leq 1, \|v\|^2 \leq 1, \|u\|_1 \leq c_1, \|v\|_1 \leq c_2 \qquad (3)$$

$\|u\|_1 \leq c_1$ and $\|v\|_1 \leq c_2$ represent the $L_1$ (or *lasso*) penalty and they result in sparse canonical vectors $u$, $v$ when the penalties $c_1$ and $c_2$, respectively, are chosen appropriately. Note that with $u$ fixed, the criterion in eq. 3 is convex in $v$, and with $v$ fixed, it is convex in $u$. Therefore, the objective function of this biconvex criterion increases in each step of an iterative algorithm [6]:

$$u \leftarrow \text{argmax}_u u^T \mathbf{X}^T \mathbf{Y} v \text{ subject to}: \|u\|^2 \leq 1, \|u\|_1 \leq c_1$$
$$v \leftarrow \text{argmax}_v u^T \mathbf{X}^T \mathbf{Y} v \text{ subject to}: \|v\|^2 \leq 1, \|v\|_1 \leq c_1 \qquad (4)$$

**A Metric to Compare Covariance Matrices.** Correlation and covariance matrices lie on the space of symmetric definite positive matrices $\mathcal{F} = Sym_p^+$. The standard Euclidean distance on matrices, the Frobenius norm, does not account for the geometry of this space. Thus, this norm is ill-suited to quantify prediction errors. However, $Sym_p^+$ can be parameterized as a Riemannian manifold using an intrinsic metric [9]:

$$d_{AI}(\mathbf{P}, \mathbf{G})^2 = tr \left( \log \mathbf{G}^{-\frac{1}{2}} \mathbf{P} \mathbf{G}^{-\frac{1}{2}} \right)^2 \qquad (5)$$

This metric has beed used successfully to build statistical frameworks of precision matrices $Sym_p^+$ [11]. $d_{AI}$ is a distance metric, invariant to affine transformations and inversion, appropriate to quantify the distance between covariance matrices from biological data successfully [10].

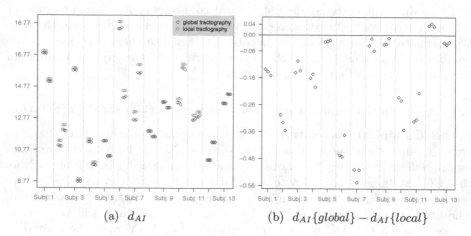

(a) $d_{AI}$               (b) $d_{AI}\{global\} - d_{AI}\{local\}$

**Fig. 1.** This plot shows how global tractography compares with local tractography for each subject and structural scan. a) Demonstrates that the distance $d_{AI}$ between the predicted and the observed functional connectivity is lower for global tractography than for local tractography. b) Shows the $d_{AI}$ metric for each difference in performance between global tractography and local tractography, per subject and structural scan, according to equation 7.

**Model Selection.** To evaluate the performance of local and global tractography, we use model selection, which is based on cross-validation. For each subject $s = 1, \ldots, S$, the SCCA model is trained based on the remaining $S - 1$ datasets. The number of components is estimated as the min of the ranks of the predictor and predicted variables in CCA. The penalty values $c_1$, $c_2$ are optimised in each cross-validation loop using an approach, which permutes the rows of both the predictor and predicted variables of the SCCA [6]. Subsequently, we use the left-out structural connectivity matrix $\mathbf{A}$ to predict the functional connectivity $\hat{\mathbf{F}}$:

$$\hat{\mathbf{F}} = (u\mathbf{A})^{-1}\mathbf{D}v^{-1} \tag{6}$$

$\mathbf{D}$ is a diagonal matrix of the canonical correlation scores. Finally, the difference between the predicted, $\hat{\mathbf{F}}$, and 'ground truth' functional connectivity matrix $\mathbf{F}$ is estimated as: $d_{AI}(\hat{\mathbf{F}}, \mathbf{F})$.

## 3   Results

Imaging data was acquired from 13 healthy adults using a Siemens Avanto 1.5 T clinical scanner using a self-shielded gradient set with maximum gradient amplitude of 40 mT m$^{-1}$ and standard 12 channel head coil. Echo-planar DWI were acquired along 60 non-collinear gradient directions at b=1000 s mm$^{-2}$, with three b=0 images for normalization. A voxel matrix of 96×96 was used and 45 contiguous axial slices acquired, each 2.5mm thick, with a 240 mm FOV,

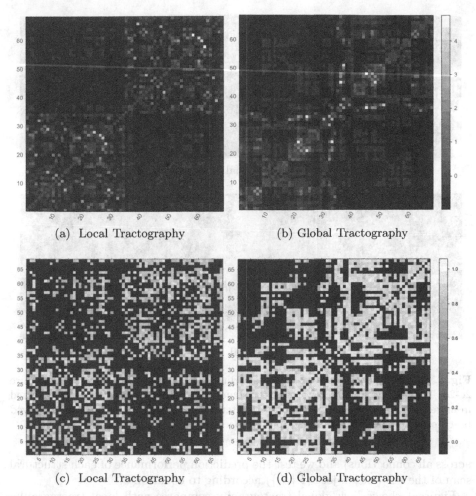

(a)  Local Tractography                    (b)  Global Tractography

(c)  Local Tractography                    (d)  Global Tractography

**Fig. 2.** The top row shows the z-scores along all structural scans for (a) local and (b) global tractography. The bottom row depicts the bootstrap results from (a) local and (b) global tractography.

voxel size of $2.5 \times 2.5 \times 2.5$ mm and TR/TE=7300/81 ms. T2*-weighted gradient-echo EPI sequence of 125 volumes was also acquired with TR/TE=3320/50 ms, 36 slices with thickness 3.0 mm, voxel size $3.0 \times 3.0 \times 3.0$ mm, flip angle 90°, FOV $192 \times 192 \times 108$ mm, voxel matrix $64 \times 64 \times 36$. High resolution T1-weighted whole-brain structural images were also obtained in all subjects.

Each of the 13 subjects' acquisition includes three structural scans that results in three structural connectivity matrices per subject and two rs-fMRI scans, which produce two functional connectivity matrices. These results in six combinations of structural-functional data per subject: $(S_i : F_j)$. From each leave-one-out cross-validation, we use data only from 12 subjects (a total of 72 samples

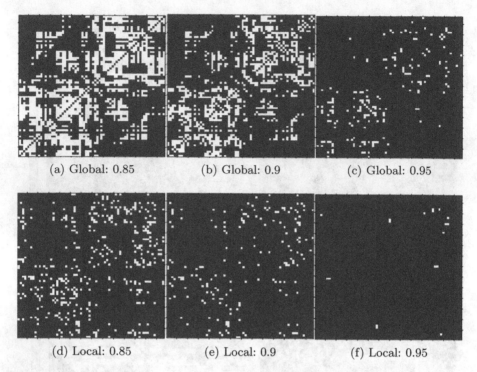

(a) Global: 0.85          (b) Global: 0.9          (c) Global: 0.95

(d) Local: 0.85          (e) Local: 0.9          (f) Local: 0.95

**Fig. 3.** Binary matrices derived by thresholding the bootstrap results shown in figure 2c-2d. The top and bottom rows show the structural connections that they are selected in more than 85%, 90% and 95% bootstrap iterations with structural networks derived based on global and local tractography, respectively.

across all connections) and we test the prediction performance of each structural scan of the left-out subject $(\hat{F}\{S_i\})$ according to equation 5.

Figure 1 shows how global tractography compares with local tractography for each subject and structural scan. Figure 1a demonstrates that the distance $d_{AI}$ between the predicted and the observed functional connectivity is lower for global tractography than for local tractography. $d_{AI}$ is a distance metric, with smaller values representing better performance. The inter-subject variability is a magnitude of order higher than the difference between the two algorithms. The prediction performance varies considerably across functional scans.

We also plot the difference in $d_{AI}$ between global and local tractography per scan, figure 1b:

$$d_{AI}(\hat{F}\{S_i{}^G\}, F_j) - d_{AI}(\hat{F}\{S_i{}^L\}, F_j) \qquad (7)$$

$S_i{}^G$ and $S_i{}^L$ corresponds to the structural brain networks derived from global and local tractography, respectively, for the same structural scan $S_i$. Note that in equation 7 the effect of variability across functional scans is cancelled.

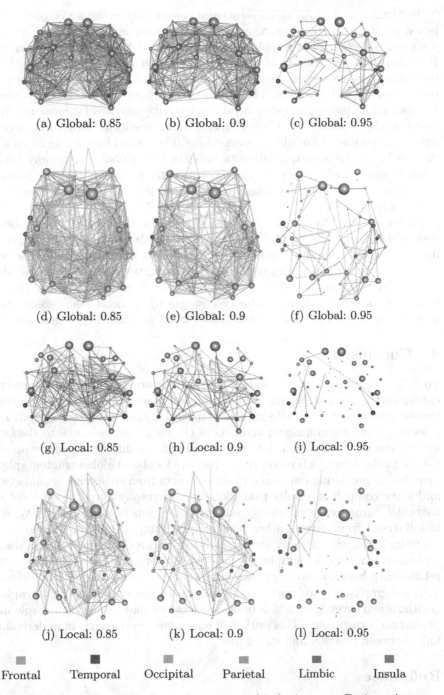

(a) Global: 0.85      (b) Global: 0.9      (c) Global: 0.95

(d) Global: 0.85      (e) Global: 0.9      (f) Global: 0.95

(g) Local: 0.85      (h) Local: 0.9      (i) Local: 0.95

(j) Local: 0.85      (k) Local: 0.9      (l) Local: 0.95

Frontal    Temporal    Occipital    Parietal    Limbic    Insula

**Fig. 4.** Thresholded matrices in figure 3 are mapped in brain space. Brain regions are represented with spheres and their radius reflect the relative size of the region.

To further investigate which structural connections are more consistently selected in each tractography method, we use bootstrap and examine the recovered $u$ vector. We resample with replacement all the available datasets and run SCCA 1000 times. The probability of a connection is estimated as the number of times the connection is selected divided by the number of bootstrap repetitions. Figure 2 summarises the results. The top row of the figure 2a-2b, demonstrates the z-scores across the original structural connectivity matrices for local and global tractography, respectively. Global tractography results in structural networks with stronger inter-hemispheric connections. The second row, figure 2c-2d shows the results of the bootstrap. Results indicate that global tractograpy leads to a higher number of connections more consistently selected across the bootstrap iterations. This is apparent when we threshold the bootstrapped connectivity matrices in figure 3.

Figure 3 shows the binary matrices derived by thresholding the bootstrap results shown in figure 2c-2d. These matrices are also mapped in brain space in figure 4. Brain regions are represented with spheres. Their centres are the center of masses of each underlying region and their radius reflect the relative size of each region. The color coding corresponds to different brain lobes: Temporal lobe (dark magenta), frontal lobe (yellow green), parietal lobe (golden road), occipital lobe (dark salmon), insula (cadet blue) and limbic (medium purple).

## 4   Conclusions

To fully understand how the brain works as a network, the physical connections through the white matter, that mediate information exchange must be accurately characterised. Global tracking may be more stable than local tractography in the presence of noise and imaging artifacts in the data. However, due to the lack of ground truth *in-vivo* tracing data direct evaluation is difficult. Here, we present a robust model selection framework to compare local and global tractography approaches in predicting functional brain networks from structural brain networks and show compelling results that global tractography outperforms local tractography. Structural connectivity only restrains functional connectivity, which is influenced from several other physiological factors. In fact, functional connectivity varies considerably across scans and it does not represent an absolute 'ground truth' for tractography. Nevertheless, we demonstrate evidence that the relationship between structure and function can capture systematic differences in tractography. Future work should aim to compare several tractography algorithms and investigate which brain connections play an important role in the prediction performance. This work is of paramount importance in understanding links between function and structure.

## References

1. van den Heuvel, M.P., et al.: Functionally linked resting-state networks reflect the underlying structural connectivity architecture of the human brain. Human Brain Mapping 30(10), 3127–3141 (2009)

2. Fillard, P., et al.: Quantitative evaluation of 10 tractography algorithms on a realistic diffusion MR phantom. NeuroImage 56(1), 220–234 (2011)
3. Behrens, T., et al.: Characterization and propagation of uncertainty in diffusion-weighted MR imaging. Magnet. Reson. Med. 50, 1077–1088 (2003)
4. Reisert, M., et al.: Global fiber reconstruction becomes practical. NeuroImage 54(2), 955–962 (2011)
5. Li, L., et al.: Quantitative assessment of a framework for creating anatomical brain networks via global tractography. NeuroImage 61(4), 1017–1030 (2012)
6. Witten, D.M., Tibshirani, R.J.: Extensions of sparse canonical correlation analysis with applications to genomic data. Stat. Appl. Genet. Mol. Biol. 8, Article 28 (2009)
7. Vounou, M., Nichols, T.E., Montana, G.: Discovering genetic associations with high-dimensional neuroimaging phenotypes: A sparse reduced-rank regression approach. NeuroImage 53(3), 1147–1159 (2010)
8. Krämer, N., Schäfer, J., Boulesteix, A.-L.: Regularized estimation of large-scale gene association networks using graphical gaussian models. BMC Bioinformatics 10, 384 (2009)
9. Förstner, W., Moonen, B.: A metric for covariance matrices. Qua Vadis Geodesia, 113 (1999)
10. Mitteroecker, P., Bookstein, F.: The ontogenetic trajectory of the phenotypic covariance matrix, with examples from craniofacial shape in rats and humans. Evolution 63(3), 727–737 (2009)
11. Deligianni, F., Varoquaux, G., Thirion, B., Robinson, E., Sharp, D.J., Edwards, A.D., Rueckert, D.: A probabilistic framework to infer brain functional connectivity from anatomical connections. In: Székely, G., Hahn, H.K. (eds.) IPMI 2011. LNCS, vol. 6801, pp. 296–307. Springer, Heidelberg (2011)
12. Deligianni, F., et al.: Inference of functional connectivity from structural brain connectivity. In: ISBI, p. 1113 (2010)
13. Desikan, R.S., et al.: An automated labeling system for subdividing the human cerebral cortex on MRI scans into gyral based regions of interest. NeuroImage 31(3), 968–980 (2006)
14. Modat, M., et al.: Fast free-form deformation using graphics processing units. Comput. Methods Programs Biomed. 98(3), 278–284 (2010)
15. Smith, S., et al.: Advances in functional and structural MR image analysis and implementation as FSL. NeuroImage 23, 208–219 (2004)
16. Clayden, J., et al.: Tractor: Magnetic resonance imaging and tractography with R. Journal of Statistical Software 44(8), 1–18 (2011)
17. Sporns, O., Tononi, G., Edelman, G.: Theoretical neuroanatomy: relating anatomical and functional connectivity in graphs and cortical connection matrices. Cereb. Cortex 10, 127–141 (2000)
18. Ledoit, O., Wolf, M.: A well-conditioned estimator for large-dimensional covariance matrices. J. Multivar. Anal. 88, 365–411 (2004)
19. Schäfer, J., Strimmer, K.: A shrinkage approach to large-scale covariance matrix estimation and implications for functional genomics. Stat. Appl. Genet. Mol. Biol. 4, Article 32 (2005)

# Multi-modal Surface-Based Alignment of Cortical Areas Using Intra-cortical T1 Contrast

Christine Lucas Tardif[1,*], Juliane Dinse[1,2], Andreas Schäfer[1], Robert Turner[1], and Pierre-Louis Bazin[1]

[1] Max Planck Institute for Human Cognitive and Brain Sciences, Leipzig, Germany
[2] Faculty of Computer Science, Otto-von-Guericke University, Magdeburg, Germany
ctardif@cbs.mpg.de

**Abstract.** The position of cortical areas in the brain is related to cortical folding patterns; however, intersubject variability remains, particularly for higher cortical areas. Current cortical surface registration techniques align cortical folding patterns using sulcal landmarks or cortical curvature, for instance. The alignment of cortical areas by these techniques is thus inherently limited by the sole use of geometric similarity metrics. Magnetic resonance imaging T1 maps show intra-cortical contrast that reflects myelin content, and thus can be used, in addition to cortical geometry, to improve the alignment of cortical areas. In this article, we present a new symmetric diffeomorphic multi-modal surface-based registration technique that works in the level-set framework. We demonstrate that the alignment of cortical areas is improved by using T1 maps. Finally, we present a unique group-average ultra-high resolution T1 map at multiple cortical depths, highlighting the registration accuracy achieved. The method can easily be extended to include other MR contrasts, such as functional data and anatomical connectivity, as well as other neuroimaging modalities.

**Keywords:** neuroimaging analysis, multi-modal, multi-contrast, surface registration, cortical areas, cortical folding, cortical curvature, cortical morphometry, myelin, quantitative T1, brain mapping, group analysis.

## 1 Introduction

In magnetic resonance imaging (MRI) studies of the cerebral cortex, surface-based registration, based on aligning the geometry of 2D manifolds, is often preferred over volume-based registration to align cortical areas between subjects or with an atlas. Cortical areas that are close in volume space may be very distant from each other along the cortical surface. The pioneering work of Brodmann [1] and recent neuroimaging studies [2,3] have analyzed the relationship between cortical folding patterns and the functional/architectonic boundaries of cortical areas, which is particularly strong for primary cortical areas. Surface-based registration driven by cortical folding patterns has been shown to improve

---

* Corresponding author.

L. Shen et al. (Eds.): MBIA 2013, LNCS 8159, pp. 222–232, 2013.
© Springer International Publishing Switzerland 2013

the statistical power and spatial specificity of group functional MRI analysis [4]. Current surface-based registration techniques use a variety of similarity metrics to describe cortical geometry: manually or automatically defined landmarks such as sulcal curves [5,6], automatic shape features such as curvature and sulcal depth [7–10], or a combination of both [11]. Pantazis et al. present a comparison of different methods [12]. Unfortunately, the relationship between cortical folding patterns and architectonic areal boundaries is complex and variable, particularly in higher cortical areas and regions of high inter-subject folding variability. Thus the alignment of cortical areas is inherently limited by the sole use of geometric similarity metrics.

Recent studies have shown intra-cortical contrast in group average T1 maps [13, 14], T2* maps [15] and T1-weighted/T2-weighted images [16]. Primary areas as well as extrastriate visual areas, which are more densely myelinated, are clearly discernible in these images mapped onto the inflated cortical surface. More discrete contrast is also visible in other regions, including the frontal lobe. We propose to use T1 maps, a quantitative index of myelin density [13], to improve the surface-based alignment of cortical areas. High-resolution T1 maps show exquisite intra-cortical contrast that varies as a function of cortical depth.

We present a novel automated surface-based registration technique for accurate surface registration, with key improvements over current methods. Our method provides a direct symmetric diffeomorphic transformation between the original surfaces. Similarly to Tosun et al. [8], we developed a multi-scale approach that is applied to partially inflated surfaces. Our multi-modal technique applies SyN [17], one of the leading non-linear volume-based registration algorithms [18], to surface information represented in volume space. We include two geometrical contrasts, the level-set representation of the cortical surface and cortical curvature, and intra-cortical T1 contrast. The method can be extended to include other MR contrasts and neuroimaging modalities instead of or in addition to T1, such as functional data.

Our surface-based registration technique can be applied to standard clinical data sets (typically 1 mm isotropic T1-weighted images) using the geometrical contrasts only, similarly to currently available methods. We chose to include ultra-high resolution T1 maps of five subjects to demonstrate the full potential of our technique. We evaluate the addition of T1 contrast to surface-based registration by comparison to our purely geometric implementation. Finally, we show the resulting group-average high-resolution T1 map at different cortical depths.

## 2   Methods

### 2.1   Data Acquisition and Pre-processing

Five subjects were scanned on a 7 Tesla (T) MR scanner with a 24-channel receive-only head coil. T1 maps were acquired using the MP2RAGE sequence ($TI_1/TI_2 = 900/2750$ ms, $TR = 5$ s, $TE = 2.45$ ms, $\alpha_1/\alpha_2 = 5°/3°$, bandwidth $= 250$ Hz/px, echo spacing $= 6.8$ ms, partial Fourier $= 6/8$) [19]. A whole brain scan was performed at 0.7 mm isotropic resolution with a GRAPPA acceleration factor of 2 (11 minutes), followed by a 0.5 mm isotropic scan (28 minutes) of each hemisphere for a total scan time of 67 minutes. In the inferior temporal lobes, the image quality was impaired due to insufficient radiofrequency transmit field provided by the coil. We do not discuss the results in this area. The B1 transmission field homogeneity could be improved by using dielectric pads in future studies [20]. A major concern at high resolutions and long scan times is subject motion. We selected subjects with previous scanning experience and detected no gross motion artifacts, such as ringing or blurring, in the images. An example of a 0.5 mm³ T1 map is shown in Fig. 1.

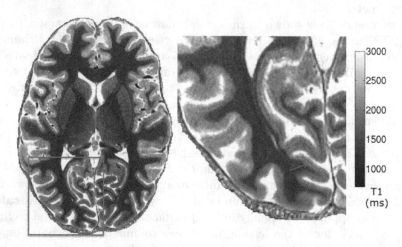

**Fig. 1.** Axial view of a co-registered and fused T1 map at 0.4 mm isotropic resolution displaying intra-cortical contrast, including layer structure such as the Stria of Gennari (red arrow)

The three T1 maps were co-registered into MNI space at 0.4 mm isotropic to minimize blurring caused by resampling, and the 0.5 mm images were fused to generate a whole brain T1 map. The resulting T1 maps were segmented [21] and the cortical surfaces of the left hemispheres reconstructed [22]. Realistic corti-cal layers (20 in number) were defined using a novel volume-preserving layering model [23], which follows the cortical laminae in areas of curvature. Cortical profiles were reconstructed perpendicularly to these layers. The level-set corre-sponding to the middle of the cortex (layer 10) was used for registration. The T1 times corresponding to the central 10 layers of the cortical profiles were aver-aged for registration. We excluded the first and last pairs of layers to minimize partial volume effects with white matter and cerebral spinal fluid, and divided the remaining 16 layers into 4 groups: Layer 1 (outer - near pial surface), Layer 2 (outer middle), Layer 3 (inner middle), and Layer 4 (deep - near white matter surface). Once the 0.4 mm isotropic T1 maps were sampled at the appropri-ate cortical depths, the images were downsampled to an isotropic resolution of 0.8 mm for the registration process. This will only affect the resolution in the tangential plane of the cortical surface.

## 2.2   Surface Registration

The surface registration algorithm we present here applies SyN, a symmetric image normalization algorithm that maximizes the cross-correlation within the space of diffeomorphic maps [17], to level-set representations of cortical surfaces and cortical features mapped onto these surfaces, curvature and T1.

We used a multi-scale approach by partially inflating the level-set surface $\varphi$ using Eq. 1, where $G$ is a Gaussian kernel and $\kappa$ is the surface curvature. Eq. 1 is applied iteratively until the desired level of inflation is reached. The four scales used in our experiments are illustrated in Fig. 2. The SyN algorithm was applied at each scale using a specific set of coarse, medium and fine iterations.

$$\frac{\partial \varphi}{\partial t} = [(\varphi - G * \varphi_0) - \kappa] \cdot |\Delta \varphi| \qquad (1)$$

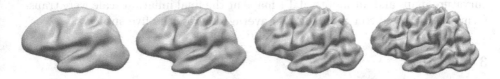

**Fig. 2.** The four cortical inflation scales at which the SyN algorithm is applied, from left to right, to gradually refine the mapping between two surfaces

The width of the level-set narrow band at each scale was equal to the maximum distance $d$ between the source and target level-sets. The level-set $\varphi$ was modulated using the sigmoid function in Eq. 2, where the slope is steepest at the intersection with the surface.

$$\tilde{\varphi} = \frac{1}{1 + e^{4\varphi/d}} \qquad (2)$$

In addition to this contrast, which is radial to the cortical surface, we used curvature and T1 as tangential image contrasts. The curvature was calculated at each inflation scale as the product of the shape index and the curvedness [24]. The T1 times were smoothed tangential to the cortical surface using a Gaussian kernel of 3 mm FWHM for the purpose of registration only. The resulting T1 times were mapped to each scale during the inflation process by coordinate tracking [25]. For both tangential contrasts, curvature and T1, the values were dilated radially from the surface to the full width of the narrow band. The tangential contrasts were linearly rescaled to the range [-0.5, 0.5]. An example of the three contrasts is shown in Fig. 3.

The radial and tangential contrasts had an equal weighting of one. We performed three surface registration experiments with different tangential contrast combinations: 1) curvature only, 2) half curvature half T1, and 3) T1 only. The three contrasts were used to measure convergence. The cortical surface of a single subject was chosen as the target. After registration, the unmodulated level-sets,

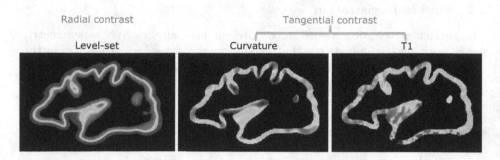

**Fig. 3.** Sagittal view of the three image contrasts used to align the partially inflated cortical surfaces: the level-set that varies radially to the surface, the curvature and T1 that vary tangentially to the surface

curvature maps and unsmoothed T1 maps at the final inflation scale were transformed using the direct mapping and averaged across the five subjects.

## 3    Results

The group-average T1 maps, corresponding to the mean of the middle 10 layers of the cortex, shown in Fig. 4. Primary areas, which are more densely myelinated, exhibit a shorter T1. The results from the three experiments using different contrast combinations are very similar. This observation agrees with previous reports that cortical areas are correlated with cortical folding. However, there are some small, yet important, differences between the averaged T1 maps which are highlighted in Fig. 4. For instance, in the average registered by T1 alone, the boundaries of the primary motor (M1) and somatosensory (S1) cortices are sharpest, mainly in the direction parallel to the central sulcus. We can also see a clearer cluster of decreased T1 times on the lateral occipital cortex corresponding to the motion-sensitive visual area V5/MT+. The frontal cortex contains more structure in the average T1 maps by using T1, including two clusters of decreased T1 in the inferior frontal gyrus corresponding to Broca's area (Brodmann areas 44 and 45, related to speech and language). The cingulate cortex, a very fine structure that is more difficult to register using smoothed data or inflated surfaces, is also better aligned using T1 contrast.

The level-set standard deviation shown in the first row of Fig. 5 represents the standard deviation of the remaining distance between the registered surfaces. These values are very low for all three experiments, and lowest for experiment 2 that combines all three contrasts for registration. This may be because the level-set has the strongest relative weighting of the three contrasts in experiment 2. There is an area of high standard deviation in the temporal lobe and near V5/MT+ where there is known to be intersubject variability in cortical

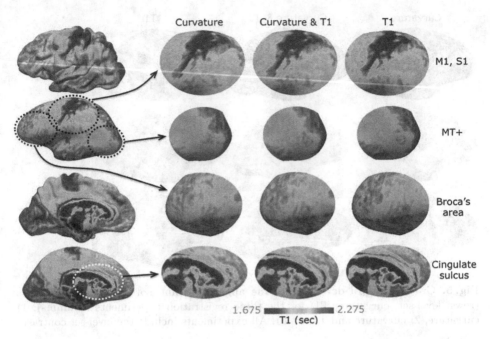

**Fig. 4.** Group-average of the aligned 0.8 mm isotropic unsmoothed T1 maps for the three tangential contrast combinations used for registration: 1) curvature, 2) curvature and T1, 3) T1. Regions of interest (ROIs) are outlined on the surfaces on the left, and zoomed-in on the right. ROIs are centred around (in vertical order): M1 and S1, MT+, Broca's area, cingulate sulcus.

folding patterns. There is also a higher standard deviation in the frontal lobe near higher cognitive areas that have a weaker relationship with cortical folding. It may therefore be more difficult to optimize both T1 and level-set alignment in these areas.

The curvature standard deviation in the second row of Fig. 5 is lowest for experiment 1, as expected. The penalty of using only T1 contrast in experiment 3 is very small. This may be because the level-sets themselves include information about the geometry of the cortex. There is a small increase in standard deviation at the sulcal fundi, where the curvature gradients are strongest, and a decrease at the gyral crowns. The increase in standard deviation in experiments 2 and 3 is indicative that the relationship between cortical areas and cortical folding is variable, as highlighted in previous studies [2].

The curvature standard deviation only highlights alignment errors perpendicular to the cortical folds. In contrast, the T1 standard deviation is a representation of the error in alignment of cortical areas, based on tissue microstructure, in all directions within the cortical surface. The T1-driven surface-based registration results from experiment 3 are characterized by a reduction in intersubject

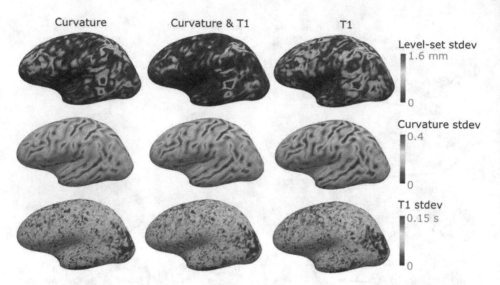

**Fig. 5.** Group-standard deviations of the aligned 0.8 mm isotropic image contrasts (rows: level-set, curvature, T1) for the three registration experiments (columns): 1) curvature, 2) curvature and T1, 3) T1. All experiments include the level-set contrast.

variability in T1 times, as shown in Fig. 5, even near the boundaries of primary areas. There is a strong decrease in T1 standard deviation in proximity to the cingulate cortex, at the eccentricity boundary of the primary visual cortex (V1) and in the frontal lobe. There is a cluster of high T1 variability on the lateral occipital and inferior parietal cortex for all three experiments, although it is most widespread for curvature-based and most focused for T1-based registration. The curvature-based registration is penalized by high intersubject variability in cortical folding patterns in this area, whereas the T1-based registration benefits from the T1 contrast arising from the highly myelinated extrastriate visual areas.

In Fig. 6, the T1 times from T1-based registration are shown for four different cortical depths, defined in Section 2.1. The T1 contrast varies significantly with cortical depth. The most striking examples are the greater contrast between M1 and S1 in Layer 3 in comparison to Layer 1, and the contrast between V5/MT+ and neighbouring cortex for deeper Layers 3 and 4 in comparison to superficial Layers 1 and 2. Brodmann areas 44 and 45 in the frontal lobe also show a distinct laminar structure, with highest contrast in Layer 2. Although these observations of the group-averaged T1 laminar structure of cortical areas are preliminary, they are in agreement with myeloarchitectonic descriptions of the cortex and indicate that careful alignment of T1 along the cortical surface can outline many cortical boundaries based on MR imaging of tissue microstructure.

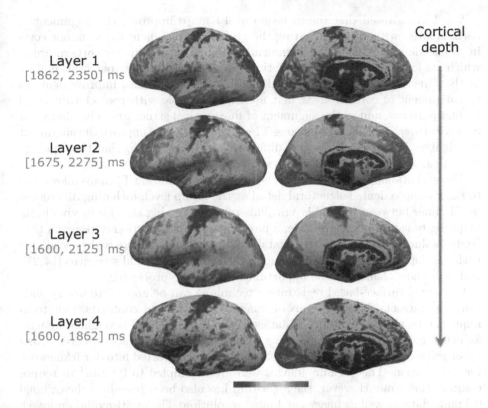

**Fig. 6.** Group-average of the aligned 0.4 mm isotropic unsmoothed T1 maps for the four cortical layers defined in Section 2.1. T1 generally becomes longer towards the pial surface, thus the T1 scales are different for each layer to highlight the inter-layer differences in T1 contrast.

## 4   Conclusion

We developed a novel surface-based registration technique that provides highly accurate symmetric diffeomorphic mappings between the original surfaces. The multi-scale approach based on partial levelset inflation improves the registration of the cortex over the SyN algorithm applied directly. This approach avoids reparametrization to a sphere and minimizes distortions. We work with the natural shape of the anatomy, making it a more general framework that is not limited to cortical surfaces. The low standard deviation of the level-sets across subjects clearly shows the high precision that was achieved. Errors in the target cortical surface could mislead the registration process, therefore future group registration experiments could alternatively be performed as an evolving group average template. Additional inflation scales can be included until complete registration or the original level-sets is achieved at the cost of processing time. This may be more suitable for morphometry as opposed to functional studies.

We demonstrated that the inclusion of T1 maps improves the alignment of cortical areas without deteriorating the geometric alignment (or at minor costs in geometric alignment). The alignment is improved for primary cortical areas, which are known to have a close relationship to cortical folding patterns, mainly in the direction parallel to the cortical folds. There are also improvements in the alignment of cortical areas that are more variable with respect to cortical folding patterns, and in the alignment of fine cortical structures. The alignment of cortical areas which exhibit strong T1 contrast may also improve the alignment of neighbouring areas with weaker differences in T1, assuming that the topology of cortical areas is consistent across subjects.

The exceptional image quality of the ultra-high resolution T1 maps allowed us to show unprecedented structural detail at the group level, including differences in T1 times between cortical layers. This represents a big step for in vivo brain mapping based on microstructure, a new and exciting direction of research [26]. High-resolution and quantitative data sets are becoming more widely available with developments in image acquisition at 3 T and higher field strengths [14,27], and bring new challenges and opportunities to image processing.

Our novel surface-based registration technique can be applied to a very wide range of datasets, both in terms of image resolution and contrasts. Our technique can be applied to standard datasets, typically $1\,mm^3$ T1-weighted images, as other cortical surface alignment tools. In addition, surfaces created using other software packages, such as FreeSurfer, can be imported into our framework for registration. The $0.4\,mm^3$ images were downsampled to $0.8\,mm^3$ to reduce computation time. However, the algorithm has also been tested on the original $0.4\,mm^3$ data as well as images at $1\,mm^3$ resolution. The multi-modal approach can be extended to include other modalities, in addition to or instead of T1, that feature intra-cortical contrast of interest for brain parcellation. Future work will include the use of other MR contrasts that reflect cortical microstructure (eg. T2* and quantitative susceptibility mapping), as well as multi-layer contrast in high-resolution images. Another interesting application would be the inclusion of functional and anatomical connectivity data.

# References

1. Brodmann, K.: Vergleichende Lokalisationslehre der Grosshirnrinde. Barth, Leipzig (1909)
2. Fischl, B., Rajendran, N., Busa, E., Augustinack, J., Hinds, O., Yeo, B.T., Mohlberg, H., Amunts, K., Zilles, K.: Cortical Folding Patterns and Predicting Cytoarchitecture. Cereb. Cortex 18, 1973–1980 (2008)
3. Frost, M.A., Goebel, R.: Measuring Structural-Functional Correspondence: Spatial Variability of Specialised Brain Regions after Macro-anatomical Alignment. NeuroImage 59, 1369–1381 (2012)
4. van Atteveldt, N., Formisano, E., Goebel, R., Blomert, L.: Integration of Letters and Speech Sounds in the Human Brain. Neuron 43, 271–282 (2004)
5. Van Essen, D.C.: A Population-Average, Landmark- and Surface-Based (PALS) Atlas of Human Cerebral Cortex. NeuroImage 28, 635–662 (2005)

6. Joshi, A.A., Shattuck, D.W., Thompson, P.M., Leahy, R.M.: Surface-Constrained Volumetric Brain Registration using Harmonic Mappings. IEEE Trans. Med. Imag. 26, 1657–1669 (2007)
7. Fischl, B., Sereno, M.I., Dale, A.M.: Cortical Surface-Based Analysis II: Inflation, Flattening, and a Surface-Base Coordinate System. NeuroImage 9, 195–207 (1999)
8. Tosun, D., Rettmann, M.E., Han, X., Tao, X., Xu, C., Resnick, S.M., Pham, D.L., Prince, J.L.: Cortical Surface Segmentation and Mapping. NeuroImage 23, S108–S118 (2004)
9. Goebel, R., Esposito, F., Formisano, E.: Analysis of Functional Image Analysis Contest (FIAC) Data with Brainvoyager QX: From Single-Subject to Cortically Aligned Group General Linear Model Analysis and Self-Organizing Group Independent Component Analysis. Hum. Brain. Map. 27, 392–401 (2006)
10. Yeo, B.T.T., Sabuncu, M.R., Vercauteren, T., Ayache, N., Fischl, B., Golland, P.: Spherical Demons: Fast Diffeomorphic Landmark-Free Surface Registration. IEEE Trans. Med. Imag. 29, 650–668 (2010)
11. Park, H., Park, J.-S., Seong, J.-K., Na, D.L., Lee, J.-M.: Cortical Surface Registration using Spherical Thin-Plate Spline with Sulcal Lines and Mean Curvature as Features. J. Neurosci. Methods 206, 46–53 (2012)
12. Pantazis, D., Joshi, A., Jiang, J., Shattuck, D.W., Bernstein, L.E., Damasio, H., Leahy, R.M.: Comparison of Landmark-Based and Automatic Methods for Cortical Surface Registration. NeuroImage 49, 2479–2493 (2010)
13. Geyer, S., Weiss, M., Reimann, K., Lohmann, G., Turner, R.: Microstructural Parcellation of the Human Cerebral Cortex - From Brodmann's Post-Mortem Map to In Vivo Mapping with High-Field Magnetic Resonance Imaging. Front. Human Neurosci. 5, 1–19 (2011)
14. Sereno, M.I., Lutti, A., Weiskopf, N., Dick, F.: Mapping the Human Cortical Surface by Combining Quantitative T1 with Retinotopy. Cereb. Cortex (2012) (in press)
15. Cohen-Adad, J., Polimeni, J.R., Helmer, K.G., Benner, T., McNab, J.A., Wald, L.L., Rosen, B.R., Mainero, C.: T2* Mapping and B0 Orientation-Dependence at 7 T Reveal Cyto- and Myeloarchitecture Organization of the Human Cortex. NeuroImage 60, 1006–1014 (2012)
16. Glasser, M.F., Van Essen, D.C.: Mapping Human Cortical Areas In Vivo Based on Myelin Content as Revealed by T1- and T2-weighted MRI. J. Neurosci. 31, 11597–11616 (2011)
17. Avants, B.B., Epstein, C.L., Grossman, M., Gee, J.C.: Symmetric Diffeomorphic Image Registration with Cross-correlation: Evaluating Automated Labeling of Elderly and Neurodegenerative Brain. Med. Imag. Anal. 12, 26–41 (2008)
18. Klein, A., Andersson, J., Ardekani, B.A., Ashburner, J., Avants, B., Chiang, M.-C., Christensen, G.E., Collins, D.L., Gee, J., Hellier, P., Song, J.H., Jenkinson, M., Lepage, C., Rueckert, D., Thompson, P., Vercauteren, T., Woods, R.P., Mann, J.J., Parsey, R.V.: Evaluation of 14 Monlinear Deformation Algorithms applied to Human Brain MRI Registration. NeuroImage 46, 786–802 (2009)
19. Marques, J.P., Kober, T., Krueger, G., van der Zwaag, W., Van de Moortele, P.F., Gruetter, R.: MP2RAGE, a Self Bias-Field Corrected Sequence for Improved Segmentation and T1-Mapping at High Field. NeuroImage 49, 1271–1281 (2010)
20. Teeuwisse, W.M., Brink, W.M., Webb, A.G.: Quantitative Assessment of the Effects of High-Permittivity Pads in 7 Tesla MRI of the Brain. Magn. Reson. Med. 67, 1285–1293 (2012)

21. Bazin, P.-L., Weiss, M., Dinse, J., Schäfer, A., Trampel, R., Turner, R.: A Computational Framework for Ultra-high Resolution Cortical Segmentation at 7 Tesla. NeuroImage (in press, 2013)
22. Han, X., Pham, D.L., Tosun, D., Rettmann, M.E., Xu, C., Prince, J.L.: CRUISE: Cortical Reconstruction using Implicit Surface Evolution. NeuroImage 23, 997–1012 (2004)
23. Waehnert, M.D., Dinse, J., Weiss, M., Streicher, M.N., Waehnert, P., Geyer, S., Turner, R., Bazin, P.-L.: Anatomically Motivated Modeling of Cortical Laminae. NeuroImage (in press, 2013)
24. Koenderink, J.J., van Doorn, A.J.: Surface Shape and Curvature Scales. Imag. Vision Comp. 10, 557–564 (1992)
25. Vemuri, B.C., Ye, J., Chen, Y., Leonard, C.M.: Image Registration via Level-Set Motion: Applications to Atlas-Based Segmentation. Med. Imag. Anal. 7, 1–20 (2003)
26. Van Essen, D.C., Glasser, M.F.: In Vivo Architectonics: A Cortical-Centric Perspective. NeuroImage (in press, 2013)
27. Van Essen, D.C., Ugurbil, K., Auerbach, E., Barch, D., Behrens, T.E.J., Bucholz, R., Chang, A., Chen, L., Corbetta, M., Curtiss, S.W., Della Penna, S., Feinberg, D., Glasser, M.F., Harel, N., Heath, A.C., Larson-Prior, L., Marcus, D., Michalareas, G., Moeller, S., Oostenveld, R., Petersen, S.E., Prior, F., Schlaggar, B.L., Smith, S.M., Snyder, A.Z., Xu, J., Yacoub, E.: The Human Connectome Project: A Data Acquisition Perspective. NeuroImage 62, 2222–2231 (2012)

# A Heat Kernel Based Cortical Thickness Estimation Algorithm

Gang Wang[1,2], Xiaofeng Zhang[1], Qingtang Su[1], Jiannong Chen[3], Lili Wang[1], Yunyan Ma[4], Qiming Liu[1], Liang Xu[2], Jie Shi[2], and Yalin Wang[2]

[1] School of Computer Science and Technology, Ludong University, P.R. China
[2] School of Computing, Informatics, and Decision Systems Engineering, Arizona State University, USA
[3] School of Physics & Photoelectric, Ludong University, P.R. China
[4] School of Mathematics & Statistics Science, Ludong University, P.R. China

**Abstract.** Cortical thickness estimation in magnetic resonance imaging (MRI) is an important technique for research on brain development and neurodegenerative diseases. This paper presents a heat kernel based cortical thickness estimation algorithm, which is driven by the graph spectrum and the heat kernel theory, to capture the grey matter geometry information in the *in vivo* brain MR images. First, we use the harmonic energy function to establish the tetrahedral mesh matching with the MR images and generate the Laplace-Beltrami operator matrix which includes the inherent geometric characteristics of the tetrahedral mesh. Second, the isothermal surfaces are computed by the finite element method with the volumetric Laplace-Beltrami operator and the direction of the steamline is obtained by tracing the maximum heat transfer probability based on the heat kernel diffusion. Thereby we can calculate the cerebral cortex thickness information between the point on the outer surface and the corresponding point on the inner surface. The method relies on intrinsic brain geometry structure and the computation is robust and accurate. To validate our algorithm, we apply it to study the thickness differences associated with Alzheimer's disease (AD) and mild cognitive impairment (MCI) on the Alzheimer's Disease Neuroimaging Initiative (ADNI) dataset. Our preliminary experimental results in 151 subjects (51 AD, 45 MCI, 55 controls) show that the new algorithm successfully detects statistically significant difference among patients of AD, MCI and healthy control subjects. The results also indicate that the new method may have better performance than the Freesurfer software.

**Keywords:** Cortical thickness, Heat Kernel, Tetrahedral Mesh, Streamline, False Discovery Rate.

## 1 Introduction

Alzheimer's disease (AD) is a common central nervous system degenerative disease. Its symptoms on clinical anatomy are the partly atrophy in the cerebral cortex of the patients. If we can accurately estimate the cortical thickness and

L. Shen et al. (Eds.): MBIA 2013, LNCS 8159, pp. 233–245, 2013.

identify out reliable different regions between patient and control groups, it may help the early detection of the disease, evaluate disease burden, progression and response to interventions. However, despite evidence that medial temporal atrophy is associated with AD progression, the MRI imaging measurement of medial temporal atrophy is still not sufficiently accurate on its own to serve as an absolute diagnostic criterion for the clinical diagnosis of AD at the mild cognitive impairment (MCI) stage.

According to the geometric properties of the measurement tools, the thickness estimation methods can be broadly divided into two categories: based on either surface or voxel characteristics (as reviewed in [1]). The measurement methods based on the surface features are aimed to establish triangular mesh models in accordance with the topological properties of the inner and outer surface, and then use the deformable evolution model to couple the two opposing surfaces. The thickness is defined as the value of the level set propagation distance between the two surfaces. This measurement accuracy can reach the sub-pixel level but requires constantly correcting the weights of various evolutionary parameters to ensure the mesh regularity. Sometimes the model can not work in the high folding regions such as the sulci. Various approaches were proposed to address this problem and increase the thickness estimation accuracy in the high curvature areas. For example, Mak-Fan et al. modeled the sulci regional by adding the cortex thickness constraints [2]. Fischl and Dale proposed to model the middle part of the sulci by imposing the self-intersection constraints [3]. Although better measurement results are achieved, the computation cost is high [4]. The voxel-based method is the measurement on a three-dimension cubic voxel grid. There is no correction of the mesh topology regularity, so the calculation is simple [5,6]. However, due to the restrictions of the grid resolution, the measurement accuracy is low and sensitive to noise [7]. The voxel-based measurement acquires the cortex thickness information by solving partial differential equations in the potential field, for example, Jones et al. [8] first used the Laplace equation to characterize the layered structure of the volume between the inner and outer surfaces and obtained the stream line. This method is known as the Lagrangian method. Hyde et al. [9] proposed the Euler method by solving the one-order linear partial differential equations for thickness calculation which can improve the computation efficiency. The main disadvantage of the voxel-based estimation method is the computational inaccuracy on the discrete grid. The limited grid resolution affects the accuracy of the thickness measurement. Some prior work, e.g.[10], used the boundary topology to initialize a sub-voxel resolution surface and correct the direction of the stream line. This method can increase the measurement accuracy.

From the above discussion, in order to improve the computational efficiency and the degree of automation, one may expect the choice of voxel-based measurement algorithm is more feasible. However, we should overcome the defect of the limited grid resolution which can not precisely characterize the curved cortical surfaces from MR images. The 3D model we need should achieve a good fitting for the cerebral cortex morphology and facilitate an effective computation on the sub-voxel resolution. The preferred model to satisfy the above requirements is a tetrahedral mesh [11], as a cubic voxel can be divided into $n$ tetrahedra according to the resolution requirement.

It is also worth noticing that the tetrahedral mesh quality will affect the accuracy of solving the partial differential equations. For example, too small dihedral angles will lead to stiffness matrix ill-posed problem in the finite element method and too large dihedral angles will lead to the interpolation and discretization errors. The common tetrahedra generation method is to revise the tetrahedra through the iterative processing. One class of methods are to divide the voxels of the MRI to tetrahedra according to the generation quality [12]. But it usually results in the loss of the original image information because of the lack of the boundary restriction conditions. Another class of methods intends to comply with the precise topology structure of the original image by adaptively adjusting the size of the tetrahedra [13], which constantly use the external force to pull the tetrahedral vertices to the boundary of the MRI. However, it neglects the quality of each tetrahedron.

There are two main contributions in our paper. First, this paper intends to generate the high-quality tetrahedral mesh suitable for the areas of the cortex with rich details on the basis of the results of the previous studies. And the tetrahedral mesh can be facilitated to analyze the potential field, which has been elaborated in many literatures, e.g. [14]. Compared with prior work [8], our PDE solving computation can achieve sub-voxel accuracy. Second, we propose a heat kernel based method to accurately estimate the streamline with the intrinsic and global cortical geometry information. In a prior work [8], the computations of the streamline by solving the partial differential equations are rooted in computational geometry to determine the streamline directions. It neglects the inherent geometric characteristics between the points in the mesh. Geometrically speaking, heat kernel determines the intrinsic Riemannian metric [15] and it can be reliably computed through the Laplace-Beltrami matrix. Recently, the surface based heat kernel methods were widely used in image shape analysis [16], classification [17], and registration [18]. However, 3D heat kernel methods are still rare in medical image analysis field. Here we propose a novel 3D heat kernel method and apply it to refine streamline computation and improve the accuracy of the cortical thickness estimation. Besides the computational efficacy and efficiency, our method also takes numerous other advantages of the spectral analysis such as the measurement invariance of inelastic deformation and the robustness of the topological noise.

## 2   Tetrahedral Mesh Generation Algorithm

The pipeline of our tetrahedral mesh generation algorithm for the MR images is shown in Fig. 1. First we fill the MRI space with the cubic background voxels and the space attribute of each vertex is determined by the point-to-boundary distance function $\phi(x)$. $\phi(x)$ is calculated using the fast marching method based on the vertex connection relationship. The sign of the $\phi(x)$ indicates the region

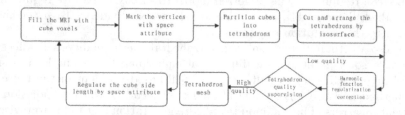

**Fig. 1.** Tetrahedral mesh generation work flow

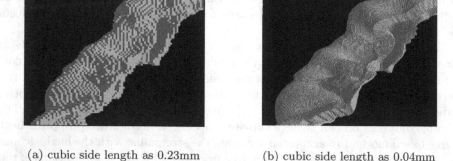

(a) cubic side length as 0.23mm        (b) cubic side length as 0.04mm

**Fig. 2.** Generated tetrahedral meshes with different cubic side lengths

where the vertex is located, and mark the square surface as the boundary where the $\phi(x)$ of vertices is equal to zero. Here we can adaptively adjust the filled cubic lengths by calculating the vertex coordinates($x$ or $y$) difference of the adjacent boundary surface with the same $z$ coordinate.

The results of different cubic length are shown in Fig. 2. We adaptively adjust the cubic side lengths to fill the MRI according to the vertices fluctuation of the cubes. On the other hand, the degree of the approximation and smoothness of the mesh can be adaptively adjusted. Secondly, the cubic voxel containing the boundary surface and the internal voxel are split into the tetrahedra according to the pyramid and the body-centered lattice forms. The details of the splitting algorithm are shown in Fig. 3. Here, the left voxel contains the boundary surface (ABCD), $O$ and $O'$ are the central points of the left and right cubic voxels, the tetrahedra (ABDO and BDCO) are the split results by the pyramid form. And the right voxel is the internal one, the tetrahedra (OO'EF and OO'GH) are the split results by the body-centered lattice form. So the cubic voxels are composed of excellent quality tetrahedra, which have dihedral angles as 60° and 90° .

On this basis, the tetrahedra near the boundary are to be cut by the iso-surface ($\phi(x) = 0$) based on the vertex space attribute and linear proportional function. Finishing the cutting, we should consider the reconstruction of the new

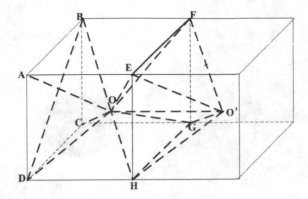

**Fig. 3.** Two kinds of forms for splitting the cubic voxels into tetrahedra

tetrahedra under the condition of the original tetrahedral collapse. In addition, if we find the cutting point of the edge is close to the holding internal vertex, the implementation of adsorption operation is required, i.e. the internal vertex will be pulled onto the isosurface. After the above operations, the original background grid is organized into the tetrahedral mesh which substantially fits the cerebral cortex geometry structure.

The obtained tetrahedral mesh needs to be corrected to improve the quality and the smoothness owing to the cutting and organization operations. We achieve it with the regularization algorithm for the boundary smoothness and tetrahedral quality improvement based on the harmonic function minimization [19]. The initial tetrahedra conforming state is given by $X$ , while the deformed state is denoted by $x$ , and the displacement vector field $v$ is given by $v = x - X$ . Then the regularized tetrahedral mesh is obtained by finding a $v$ that minimizes an energy $G(v)$ . $G(v)$ is composed of three additive terms, an elastic term $E(v)$, a smoothness term $S(v)$ and a fidelity term $B(v)$ . The details of this algorithm can be referred to [19].

## 3   Thickness Measurement Algorithm Based on the Heat Kernel Diffusion

### 3.1   Heat Kernel

Let $f$ be a real-valued function, with $f \in \mathbb{C}^2$, defined on a tetrahedral mesh $K$. We use the volumetric Laplace-Beltrami operator proposed in a prior work [20]. We define the piecewise Laplace-Beltrami operator as the linear operator $\Delta_K$ : $C^{PL} \to C^{PL}$ on the space of piecewise linear function $f$, on $K$, which is defined as

$$\Delta_K(f) = \Sigma_{\{u,v\}\in K} k(u,v)(f(u) - f(v)) \tag{1}$$

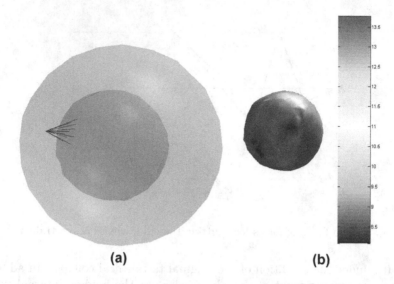

**Fig. 4.** The heat transition paths and the values of the from the specific point on the outer isothermal surface (0.95°) to the different points on the inner isothermal surface (0.90°)

where $k(u,v) = \frac{1}{12}\Sigma_{i=1}^{n} l_i \cot(\theta_i)$, $\theta_i$ is the associated dihedral angle and $l_i$ is the length of an edge to which edge $\{u,v\}$ is against in a tetrahedron model. Compared with other rasterization-based Laplace-Beltrami operator computation methods, because of the multi-resolution nature of the tetrahedral mesh, our method may capture and quantify local volumetric geometric structure more accurately.

The heat kernel diffusion on differentiable manifold with Riemannian metric is governed by the heat equation:

$$\Delta_K f(x,t) = \frac{\partial f(x,t)}{\partial t} \tag{2}$$

where $f(x,t)$ is the heat distribution of the volume at the given time $t$. We know that the heat diffusion process can be represented by its time dependent and its spatially dependent parts.

$$f(x,t) = F(x)T(t) \tag{3}$$

When Eq. 3 is substituted to Eq. 2, we can get the Helmholtz equation to describe the heat vibration modes in the spatial domain.

$$\Delta F(x) = -\lambda F(x) \tag{4}$$

Eq. 4 can be treated as the Laplacian eigenvalue problem with infinite number of eigenvalue $\lambda_i$ and eigenfunction $F_i$ pairs. The solution of equation above can be interpreted to the superposition of the harmonic functions in the given spatial position and time. Given an initial heat distribution $F : K \to \mathbb{R}$, let $H_t(F)$

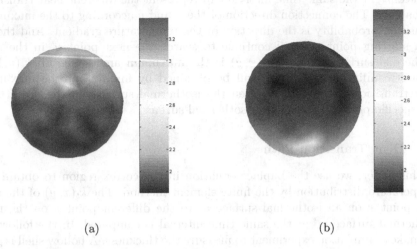

(a)                                                                   (b)

**Fig. 5.** The thickness measurement result from Fig. 4. (a) shows that the half outer surface which is far from the inner hole and (b) shows the half outer surface which is close to the inner hole. The colormap information represents the size of the thickness.

denote the heat distribution at time $t$, and $\lim_{t\to 0} H_t(F) = F$. $H_t$ is called the heat operator. Both $\Delta_K$ and $H_t$ share the same eigenfunctions, and if $\lambda_i$ is an eigenvalue of $\Delta_K$, then $e^{-\lambda_i t}$ is an eigenvalue of $H_t$ corresponding to the same eigenfunction.

For any compact Riemannian manifold, there exists a function $k_t(x, y) : \mathbb{R}^+ \times M \times M \to \mathbb{R}$, satisfy the formula

$$H_t F(x) = \int_K k_t(x, y) F(y) dy \qquad (5)$$

where $dy$ is the volume form at $y \in K$. The minimum function $k_t(x, y)$ that satisfies Eq. 5 is called the *heat kernel*, and can be considered as the amount of heat that is transferred from $x$ to $y$ in time $t$ given a unit heat source at $x$. According to the theory of the spectral analysis, the heat kernel has the following eigen-decomposition heat diffusion distance:

$$k_t(x, y) = \Sigma_{i=0}^{\infty} e^{-\lambda_i t} \phi_i(x) \phi_i(y) \qquad (6)$$

where $\lambda_i$ and $\phi_i$ are $i$th the eigenvalue and eigenfunction of the Laplace-Beltrami operator, respectively. So we can see that the heat kernel can be completely represented by the eigenvalues and eigenfunctions of the Laplace-Beltrami operator. At the same time, the heat kernel $k_t(x, y)$ can be interpreted as the transition probability of the Brownian motion on the manifold and has significant applications in computer vision and machine learning fields. The $k_t(x, y)$ of the specific point $x$ on an isothermal surface $m$ to the different point $y$ on the next isothermal surface $m'$ at the same time interval can represent the different heat transition probability. The connection direction of the $x$ and $y$ according to the maximum transition probability is the direction of the temperature gradient. And then $y$ as a starting point, we will continue to search the next point $y'$ in the next isothermal surface $n$ whose $k_t(x, y)$ is the maximum among the all $k_t(y, \mathbb{R})$ . So a streamline of the cortex will be obtained by finding out the maximum heat transition probability between the isothermal surfaces in the order from the specific point on the highest isothermal surface.

## 3.2    Heat Transition Path

In this paper, we use the Laplace equation in the cortex region to obtain the temperature distribution by the finite element method. The $k_t(x, y)$ of the specific point $x$ on an isothermal surface $m$ to the different point $y$ on the next isothermal surface $m'$ at the same time interval is computed. In the following, we make a simulation experiment to measure the thickness. A hollow shell is generated by our tetrahedron mesh generation algorithm. The outer surface center is located in $(-0, 0, 0)$ and the inner surface center is $(-0.5, 0, 0)$, the outer surface and the hole surface are the irregular spherical surfaces. First we set the temperature value of the outer surface as $1°$ and inner surface as $0°$. Through the finite element method, the temperature distribution and the isothermal surface in the mesh can be acquired. Fig. 4(a) shows that the coordinates of $x$ are $(-3.9669, 0.49833, 0.12544)$ on the outer isothermal surface $m$ whose temperature is $0.95°$, and the inner isothermal surface $m'$ is the surface of temperature of $0.90°$. The part of heat transition paths from $x$ to the isothermal surface $m'$ are represented by the blue lines. Where the red line represents the path from $x$ to $y$ whose coordinates are $(-1.9645, 0.26586, 1.0978)$ and the maximum $k_t(x, y)$ is 13.081 as the time interval is 0.02. And the important point is that the red line is perpendicular to the two isothermal surfaces approximately. In order to clearly show the heat transition paths, the interval distance between the two isothermal surfaces is enlarged to display. Fig. 4 (b) shows the values of the $k_t(x, y)$ on the inner isothermal surface from $x$ to the different $y$. As shown in Fig. 4 (a) and (b), we can see that the values of $k_t(x, \mathbb{R})$ increase as the colors go from blue to yellow and to red. This means the geometry and topology relationships from $x$ to the different points on the next isothermal surface. With this simple example, we visualize the fact that eigenvalues and eigenfunctions of the Laplace-Beltrami Operator can represent the intrinsic volume geometry characteristics.

Some thickness measurement results from Fig. 4 are shown in Fig. 5. Here the step size is chosen as 0.2 which means that the isothermal interval is $0.2°$. We add the length of all the segment lines between the isothermal surfaces which represent the maximum heat transition and obtain the thicknesses of the vertices on the outer surface. Fig. 5 (a) shows that the half outer surface which is far from the hole and (b) shows the half outer surface which is close to the hole. The colormap information represents the size of the thickness.

## 4    Statistical Maps and Multiple Comparison

The experiments in this work were performed on T1 image data (AD=51, MCI=45, control=55) from the Alzheimer's Disease Neuroimaging Initiative (ADNI) [21]. As a proof-of-principle work, our analysis was focused on the medial temporal lobe of the left brain hemisphere. The grey matter segmentation, surface reconstruction, surface correspondence, region of interest (ROI) extraction on white matter and pial surfaces were computed by Freesurfer software [22].

With the segmented brain images, the acquired data was interpolated to form cubic voxels with an edge length of 0.2mm. The minimum dihedral angle of the generated tetrahedron mesh is 12 degree and maximum dihedral angle is 130 degree. The maximum edge ratio is set as 5.0. Then the thickness measurement based on heat kernel is applied on the extracted ROI. We applied the Student's $t$ test on sets of thickness values measured on corresponding surface points to study the statistical group difference. Given each matching surface point, we measure the difference between the mean thickness of three different groups (AD vs. control, MCI vs. control and AD vs. MCI) by

$$ t = \frac{\bar{U} - \bar{V}}{\sqrt{\frac{2}{n}} S_{UV}} \tag{7} $$

where $\bar{U}$ and $\bar{V}$ are the thickness means of the two groups and $S_{UV}$ is the grand standard deviation. The denominator of $t$ is the standard error of the difference between two means. For multiple comparison, we ran a permutation test with 15,000 random assignments of subjects to groups to estimate the statistical significance of the thickness with group differences. The covariate was permuted 15,000 times. The probability was later color coded on each surface template point as the statistical $p$-map of group difference. Fig. 6 shows the $p$-maps of group difference detected between AD and control, AD and MCI, control and MCI groups, respectively, and the significant level at each surface template point as 0.05. Fig. 6 (a), (c) and (e) are the statistical $p$-map results with Heat Diffusion; (b), (d) and (f) are those with Freesurfer. All group difference $p$-maps were corrected for multiple comparisons using the widely-used false discovery rate method (FDR) [23]. The FDR method decides whether a threshold can be assigned to the statistical map that keeps the expected false discovery rate below 5% (i.e., no more than 5% of the voxels are false positive findings). In Fig. 6, the non-blue color areas denote the statistically significant difference areas between two groups. Fig. 7 (a)-(c) are the cumulative distribution function (CDF) plots showing the uncorrected $p$-values (as in a conventional FDR analysis). The $x$ value at which the CDF plot intersects the $y = 20x$ line represents the FDR-corrected $p$-value or $q$-value. It is the highest statistical threshold that can be applied to the data, for which at most 5% false positives are expected in the map. In general, a larger $q$-value indicates a more significant difference in the sense that there is a broader range of statistic threshold that can be used to limit the rate of false positives to at most 5% [24]. The use of the $y = 20x$ line is

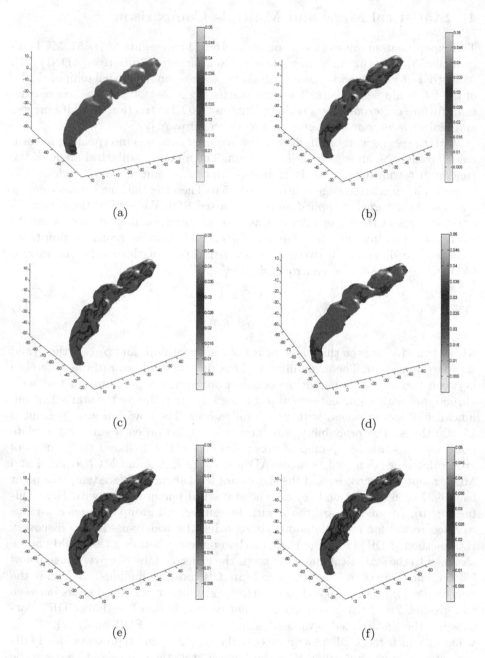

**Fig. 6.** Statistical p-map results of Heat Diffusion and Freesurfer show group differences among three different groups, (a), (c), (e) are the results of our method, (b), (d), (f) are results of Freesurfer software on group difference between AD and control, control and MCI, AD and MCI, respectively

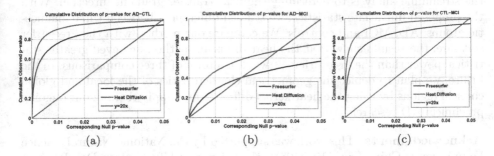

**Fig. 7.** The cumulative distributions of p-values comparison for difference detected between three groups (AD, MCI, CTL). In the CDF, the q-values are the intersection point of the curve and the $y = 20x$ line. In a total of 3 comparisons, the heat diffusion method achieved the highest q-values.

**Table 1.** The FDR corrected $p$-value ($q$-value) comparison

|  | Heat kernel diffusion | Freesurfer |
| --- | --- | --- |
| AD-CTL | 0.0492 | 0.0459 |
| AD-MCI | 0.0347 | 0.0201 |
| CTL-MCI | 0.0425 | 0.0348 |

related to the fact that significance is declared when the volume of suprathreshold statistics is more than 20 times that expected under the null hypothesis.

With the proposed univariate statistics, we studied differences between three diagnostic groups: AD, MCI and controls. As expected, we found relatively strong thickness differences between AD and control groups ($q$-value: 0.0492 with heat diffusion method and 0.0459 with Freesurfer software) and strong thickness differences between MCI and control groups ($q$-value: 0.0425 with heat diffusion method and 0.0348 with Freesurfer software), the details are in Fig. 6 and Fig. 7. We compared the statistical power (determined by FDR corrected overall significant values) with the two thickness methods, our method demonstrated the strongest or comparable statistical power for the three group comparisons (detailed in Table 1). Although more validation is certainly necessary, the current results suggest that the heat diffusion measure may offer greater statistical power than the Freesurfer software.

## 5    Conclusion

In this paper, we present a heat kernel based thickness estimation algorithm which can improve the computational efficiency and accuracy for *in vivo* MR image cortical thickness estimation. Through establishing the tetrahedral mesh matching with the MRI by the harmonic energy function, we can reduce the limited grid resolution effects. At the same time, we introduce the heat kernel to the streamline analysis to determine the heat transfer gradient direction. With the proposed univariate statistics, we studied differences between three diagnostic groups: AD, MCI and controls. We compare our method with the Freesurfer software, the results show that the heat diffusion method achieved greater statistical power than the Freesurfer software in a total of three comparisons. In the future, we plan to depict the geometrical characteristics of the local and global cortical regions by using the heat kernel diffusion and apply them in our ongoing preclinical AD research.

**Acknowledgments.** This work was supported by the National Natural Science Foundation of China (No. 11074105), , the Science and Technology Development Program of Shandong Province (No. 2011YD01078), the Natural Science Foundation of Shandong Province (No. ZR2012FL21). the School-Enterprise Fund of Ludong University (No. 2010HX007).

# References

1. Clarkson, M.J., Cardoso, M.J., Ridgway, G.R., Modat, M., Leung, K.K., Rohrer, J.D., Fox, N.C., Ourselin, S.: A comparison of voxel and surface based cortical thickness estimation methods. Neuroimage 57(3), 856–865 (2011)
2. Mak-Fan, K.M., Taylor, M.J., Roberts, W., Lerch, J.P.: Measures of cortical grey matter structure and development in children with autism spectrum disorder. J. Autism Dev. Disord. 42(3), 419–427 (2012)
3. Fischl, B., Dale, A.M.: Measuring the thickness of the human cerebral cortex from magnetic resonance images. Proc. Natl. Acad. Sci. U.S.A. 97(20), 11050–11055 (2000)
4. Dahnke, R., Yotter, R.A., Gaser, C.: Cortical thickness and central surface estimation. Neuroimage 65, 336–348 (2013)
5. Cardoso, M.J., Clarkson, M.J., Ridgway, G.R., Modat, M., Fox, N.C., Ourselin, S.: LoAd: a locally adaptive cortical segmentation algorithm. Neuroimage 56(3), 1386–1397 (2011)
6. Scott, M.L., Bromiley, P.A., Thacker, N.A., Hutchinson, C.E., Jackson, A.: A fast, model-independent method for cerebral cortical thickness estimation using MRI. Med. Image Anal. 13(2), 269–285 (2009)
7. Das, S.R., Avants, B.B., Grossman, M., Gee, J.C.: Registration based cortical thickness measurement. Neuroimage 45(3), 867–879 (2009)
8. Jones, S.E., Buchbinder, B.R., Aharon, I.: Three-dimensional mapping of cortical thickness using Laplace's equation. Hum. Brain Mapp. 11(1), 12–32 (2000)
9. Hyde, D.E., Duffy, F.H., Warfield, S.K.: Anisotropic partial volume CSF modeling for EEG source localization. Neuroimage 62(3), 2161–2170 (2012)
10. Jones, G., Chapman, S.: Modeling growth in biological materials. SIAM Review 54(1), 52–118 (2012)
11. Cassidy, J., Lilge, L., Betz, V.: Fullmonte: a framework for high-performance monte carlo simulation of light through turbid media with complex geometry, pp. 85920H-1–85920H-14 (2013)
12. Liu, Y., Xing, H.: A boundary focused quadrilateral mesh generation algorithm for multi-material structures. Journal of Computational Physics 232(1), 516–528 (2013)

13. Lederman, C., Joshi, A., Dinov, I.: Tetrahedral mesh generation for medical images with multiple regions using active surfaces. In: Proc. IEEE Int. Symp. Biomed. Imaging, pp. 436–439 (2010)
14. Liu, Y., Foteinos, P.A., Chernikov, A.N., Chrisochoides, N.: Mesh deformation-based multi-tissue mesh generation for brain images. Eng. Comput. 28(4), 305–318 (2012)
15. Zeng, W., Guo, R., Luo, F., Gu, X.: Discrete heat kernel determines discrete riemannian metric. Graph. Models 74(4), 121–129 (2012)
16. Chung, M.K., Robbins, S.M., Dalton, K.M., Davidson, R.J., Alexander, A.L., Evans, A.C.: Cortical thickness analysis in autism with heat kernel smoothing. NeuroImage 25(4), 1256–1265 (2005)
17. Bronstein, M.M., Bronstein, A.M.: Shape recognition with spectral distances. IEEE Trans. Pattern Anal. Mach. Intell. 33(5), 1065–1071 (2011)
18. Sharma, A., Horaud, R.P., Mateus, D.: 3D shape registration using spectral graph embedding and probabilistic matching. Image Processing and Analysing With Graphs: Theory and Practice, 441–474 (2012)
19. Lederman, C., Joshi, A., Dinov, I., Vese, L., Toga, A., Van Horn, J.D.: The generation of tetrahedral mesh models for neuroanatomical MRI. Neuroimage 55(1), 153–164 (2011)
20. Wang, Y., Gu, X., Chan, T.F., Thompson, P.M., Yau, S.T.: Volumetric harmonic brain mapping. In: IEEE International Symposium on Biomedical Imaging: From Nano to Macro, ISBI 2004, pp. 1275–1278 (2004)
21. Mueller, S.G., Weiner, M.W., Thal, L.J., Petersen, R.C., Jack, C., Jagust, W., Trojanowski, J.Q., Toga, A.W., Beckett, L.: The Alzheimer's disease neuroimaging initiative. Neuroimaging Clin. N. Am. 15(4), 869–877 (2005)
22. Fischl, B., Sereno, M.I., Dale, A.M.: Cortical surface-based analysis II: Inflation, flattening, and a surface-based coordinate system. NeuroImage 9(2), 195–207 (1999)
23. Nichols, T., Hayasaka, S.: Controlling the familywise error rate in functional neuroimaging: a comparative review. Stat. Methods Med. Res. 12(5), 419–446 (2003)
24. Wang, Y., Shi, J., Yin, X., Gu, X., Chan, T.F., Yau, S.T., Toga, A.W., Thompson, P.M.: Brain surface conformal parameterization with the Ricci flow. IEEE Trans. Med. Imaging 31(2), 251–264 (2012)

# A Family of Fast Spherical Registration Algorithms for Cortical Shapes

Boris A. Gutman, Sarah K. Madsen, Arthur W. Toga, and Paul M. Thompson

Imaging Genetics Center, Laboratory of Neuro Imaging, University of California, Los Angeles

**Abstract.** We introduce a family of fast spherical registration algorithms: a spherical fluid model and several modifications of the spherical demons algorithm introduced in [1]. Our algorithms are based on fast convolution of tangential spherical vector fields in the spectral domain. Using the vector harmonic representation of spherical fields, we derive a more principled approach for kernel smoothing via Mercer's theorem and the diffusion equation. This is a non-trivial extension of scalar spherical convolution, as the vector harmonics do not generalize directly from scalar harmonics on the sphere, as in the Euclidean case. The fluid algorithm is optimized in the Eulerian frame, leading to a very efficient optimization. Several new adaptations of the demons algorithm are presented, including compositive and diffeomorphic demons, as well as fluid-like and diffusion-like regularization. The resulting algorithms are all significantly faster than [1], while also retaining greater flexibility. Our algorithms are validated and compared using cortical surface models.

**Keywords:** Shape Registration, Spherical Mapping, Diffeomorphic Demons, Fluid Registration, Vector Spherical Harmonics.

## 1 Introduction

Non-rigid shape registration represents an important area of research in medical imaging, in particular for cortical shape analysis. The highly variable, convoluted geometry of the cortical boundary together with an abundance of MR data present a significant challenge for fully automating reliable correspondence searches. Current methods for parametric shape registration range from conformal maps and intrinsic embeddings via the Laplace-Beltrami (LB) operator [2-4] to the more direct adaptations of image registration algorithms in the Euclidian domain. The latter approach is appealing, as non-linear medical image registration has by now become a mature field with several well-validated methods. For example, an approach taken by [5] maps subcortical shapes directly to the 2D plane, and performs the usual fluid registration of mean curvature and conformal factor features following [6] to achieve final correspondence. The method is fast and reliable, provided a consistent set of boundaries is introduced to enable the initial parameterization. The boundary constraint requires a strong prior on the final correspondence search, before any registration can be attempted at all.

This illustrates the significant advantage that using a parametric domain of the same topology as the shape – for example the 2-sphere – offers compared to the Euclidian

L. Shen et al. (Eds.): MBIA 2013, LNCS 8159, pp. 246–257, 2013.

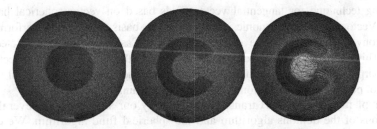

**Fig. 1.** Smooth spherical circle to C. No registration paper is complete without the "circle to C." Here, we used diffeomorphic demons with fluid- and diffusion-like regularization.

domain. In effect, using the spherical domain enables truly automated parametric registration of genus-zero shapes. As a result, several adaptations of Euclidian registration to the sphere have been proposed. Thompson et al. [7] proposed elastic matching based on sulcal landmarks, constraining the curve-induced flow by the Cauchy-Navier differential operator, and correcting explicitly for metric distortions. In [4, 8], the authors extend Miller's LDDMM framework [9] to point and curve-set registration on the sphere. Closer to this work, in [10, 11] the authors propose landmark-free methods on the sphere, minimizing the sum of squared distances (SSD) between corresponding curvature maps and curvature-derived feature functions. The optical flow algorithm is adapted to the sphere in [10], and solved using a narrow band approach, while in [11] a straight-forward optimization of coordinates is performed directly on the surface. In a more recent effort, Yeo extended the very efficient diffeomorphic demons algorithm [12, 13] to spherical images, and showed that registering curvature and thickness features of the cortex leads to robust shape registration [1]. The resulting algorithm can accurately register two cortical surfaces of high resolution (150K vertices) in under 5 minutes, while maintaining invertible warps. This is quite an impressive result, since FreeSurfer [11], perhaps the most popular tool for cortical surface alignment, takes on the order of 1 hour.

Inspired by the recent work on spherical shape registration, we revisit the spherical registration problem from the perspective of adapting well-known Euclidean registration approaches. At the heart of many image registration algorithms, one finds a Gaussian convolution of either the displacement field itself, or the update step/instantaneous velocity of the field. On the other hand, it is often convenient to decompose the velocity or the displacement over an orthogonal basis, formed by the eigenfunctions of a suitable differential operator. As the most basic example, Gaussian convolution can be performed quickly in the Fourier domain; this is often used to approximate the solution to the fluid equation [14]. A more precise solution is offered in [15], where the decomposition is in eigenfunctions of the fluid operator itself. The many variants of the demons algorithm likewise require a convolution of the field ("diffusion-like" demons) or the update step ("fluid-like" demons) with a smoothing kernel for regularization, which is typically done in the Fourier domain [13]. However, the adaptation of this idea to the sphere is not trivial, since the well-known scalar spherical harmonics cannot be applied directly to canonical coordinates of tangential vector fields. To mitigate this problem, Yeo et al. [1] use a straightforward recursive smoothing scheme. This limits the possible kernel range, as the execution time depends directly on the size of the kernel. In this work, we derive a smoothing technique for tangential vector fields based on *vector* spherical harmonics (VSH). Vector spherical harmonics form a suitable basis in which to perform the required convolution, as they are eigenfields of the Casimir operator restricted to the sphere. This allows for a natural extension of Mercer's theorem to spherical vector fields for the purpose of fast spherical field regularization. Such an approach has all the usual benefits of performing convolution in the spectral domain.

We implement a fast VSH transform, and apply our smoothing in several natural adaptations of the demons algorithm and the spherical fluid algorithm. We compare the performance of the proposed algorithms based on 100 white matter (WM) surfaces, using both synthetic warps and true cross-subject registration. We conclude that the combined fluid- and diffusion-like diffeomorphic demons offer the best accuracy, followed closely by the fluid algorithm. Both of these approaches significantly outperform compositive demons, as well as diffeomorphic demons with only fluid-like or diffusion-like regularization, such as implemented in [1].

The remainder of the paper is organized as follows. The first section describes fast heat kernel smoothing for spherical fields. The second and third sections outline the demons and fluid adaptations to the sphere based on the proposed vector smoothing. The fourth section describes some implementation details. The fifth section compares the results across our methods, and the sixth concludes the paper.

## 2    Heat Kernel for Spherical Vector Fields

In direct analogue to Fourier series on $\mathbb{R}^n$, and scalar spherical harmonics – the eigenfunctions of the Laplacian and the scalar LB operator on $\mathbb{S}^2$, VSH can be derived from the Casimir operator, or the Laplacian operator on spherical tangential fields. The curvature of the sphere implies a non-trivial parallel transport, which complicates the vector Laplacian form and distinguishes it from the scalar case. In canonical coordinates, the vector Laplacian of $\mathbf{v} = v_\theta e_\theta + v_\varphi e_\varphi$ is written as

$$
\Delta \mathbf{v} = \left[ -\left( \frac{\partial^2}{\partial \theta^2} + \cot\theta \frac{\partial}{\partial \theta} + \frac{1}{\sin^2\theta} \frac{\partial^2}{\partial \varphi^2} - \frac{1}{\sin^2\theta} \right) v_\theta + \frac{2\cot\theta}{\sin\theta} \frac{\partial v_\varphi}{\partial \varphi} \right] e_\theta
$$
$$
+ \left[ -\left( \frac{\partial^2}{\partial \theta^2} + \cot\theta \frac{\partial}{\partial \theta} + \frac{1}{\sin^2\theta} \frac{\partial^2}{\partial \varphi^2} - \frac{1}{\sin^2\theta} \right) v_\varphi - \frac{2\cot\theta}{\sin\theta} \frac{\partial v_\theta}{\partial \varphi} \right] e_\varphi. \tag{1}
$$

Vector spherical harmonics satisfy $\Delta \mathbf{A}_{lm} = l(l+1)\mathbf{A}_{lm}$, and can be defined as the gradient of the scalar harmonics $Y_{lm}$, and its orthogonal complement (see, e.g. [16]).

$$
\mathbf{B}_{lm} = \frac{1}{\sqrt{l(l+1)}} \left[ \frac{\partial Y_{lm}}{\partial \theta} e_\theta + \frac{1}{\sin\theta} \frac{\partial Y_{lm}}{\partial \varphi} e_\theta \right], \tag{2}
$$

$$
\mathbf{C}_{lm} = -e_r \times \mathbf{B}_{lm}.
$$

This leads to harmonic decomposition of a spherical vector field into

$$
\mathbf{v} = \sum_{\substack{l=1 \\ |m|\le l}}^{\infty} [\mathbf{B}_{lm} f^B(l,m) + \mathbf{C}_{lm} f^C(l,m)], \quad f^A(l,m) = \langle \mathbf{v}, \mathbf{A}_{lm} \rangle_{L^2(T\mathbb{S}^2)} \tag{3}
$$

Taking advantage of the eigenfields, we can extend Mercer's Theorem [17] to spherical fields, and define the heat kernel as

$$K_\sigma(p,q) = \sum_{l=1}^{\infty} e^{-l(l+1)\sigma} \sum_{m=-l}^{l} \mathbf{B}_{lm}(p) \otimes \mathbf{B}_{lm}(q) + \mathbf{C}_{lm}(p) \otimes \mathbf{C}_{lm}(q), \quad (4)$$

where $\otimes$ is the tensor product. The kernel in (5) represents Green's function of the vector isotropic diffusion equation $\frac{\partial v}{\partial t} = -\Delta v$, $\sigma = \sqrt{2t}$. Applying the kernel to a field leads to an expression which is similar to the scalar harmonics case [18]:

$$\mathbf{K}_\sigma * \mathbf{v}(p) \quad = \quad \sum_{\substack{l=1 \\ |m| \le l}}^{\infty} e^{-l(l+1)\sigma} \left[ \mathbf{B}_{lm}(p) \int_{\mathbb{S}^2} \mathbf{B}_{lm}(q)\mathbf{v}(q)d\mu(q) \right.$$

$$\left. + \quad \mathbf{C}_{lm}(p) \int_{\mathbb{S}^2} \mathbf{C}_{lm}(q)\mathbf{v}(q)d\mu(q) \right]. \quad (5)$$

It is easy to see that all that is required for an efficient heat kernel smoothing of a spherical field is a forward harmonic transform followed by an $O(n)$ operation and an inverse transform.

## 3    Spherical Demons

The general idea behind a demons approach [12] is a two-step optimization, in which the first step represents a search for the update direction of the current warp, and the second – the regularization of the new warp resulting from this update. Thus, for fields $u, g, G: \mathbb{R}^n \to \mathbb{R}^n$, we have the following optimization problems.

$$u = \arg \min_u \left( \|S - T * \{g * u\}\|_2^2 + \frac{1}{\sigma} \text{dist}(g, \{g * u\}) \right), \quad (6)$$

where $u$ is a "hidden" transformation, and the regularization

$$G = \arg \min_G \left( \frac{1}{\sigma_G} R(G) + \frac{1}{\sigma} \text{dist}(G, \{g * u\}) \right), \quad (7)$$

with the update $g_{t+1} = G_t$. Here $S, T$ are fixed and moving images with $T *$ $g: \mathbb{R}^n \to \mathbb{R}$ defined using the Lagrangian frame by $\{T * g\}[x + g(x)] = T[x]$. The optimized field $g$ is the warp bringing the two images into correspondence. The regularization term $R(G)$ is generally taken as a norm of a differential operator, so that the minimization can be achieved with a convolution. A well-known example, minimizing the harmonic energy in $\mathbb{R}^n$ is equivalent to a Gaussian smoothing of the displacement field $G$. Likewise, the second term in the first equation (6) can be interpreted as a penalty on the harmonic energy of $u$, as well as its norm, and can be smoothed with a Gaussian kernel. Smoothing the displacement field is often termed "diffusion-like regularization" , and  smoothing the update, "fluid-like regularization" [13]. The unique advantage of the demons family of algorithms is precisely the separation of the two optimization problems: each cost can be optimized very efficiently with either a linear approximation or a fast convolution. Lastly, a more recent modification of the demons framework [13] introduced the idea of maintaining diffeomorphic warps by passing each update step $u$ through the exponential $u \rightarrow exp(u)$, thus ensuring invertibiliy. Since diffeomorphisms form a Lie group under composition, this approach guarantees a smooth invertible final warp $g$.

Adapting the demons approach to spherical images $S, T: \mathbb{S}^2 \rightarrow \mathbb{R}$, we optimize over $u, g, G: \mathbb{S}^2 \rightarrow T_x\mathbb{S}^2$, and following the convention in [1], define $T * g$ by $\{T * g\}[p(x, g\{x\})] = T[x]$, where

$$p(x, g\{x\}) = x\sqrt{1 - \|g\{x\}\|^2} + g\{x\}. \tag{8}$$

Although such a parameterization of the warp contains a nonlinearity, as the geodesic length of the displacement is the arcsine of $\|g\{x\}\|$, it leads to significantly simpler computations than an arc length parameterization. Indeed, given $p(x, g\{x\})$, it is easy to compute $g\{x\}$ by $g\{x\} = -G^2(x)p(x, g\{x\})$, where $G$ is the cross-product matrix, as suggested in [1]. In solving the first optimization problem (6), we deviate from [1], who optimize the problem directly in the original image space, and follow [13] more closely: we reformulate the problem as

$$u = \arg \min_u \left( \|S - [T * g] * u\|_2^2 + \frac{1}{\sigma}\|u\|^2 \right). \tag{9}$$

This leads to a straightforward linear problem, following the linearization of $\|S - T * \{g\} * \{u\}\|_2^2$, which can be solved separately for every point on $\mathbb{S}^2$.

$$u\{p\} = \frac{S\{p\} - [T * g] * u\{p\}}{\left\|\vec{\nabla}[T * g]\{p\}\right\|^2 + \frac{1}{\sigma^2\{p\}}} \vec{\nabla}[T * g]\{p\}, \tag{10}$$

where $\sigma^2\{p\}$ is a normalization term controlling for image noise. Note that we have omitted the matrix $\frac{\partial p(x,u)}{\partial u}$, because at $u = 0$ it is simply the identity.

The second optimization step consists entirely in applying a smoothing kernel to the composition $g_t * u_{t+1}$. In this sense, the energetic norm used in $R(G)$ is in practice defined by the kernel of choice, rather than the other way around [4]. However, as mentioned earlier, convolving tangential vector fields on the sphere does not generalize directly from scalar convolution as in $\mathbb{R}^n$ due to the non-trivial parallel transport operator $T(p, q): T_p\mathbb{S}^2 \rightarrow T_q\mathbb{S}^2$. A straightforward solution is to recursively approximate the kernel by repeated application of $T(p, q)$ over some neighborhood for each vertex on a mesh. In this case, the effective size of the kernel depends directly on the number of smoothing iterations performed. This is an approach taken in [1], and allows one to create custom kernels depending on the weighting function. Thus, equation (7) is approximately solved by

$$\widetilde{G}(p) = \sum_{q \in \mathcal{N}(p)} \lambda(p, q)T(p, q) * \{g * u\}(q), \tag{11}$$

where $\mathcal{N}(p)$ is the 1-ring of the vertex $p$, and $\lambda(p, q)[\sigma]$ is normalized to add up to 1 over the 1-ring, and monotonically increasing with $\sigma$. While this appears to work well in practice, the approach can only be applied to kernels of a limited size. We replace this with vector heat kernel smoothing via the VSH, which eliminates the limitation on the kernel size and speeds up the process considerably. Further, the energy minimized can actually be defined in closed form, and computed essentially for free as part of the VSH transform. One additional advantage of having a low-cost smoothing technique for spherical fields is that it enables us to naturally extend the fluid-like regularization of Euclidean demons to the sphere. This modification turns out crucial for improving cortical correspondence accuracy, as we will see shortly. We thus have our final demons algorithm family:

**Algorithm 1 (VSH-based spherical demons)**
Given images $S, T : \mathbb{S}^2 \to \mathbb{R}$, max step $R_{max}$, tolerance
   Initialize $u, g_0 : \mathbb{S}^2 \to T_x \mathbb{S}^2$ to be uniformly 0.
   While(t < max_iterations AND $\frac{\|S - T*\{g_{t-1}\}\|_2^2 - \|S - T*\{g_t\}\|_2^2}{\|S - T*\{g_0\}\|_2^2}$ > tol.)

   1. Compute update $u$ using (10)
   2. Find $\sigma^2$, so that $R_{max} \leq \|u(p)\| \, \forall p \in \mathbb{S}^2$ [13]
   3. For fluid-like registration, $u \to \mathbf{K}_{\sigma\,\text{fluid}} * u$ using (5)
   4. For diffeomorphic registration, $u \to exp(u)$ [1]
   5. Compute $g_{t+1}\{x\} = -\mathcal{G}^2(x)p(x, g_t\{x\} * u)$
   6. For diffusion-like regularization, $g_{t+1} \to \mathbf{K}_{\sigma\,\text{diff}} * g_{t+1}$
   End While
Return $g$

## 4    Spherical Fluid Registration

The fluid registration paradigm, first introduced in [6], differs markedly from the demons family in that the fidelity term $\|S - T * g\|_2^2$ is only represented as defining the body force $F(g)$ of the simplified Navier-Stokes equation

$$\mu\Delta u + (\lambda + \mu)\vec{\nabla}(\vec{\nabla} \cdot u) = -F(g)$$
$$F[x, g(x, t)] = (S[x] - T[\, p(x, -g\{x, t\})])\vec{\nabla}T[\, p(x, -g\{x, t\})]. \tag{12}$$

The equations model the behavior of a viscous fluid, driven by the instantaneous forces resulting from image mismatch. Unlike demons, the fluid regularization has no memory of the previous step. Instead, the instantaneous velocity is explicitly integrated over time, allowing for very large deformations. The power and popularity of the fluid framework are largely due to this flexibility.

Optimization is performed in the Eulerian reference frame. In this frame, the velocity $u(x, t)$ describes the motion of the particle at position $x$ and time $t$. The field $g(x, t)$ implies that from time 0, this particle underwent a transformation parameterized by $T(x, x_0) * g(x, t)$, using our convention (8). It is easy to see that $x_0 = p(x, -g\{x, t\})$.

The algorithm's only memory of previous iterations is expressed in the material derivative, which accounts for the field Jacobian $Dg$ to update the displacement.

$$\frac{\partial \boldsymbol{g}}{\partial t} = [Id - D\boldsymbol{g}]\boldsymbol{u}. \tag{13}$$

To update the field in the spherical domain, one must also account for the non-linearity in the displacement parameterization. Since the particle to reside at $x$ after applying $\delta \boldsymbol{g} = \delta t \frac{\partial \boldsymbol{g}}{\partial t}$ is to be found at $p[r, -\boldsymbol{T}(x, r) * \delta \boldsymbol{g}]$ in the original image, where for clarity we mean $r = p(x, -\boldsymbol{g}\{x, t\})$, we must update the field by

$$\boldsymbol{g}(x, t + \delta t) = \mathcal{G}^2(x)p[r, -\boldsymbol{T}(x, r) * \delta \boldsymbol{g}]. \tag{14}$$

Because the field is updated at fixed coordinate points on the sphere, the matrices $\mathcal{G}(x)$ can be pre-computed offline just as in the demons algorithm.

The most computationally intensive aspect of the fluid registration approach is solving for the velocity $\boldsymbol{u}$, given the body force. In the original formulation [6], the successive over-relaxation (SOR) approach was used, which, while accurate, proved prohibitively computationally expensive. A significant improvement on speed was achieved in [15], where the authors derived and applied eigenfunctions of the operator (12). However, the most common simplification of this problem in $\mathbb{R}^n$ is to apply a Gaussian filter to the field, which can be shown [14, 19] to approximate (12). Following similar arguments, we propose an analogue of fluid approximation on the sphere, using VSH-based vector heat kernel smoothing.

**Algorithm 2 (spherical fluid registration)**
```
Given images S,T:S² → ℝ, max step R_max, tolerance
Initialize u,g:S² → T_xS² to be uniformly 0. n = 0.
  While(n < max_iterations AND
```
$$\frac{\|S[x] - T[p(x, -g\{x,t\})]\|_2^2 - \|S[x] - T[p(x, -g\{x, t + \delta t\})]\|_2^2}{\|S[x] - T[p(x,0)]\|_2^2} > \text{tolerance})$$
```
    1. Compute body force F using (12)
    2. Set u → -K_σ * F
```
    3. Compute $\frac{\partial g}{\partial t}$ using (13), set $\delta t = R_{max}/\max\left(\left\|\frac{\partial g}{\partial t}\right\|\right)$
```
    4. Compute g(x,t+δt) using (14), set n = n + 1
  End While
Return g
```

# 5    Implementation Issues

## 5.1    VSH Computation

We apply the exact quadrature method for spherical harmonics sampled at regular canonical coordinates [16]. We vectorize the SpharmonicKit implementation [20] following [16], except normalizing vector and scalar harmonics $\|\mathbf{B}_{lm}\|, \|\mathbf{C}_{lm}\|, \|Y_{lm}\| = 1$. This results in slightly different weights for computing the vector coefficients from the scalar ones. Setting the auxiliary scalar coefficients as in [16], $g^{\theta,\varphi}(l, m) = \langle \frac{1}{\sin\theta} V_{\theta,\varphi}, Y_{lm}\rangle_{L^2(\mathbb{S}^2)}$, the vector coefficients can be obtained from

$$f^B(l,m) = \sum_{n=-1}^{1} W_1(l,m,n)g^\theta(l+n,m) + W_2(l,m)g^\varphi(l,m) \tag{15}$$

$$f^C(l,m) = \sum_{n=-1}^{1} -W_1(l,m,n)g^\varphi(l+n,m) + W_2(l,m)g^\theta(l,m),$$

with the weights $W_1, W_2$ pre-computed offline for repeated use. An analogous expression can be obtained for computing the auxiliary vector coefficients back from the VSH coefficients. The resulting convolution algorithm requires only two forward and two inverse scalar spherical harmonic transforms, with an $O(n)$ operation. For a bandwidth of 256, which corresponds to a grid of 512x512 vertices, typical execution time for the full convolution is around a tenth of a second.

The requirement that the fields be defined at regular spherical coordinates suggests performing the entire registration on the regular grid, only interpolating the final warp back to the original mesh coordinates. This proves faster and more stable than performing forward and reverse sampling of a field at every iteration. Further, sampling on this regular grid is denser than the typical FreeSurfer resolution of 150K vertices.

### 5.2   Demons Optimization

Some notable differences exist between our implementation of spherical demons and [1]. We choose to interpolate the moving image at regular coordinates, computing the update step from the currently warped image. Thus, there is no need to interpolate the gradient or compute the field Jacobian. However, in our implementation we use only a first order estimate of the update, while Yeo et al. use the Gauss-Newton scheme. The latter relies on empirically estimating the Hessian. Thus, in [1] there is a heavier computational burden for each iteration, but fewer iterations are required. We note that a Gauss-Newton scheme could be applied directly to our framework as well. Also unlike [1], we follow [13] in setting the gradient term in (10) to be the symmetric gradient. This was found to improve convergence.

An additional aspect of the diffeomorphic demons approach is the "scaling and squaring" procedure. We follow [1], but perform the procedure based on regular spherical grids. The advantage of this approach is that sampling from a regular grid onto an irregular one is an $O(1)$ operation per vertex, whereas sampling the other way generally grows with the number of triangles even for fast samplers. The repeated sampling during "scaling and squaring" means that using a warp defined on a regular grid leads to faster exponentiation. We note also that the "slow" kind of spherical sampling (irregular to regular) must still be done at least once per iteration in the demons pipeline. For this, our in-house fast sampling algorithm performs roughly 2.5 triangle intersection checks per vertex for the spherical grids we use, leading to compute times less than 1 second.

### 5.3   Fluid Optimization

Our fluid registration is adapted to the sphere to be very close to [14], with the exception of the fidelity term (here, SSD). The other main difference lies in not using regridding during our optimization. In [6, 14], the authors restart the optimization process setting

$T[x] \rightarrow T[\,p(x, -\boldsymbol{g}\{x, t\})]$, $\boldsymbol{g} = \boldsymbol{0}$, if the Jacobian determinant $|D\boldsymbol{g}|$ falls below some threshold. This "regridding" step is used to alleviate problems caused by discretization, which can make the warp non-invertible. The final output warp $\boldsymbol{g}$ is then the composition of all the intermediate warps. Here, we chose not to do this for a more fair comparison to the demons algorithm, where regridding is not customary.

A significant advantage of the fluid algorithm over the demons specifically on $\mathbb{S}^2$ is that there is no need for "slow" sampling, as we only interpolate the original image $T$. This is due to the choice of the Eulerian frame, and leads to significantly faster compute times per iteration.

## 6    Experiments

For our experiments, we used 100 left white matter surfaces extracted using FreeSurfer from the ADNI dataset. The initial spherical map was computed as in [21]. Throughout the experiments, we use only mean curvature as the feature function. We apply a 3-level multi-resolution scheme, smoothing the curvature maps [18] and regularizing the registration more at the first level, and relaxing both at subsequent levels. A rotational pre-registration step was applied based on fast spherical cross-correlation of the smoothed curvature [22].

Three sets of experiments were done on the cortical shapes: (1) Recovering a synthetic warp, (2) Pairwise registration, and (3) All-to-one registration. In the first experiment each subject's spherical map underwent a unique synthetic spherical warp. To synthesize a relatively large warp smooth, we first randomly seeded a warp field by its VSH coefficients and computed a smoothed inverse. This was then composed with a spherical MRF that was passed through an exponential, as in [13]. The result was a diffeomorphic deformation that was both large and highly non-linear. Further, some noise was added to the original shapes. The SSD and Laplacian norm of the warps are plotted in Figure 2. Table 1 shows the relative error and normalized cross-correlation with the original warps for each method.

In the second experiment, shapes were randomly paired and 50 registrations were performed for each pair. The SSD and Laplacian norm of the warp are plotted in Figure 3. For ease of reading, here we only compare the diffeomorphic variants of the demons algorithm and the fluid algorithm.

In the third experiment, we mapped all subjects to a random target brain, using the combined diffeomorphic demons approach, and the fluid approach. We computed the resulting brain averages and compared the result to using only rotational registration. The resulting averages are shown in Figure 4. Step size, $\sigma_{fluid}$ and $\sigma_{diff}$ were tuned experimentally to maximize agreement between recovered warp and synthetic warps. This was done separately for each method with one exception. For "fluid-like" demons, parameters were set as in the fluid registration for fair comparison. In general we found that the diffeomorphic demons favors larger step size than fluid registration. For the combined demons algorithm, the optimal $\sigma_{fluid}$ and $\sigma_{diff}$ were lower than the corresponding $\sigma_{fluid}$ and $\sigma_{diff}$ in "fluid-like" and "diffusion-like" versions. Overall, we found that the fluid algorithm recovered synthetic warps most accurately. However, combined demons approach resulted in visually better results for pair-wise and all-to-one registration, as well as lower final SSD.

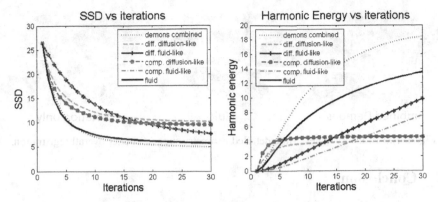

**Fig. 2.** Synthetic warp results. "Harmonic energy" is the vector Laplacian norm.

All diffeomorphic approaches and the fluid approach resulted in invertible warps with no triangle flips. Execution time per iteration was roughly 0.5 seconds for the fluid approach and 1.5 seconds per iteration for diffeomorphic demons. Thus, registration can be achieved in as little as 10 seconds per resolution level, which is an order of magnitude improvement over [1].

**Table 1.** Accuracy of synthetic warp recovery. Relative mean squared error and cross-correlation, averaged over 100 trials, with standard deviation. DF1 and FL1 stand for diffusion- and fluid-like diffeomorphic methods. DF2 and FL2 are the compositive versions.

|  | Combo | DF1 | FL1 | DF2 | FL2 | Fluid |
|---|---|---|---|---|---|---|
| $\dfrac{MSE}{\|g_{true}\|}$ | 0.192 +/-0.11 | 0.216 +/-0.11 | 0.181 +/-0.086 | 0.236 +/-0.11 | 0.181 +/-0.086 | **0.162 +/-0.063** |
| CC | 0.875 +/-0.086 | 0.833 +/-0.099 | 0.884 +/-0.062 | 0.807 +/-0.11 | 0.884 +/-0.062 | **0.890 +/-0.046** |

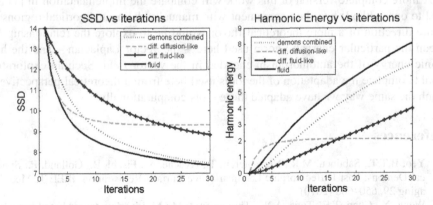

**Fig. 3.** Pair-wise warp results. "Harmonic energy" is the vector Laplacian norm.

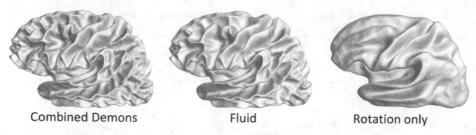

Combined Demons          Fluid          Rotation only

**Fig. 4.** 100-Brain Averages. More detailed geometry suggests better overall registration.

## 7    Conclusion

We presented a family of fast spherical registration tools for registering cortical surfaces, adapting several well-known image registration algorithms to the sphere. The full gamut of the demons approaches as well as the large deformation fluid approach are generalized to the 2-sphere, the latter being the first such adaptation. Our methods are based on fast convolution of spherical vector fields in the spectral domain, leading to perhaps some of the most efficient landmark-free cortical surface registration algorithms. The algorithms are validated on synthetic spherical warps, achieving an average normalized cross-correlation of nearly 0.9, where 1 would be a perfect recovery. Registration between pairs of real brains also shows promising results, leading to robust diffeomorphic registration in as little as 30 seconds.

A comparison of our methods reveals that the combined diffeomorphic demons and the fluid registration outperform the others in terms of minimizing geometric and image mismatch. A limitation of the tools tested here is their reliance on auxiliary measures of shapes, such as mean curvature. We recognize that an explicit correction for geometric distortion may improve our results. In particular, the fluid algorithm is flexible enough to handle any geometry-driven mismatch function without any additional modification.

A more complete version of this work will compare the implementation in [1] and [11] to our methods based on agreement with manually delineated cortical regions. A future direction of a more theoretical flavor would be to explore the relationship between the particular energetic norm used here – the vector Laplacian – and the harmonic energy of the automorphism encoded in the vector field. Such an exploration would complete the adaptation of the tools used here from a theoretical perspective in much the same way we have adapted these tools computationally.

## References

1. Yeo, B.T.T., Sabuncu, M.R., Vercauteren, T., Ayache, N., Fischl, B., Golland, P.: Spherical Demons: Fast Diffeomorphic Landmark-Free Surface Registration. IEEE T. Med. Imaging 29, 650–668 (2010)
2. Wang, Y., Chan, T.F., Toga, A.W., Thompson, P.M.: Multivariate tensor-based brain anatomical surface morphometry via holomorphic one-forms. In: Yang, G.-Z., Hawkes, D., Rueckert, D., Noble, A., Taylor, C. (eds.) MICCAI 2009, Part I. LNCS, vol. 5761, pp. 337–344. Springer, Heidelberg (2009)

3. Shi, Y., Morra, J.H., Thompson, P.M., Toga, A.W.: Inverse-consistent surface mapping with Laplace-Beltrami eigen-features. In: Prince, J.L., Pham, D.L., Myers, K.J. (eds.) IPMI 2009. LNCS, vol. 5636, pp. 467–478. Springer, Heidelberg (2009)
4. Glaunes, J., Vaillant, M., Miller, M.I.: Landmark matching via large deformation diffeomorphisms on the sphere. Journal of Mathematical Imaging and Vision 20, 179–200 (2004)
5. Shi, J., Thompson, P.M., Gutman, B., Wang, Y.: Surface fluid registration of conformal representation: Application to detect disease burden and genetic influence on hippocampus. Neuroimage 78, 111–134 (2013)
6. Christensen, G.E., Rabbitt, R.D., Miller, M.I.: Deformable templates using large deformation kinematics. IEEE Transactions on Image Processing 5, 1435–1447 (1996)
7. Thompson, P.M., Woods, R.P., Mega, M.S., Toga, A.W.: Mathematical/computational challenges in creating deformable and probabilistic atlases of the human brain. Human Brain Mapping 9, 81–92 (2000)
8. Lepore, N., Leow, A., Thompson, P.: Landmark matching on the sphere using distance functions. In: 3rd IEEE International Symposium on Biomedical Imaging: Nano to Macro, pp. 450–453 (2006)
9. Miller, M.I., Younes, L.: Group Actions, Homeomorphisms, and Matching: A General Framework. Int. J. Comput. Vision 41, 61–84 (2001)
10. Tosun, D., Prince, J.L.: Cortical surface alignment using geometry driven multispectral optical flow. In: Christensen, G.E., Sonka, M. (eds.) IPMI 2005. LNCS, vol. 3565, pp. 480–492. Springer, Heidelberg (2005)
11. Fischl, B., Sereno, M., Tootell, R., Dale, A.: High-resolution intersubject averaging and a coordinate system for the cortical surface. Human Brain Mapping 8, 272–284 (1999)
12. Thirion, J.P.: Image matching as a diffusion process: an analogy with Maxwell's demons. Medical Image Analysis 2, 243–260 (1998)
13. Vercauteren, T., Pennec, X., Perchant, A., Ayache, N.: Diffeomorphic demons: Efficient non-parametric image registration. Neuroimage 45, S61–S72 (2009)
14. D'Agostino, E., Maes, F., Vandermeulen, D., Suetens, P.: A viscous fluid model for multimodal non-rigid image registration using mutual information. Medical Image Analysis 7, 565–575 (2003)
15. Bro-Nielsen, M., Gramkow, C.: Fast Fluid Registration of Medical Images. In: Höhne, K.H., Kikinis, R. (eds.) VBC 1996. LNCS, vol. 1131, pp. 267–276. Springer, Heidelberg (1996)
16. Kostelec, P.J., Maslen, D.K., Healy, D.M., Rockmore, D.N.: Computational harmonic analysis for tensor fields on the two-sphere. J. Comput. Phys. 162, 514–535 (2000)
17. Courant, R., Hilbert, D.: Methods of mathematical physics. Interscience Publishers, New York (1953)
18. Chung, M.K., Hartley, R., Dalton, K.M., Davidson, R.J.: Encoding Cortical Surface by Spherical Harmonics. Stat. Sinica 18, 1269–1291 (2008)
19. Cachier, P., Ayache, N.: Isotropic Energies, Filters and Splines for Vector Field Regularization. J. Math. Imaging Vis. 20, 251–265 (2004)
20. Healy, D.M., Rockmore, D.N., Kostelec, P.J., Moore, S.: FFTs for the 2-sphere-improvements and variations. J. Fourier Anal. Appl. 9, 341–385 (2003)
21. Friedel, I., Schroeder, P., Desbrun, M.: Unconstrained spherical parameterization. In: ACM SIGGRAPH 2005 Sketches, p. 134. ACM, Los Angeles (2005)
22. Gutman, B., Wang, Y., Lui, L.M., Chan, T.F., Thompson, P.M., Toga, A.W.: Shape Registration with Spherical Cross Correlation. In: MICCAI Workshop on Mathematical Foundations in Computational Anatomy, MFCA 2008 (2008)

# Author Index